Clinical Communication iı

This book is dedicated to all those who experience healthcare.

Clinical Communication in Medicine

EDITED BY

Dr Jo Brown

Reader in Medical Education, Academic Director of the Student Experience, Head of Clinical Communication, National Teaching Fellow, St George's University of London, London, UK

Dr Lorraine M. Noble

Senior Lecturer in Clinical Communication, University College London Medical School, London, UK

Dr Alexia Papageorgiou

Associate Professor in Clinical Communication, University of Nicosia Medical School, Nicosia, Cyprus

Dr Jane Kidd

Undergraduate Quality Manager, Education Training and Research, University Hospitals Coventry and Warwickshire NHS Trust; External tutor, Institute of Medical and Biomedical Education, St George's University of London, London, UK

On behalf of the UK Council of Clinical Communication in Undergraduate Medical Education

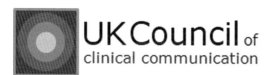

The UK Council of Clinical Communication in Undergraduate Medical Education is a representative body of the communication teaching leads from all of the medical schools in the UK. The UK Council aims to share good teaching practice, and encourages research and development of effective clinical communication teaching in the UK.
www.ukccc.org.uk

WILEY Blackwell

Contents

List of Contributors

Lucy Ambrose
General Practitioner, The Tutbury Practice, Tutbury, Staffordshire, UK

Jennifer Balls
Consultant in Palliative Medicine, Saint Francis Hospice, Romford, Essex, UK

Victoria Bates
Lecturer in Modern History, University of Bristol, Bristol, UK

Jo Brown
Reader in Medical Education, Academic Director of the Student Experience, Head of Clinical Communication, National Teaching Fellow, St George's University of London, London, UK

Xavier Coll
Honorary Senior Lecturer at the Norwich Medical School, University of East Anglia; Consultant Child and Adolescent Psychiatrist at the Children, Families, and Young People Service, Norwich, Norfolk, UK

Costas S. Constantinou
Assistant Professor, University of Nicosia Medical School, Nicosia, Cyprus

Annie Cushing
Professor of Clinical Communication, Barts and the London School of Medicine and Dentistry, Queen Mary, University of London, London, UK

Jill Dales
Communication Skills Lead & Director (retired), roleplaynorth communication skills, School of Medical Education, Faculty of Medical Sciences, Newcastle University, Newcastle, UK

Nisha Dogra
Professor of Psychiatry Education and Honorary Consultant in Child and Adolescent Psychiatry, University of Leicester, Leicester, UK

Eva Doherty
Director of Human Factors and Patient Safety, Royal College of Surgeons in Ireland, Dublin, Ireland

Rosie Illingworth
Senior Lecturer in Clinical Communication, Manchester Medical School, University of Manchester, Manchester, UK

Katherine Joekes
Senior Lecturer in Clinical Communication, St George's University of London, London, UK

Theano V. Kalavana
Assistant Professor in Clinical Communication, University of Nicosia Medical School, Nicosia, Cyprus

Jane Kidd
Undergraduate Quality Manager, Education Training and Research, University Hospitals Coventry and Warwickshire NHS Trust, Coventry; External tutor, Institute of Medical and Biomedical Education, St George's University of London, London, UK

Rob Lane
Head of Clinical Communication Skills, School of Medicine, University of Leeds, Leeds, UK

Janet Lefroy
Senior Lecturer in Medical Education, School of Medicine, Keele University, Staffordshire, UK

Susanne Lindqvist
Senior Lecturer in Interprofessional Practice and Director of Centre for Interprofessional Practice, Norwich Medical School, University of East Anglia, Norfolk, UK

Gregory Makoul
CEO, PatientWisdom, Chicago, IL; Founding Director, Connecticut Institute for Primary Care Innovation, Hartford, CT; Professor of Medicine, University of Connecticut School of Medicine, Farmington, CT, USA

Vinnie Nambisan
Consultant in Palliative Medicine, Saint Francis Hospice, Romford, Essex; Tutor in Medical Ethics and Law, University College London Medical School, London, UK

Lorraine M. Noble
Senior Lecturer in Clinical Communication, UCL Medical School, UCL, London, UK

Alexia Papageorgiou
Associate Professor in Clinical Communication, University of Nicosia Medical School, Nicosia, Cyprus

Lindsey Pope
Clinical University Teacher, Undergraduate Medical School, College of Medical, Veterinary and Life Sciences, University of Glasgow, Glasgow, UK

Sally Quilligan
Lecturer in Clinical Communication, School of Clinical Medicine, Cambridge, UK

Jonathan Reinarz
Professor in the History of Medicine, University of Birmingham, Birmingham, UK

Wesley Scott-Smith
Senior Clinical Teaching Fellow and Course Lead in Simulation, Brighton and Sussex Medical School, East Sussex, UK

Jonathan Silverman
Honorary Visiting Senior Fellow, University of Cambridge School of Clinical Medicine, Cambridge; President, European Association for Communication in Healthcare, Salisbury, UK

John Skelton
Professor of Clinical Communication, University of Birmingham, Birmingham, UK

John Spencer
Professor of Primary Care and Clinical Education, School of Medical Sciences Education Development, Faculty of Medical Sciences, Newcastle University, Newcastle, UK

Andrew Tarbuck
Consultant in Old Age Psychiatry, Norfolk and Suffolk NHS Foundation Trust; Honorary Senior Lecturer, University of East Anglia; Dementias & Neurodegenerative Diseases Local Research Network in East Anglia, Norfolk, UK

Margot Turner
Senior Lecturer in Community Medical Education with special responsibility for embedding diversity in the curriculum, St George's University of London, London, UK

Jan van Dalen
Co-ordinator of Communication Training and Assessment, School of Health Professions Education, Maastricht University, Maastricht, the Netherlands

Sandra van Dulmen
Programme Co-ordinator Communication in Health Care, Netherlands Institute for Health Services Research (NIVEL), Utrecht; Professor in Communication in Healthcare, Department of Primary and Community Care, Radboud University Medical Center, Nijmegen, the Netherlands; Professor II, Faculty of Health Sciences, Buskerud and Vestfold University College, Drammen, Norway

Catherine J. Williamson
Director of Clinical Learning, Phase 1 Medicine, School of Medicine, Pharmacy and Health, Durham University, Stockton, UK

Jonathan Wilson
Clinical Senior Lecturer, University of East Anglia, Norfolk, UK; Associate Professor, St George's University, New York, USA; Consultant Psychiatrist, Consultant Psychotherapist (Early intervention/Youth), Child Family and Young Person Service, Norfolk, UK

Connie Wiskin
Senior Lecturer, Co-Director ISU, College of Medical and Dental Sciences, University of Birmingham, Birmingham, UK

Foreword

In these utilitarian times our eyes are sadly deviated from our patients as 'individuals' to the hustle and bustle of treating large numbers of people. Yet, the everyday practice of medicine for all healthcare workers is about communicating well with individual people and being able to reach a satisfactory and true account of a problem to enable a correct diagnosis to be made.

The theories on medical education and the ways of its delivery have changed enormously over the last few decades. New curricula have come and been modified, but gone are the days of the 'see one, do one, and teach one' concept that many of us were brought up on. Now, medical education is based on robust concepts of competence and knowledge, but above all and central to everything is the role of doctors in their daily communication with patients.

There are many books on the market about clinical communication, so why is this book different from the others? First, it is unique, as it gives a historical background as well as an evidence base for how theories have developed. Second, it has been written by a group representing clinical communication teaching in the UK, and most of them are members of the UK Council of Clinical Communication in Undergraduate Medical Education.

The book is essentially divided into three parts. The first part introduces the reader to the doctor–patient relationship, probing into consultation models dating back to 1850. It discusses the term 'patient-centredness', a term that has crept into our everyday practice, and explores what it will mean for us all in the future.

The second part goes into detail about the various components of communication, such as the core skills – for example, sharing bad news, or responding to medical errors and complaints. It also explores topics we all find difficult to communicate to patients, such as explaining risk and talking about the harm/benefit equation when dealing with uncertainty.

Each of these is dissected out and gives helpful comments on how to approach the subject. I was pleased to see that it also looked at diversity issues, such as age, end of life and mental health problems; all difficult issues to deal with in real life.

The third part discusses the various models of learning such as situational, experiential and transformative learning. A lot of educational jargon...but clearly explained! There is also a section on the assessment of communication and the various types of assessment available. Clearly there would be little point in teaching if we cannot assess how well a student has learned, but also exploring what the correct tools are for this assessment.

So, we have come a long way from the 'seeing, doing and teaching one' concept, to the 'knowing, knowing how, showing how, and only at the end when a student is ready, doing'. Hopefully this should result in fewer mistakes and better care for our patients.

This book is written by authors who are all currently active in teaching, and this gives it its authenticity. The editors have brought together a group of 35 authors, mainly from UK universities but also from the USA, Holland and other European countries. It should be read by all medical teachers, researchers and students. In fact, it forms a core thesis for all professions, as the science and art of clinical communication is generic to all.

Parveen J. Kumar CBE, BSc, MD, FRCP, FRCPE, FRCPath
Professor of Medicine and Education
Barts and the London School of Medicine and Dentistry
Queen Mary University of London

CHAPTER 1

Introduction

Jane Kidd

University Hospitals Coventry and Warwickshire NHS Trust, Coventry; Institute of Medical and Biomedical Education, St George's University of London, London, UK

We believe this book is unique, in that it presents the evidence that underpins effective clinical communication. It covers the theories that inform the patient-centred approach, the topics that are taught, how they are taught and how they are assessed.

We know many books exist about how to teach clinical communication or what to include in a clinical communication curriculum, but no other book on communication in the healthcare setting takes the approach of tracing the subject to its primary disciplinary origins, looking at how it is practised, taught and learned today, as well as considering future directions.

Inspiration for the book drew on our experience in teaching clinical communication, in conversation with our colleagues, both teachers and clinicians, which in turn identified a concern that the wide and disparate evidence base for the subject had not been effectively acknowledged, collated and presented.

The book aims to enhance understanding of effective clinical communication by discussing the theories, models and evidence in each of three areas:
• the doctor-patient relationship;
• key components of clinical communication; and
• effective teaching and assessment of clinical communication.

We hope that this will prove to be an important text for teachers, researchers, academics, learners, practitioners and policymakers alike.

Reading this book, you will find yourself introduced to, or possibly reminded of, theories and models from a wide range of disciplines that support effective communication. We believe that in the absence of this knowledge, learning clinical communication can often be superficial, as students learn simply to copy certain statements or behaviours, without a deep understanding of which approaches are effective and why.

We hope that by linking the evidence to the various facets of clinical communication you will understand both the principles and practice of effective communication and how these have come about in the modern world. For educators it may enhance practice both in the teaching and assessment of the subject, learners may more fully appreciate what they are being asked to learn, and as a consequence patients, carers and colleagues may benefit from the changes resulting from this deeper understanding. We hope mostly, however, that this book will stimulate debate, the foundation of healthy academic development of any discipline.

The book is designed so that you can dip in and out as you wish, or you can simply start at the beginning and read through. The chapters begin by providing historical

Clinical Communication in Medicine, First Edition. Edited by Jo Brown, Lorraine M. Noble,
Alexia Papageorgiou and Jane Kidd.
© 2016 John Wiley & Sons, Ltd. Published 2016 by John Wiley & Sons, Ltd.

context before describing current practice, providing you with an appreciation of the depth of the evidence supporting the various components covered. Each chapter concludes with a personal view from the chapter's author on what the future might hold, given the changing context of the healthcare system, the complexity of the learning environment and the evolving roles of the professional and the patient.

We hope that you enjoy the book, that you learn something that you did not know when you picked it up, and that even if you do not agree with the ideas on what the future might hold for this infinitely complex topic, it challenges you to think about the subject and open it up for discussion.

PART 1
The Doctor-Patient Relationship

Section Lead Editor: Lorraine Noble

CHAPTER 2

Introduction to the Doctor–Patient Relationship

Lorraine M. Noble

University College London Medical School, London, UK

The relationship between the doctor and the patient is fundamental to clinical communication. The perceived role of the doctor – as a healer, service provider, professional or evidence-based practitioner – creates an implicit contract that drives expectations, not only about clinical tasks to be accomplished but about the parameters of how doctors approach and respond to patients.

In this section, the historical development of the role of the doctor will be described, including milestones such as the birth of professionalism and the impact of evidence-based medicine. The influence of the context and practice of healthcare on the relationship will be considered, with its consequent implications for doctor–patient communication.

Models of the doctor–patient relationship will be discussed, exploring the changing notions of expertise and power and the focus on the patient as a person. Models of the doctor–patient consultation will be described, highlighting key frameworks that have influenced research, training and healthcare practice. As a backdrop to this discussion, key milestones arising from the research evidence about doctor–patient communication and the synthesis of evidence and practice will be considered, to summarise the current understanding of what constitutes an effective doctor–patient relationship and effective clinical communication.

The current focus on patient-centredness as an approach will be discussed, including the complexities of its definition and use in practice. The impact of current teaching and assessment on the present and next generation of doctors will be considered, including factors affecting the transfer of what is learned to the healthcare environment. The implications for learners of construing communication as a 'set of skills' and relationship building as a 'skill' will be explored.

The effects of changing healthcare practices and societal expectations about the roles of doctors and patients will be considered, including a discussion about what patients want, the impact of a team- or systems-based approach to care, and the role of technology. The section will conclude by speculating on what the future holds for the doctor–patient relationship in an electronic world.

Clinical Communication in Medicine, First Edition. Edited by Jo Brown, Lorraine M. Noble, Alexia Papageorgiou and Jane Kidd.
© 2016 John Wiley & Sons, Ltd. Published 2016 by John Wiley & Sons, Ltd.

CHAPTER 3

History of the Doctor–Patient Relationship

Annie Cushing

Barts and the London School of Medicine and Dentistry, Queen Mary, University of London, London, UK

At the very heart of communication in healthcare lies the expectation of the doctor–patient relationship. The doctor is a healer, witness to suffering, interpreter of symptoms, educator, advocate, and a provider of treatment, comfort and access to services. Whilst the Hippocratic Oath of ancient times embodies the virtues and values within the relationship, the 'medical ideal' is varyingly shaped by the social, scientific, technological and political contexts of the day (Sigerist 1933).

From a trade to a profession

Historically medicine was more like a trade, and doctors were little more than superior servants of the rich who could afford their services. The latter shopped around and decided what they wanted, whilst the doctor complied with issuing treatments (Porter 1997). This was akin to a consumerist model for those who could afford it, whilst the doctor's success depended on the ability to attract patrons. Without standards of practice, quality control or accountability, the patient was vulnerable to quackery.

The birth of the profession in the UK came about through restricted practice with a set of standards established by the Royal Colleges in the 16th century (Warren 2000). Surgeons separated from barber-surgeons and became university educated when the London College of Surgeons was founded in 1745 (Science Museum 2014). These developments recognised academic rigour of physicians and surgeons, in contrast to a trade guild, but there was no 'social contract' with patients, and in fact doctors were more likely to flee epidemics during the 17th century than see any social obligation to stay and treat patients (Wynia 2008).

The modern use of the term 'professionalism' as a basis for the doctor's role towards individuals and society was first mooted in England by Dr Thomas Percival in 1803, but not until 1847 in the USA was it enshrined as a social contract demanding altruism, civic-mindedness, devotion to scientific ideals and a promise of competence and quality assurance through self-regulation (Wynia 2008). Interestingly it was accompanied by expectations that patients should communicate their problem, but not 'weary' the physician with 'tedious detail', and would obey the prescriptions of the physician (Baker *et al.* 1999).

Clinical Communication in Medicine, First Edition. Edited by Jo Brown, Lorraine M. Noble,
Alexia Papageorgiou and Jane Kidd.
© 2016 John Wiley & Sons, Ltd. Published 2016 by John Wiley & Sons, Ltd.

The paradigm of illness underlying the practice of medicine has been dominated since the 17th century by the dualism of mind and body, attributed to the French philosopher René Descartes. Originally his ideas were motivated by religious intentions, in which he argued for the soul's immortality and maintained that the mind or soul *can* exist without the body (Skirry 2006). However, Cartesian Mind-Body dualism came to influence the systems-based approach to medicine and underpin the prevailing discourse within the doctor–patient relationship.

Rise of the scientific paradigm and dominance of the biomedical model

The scientific approach to medicine during the 19th century had a major impact on the role of the doctor. Medical care was revolutionised by the discoveries of the circulation of the heart and vascular system, the germ theory of disease and cell theory with its application to the effects of disease on tissues and organs (Hahn & Kleinman 1983). Doctors' status rose with their scientific knowledge, specialist equipment and professional code. Classifications based on the signs and symptoms of disease became the primary focus. The body was increasingly seen as a machine, and the disease, not the patient's experience of illness, became the object of study and treatment. The relationship was that of an expert doctor, with loss of humility and increased hubris (Wynia 2008), and the patient as a passive recipient of care.

The patient's account of his or her illness was subject to the same systematic approach and became known as 'the medical history'. Its importance in the diagnostic process was recognised by the Canadian physician William Osler, who revolutionised training by insisting that students learned from seeing and talking to patients on the wards. His admonition *'listen to your patient, he is telling you the diagnosis'* highlighted the central role of the patient's narrative (Osler 1914). 'Taking a medical history' became part of clinical reasoning in establishing the causation of disease.

Biomedicine was the predominant model, based essentially on the belief that abnormalities in the body result in symptoms, and that health is the absence of disease (Hahn & Kleinman 1983). By embracing reductionism, the importance of the psychosocial aspect of illness and the patient's perspective went unrecognised and unacknowledged. As the patient's views were unimportant in this biomedical model, informed consent was also a nonexistent phenomenon.

From the late 19th century, psychoanalysis and talking therapies emerged to study the mind and explain conversion of psychological traumas to physical symptoms and expressions of unhappiness (European Graduate School n.d.). Whilst therapeutic alliance in the doctor–patient relationship was crucial to the healing process, the power resided with the doctor.

Healthcare as a right

In the UK in 1945, the creation of a National Health Service (NHS) by Aneurin Bevan brought about healthcare free at the point of need. The benign paternalism of the welfare state provided for the population 'from the cradle to the grave' (Beveridge 1942). This was a hugely significant historical moment, enshrining health as a right, and consultation rates increased enormously (Rivett 1998). Doctors now treated people from all socio-economic groups who were grateful, powerless and uncritical. The formers' success was dependent on approval from hospital superiors and not patients. The medical profession was reluctantly drawn into practising within an NHS, initially fearing control by the state, but they still had enormous freedom with state-sanctioned power and deferential patients.

Challenges to the biomedical model and rise of the biopsychosocial model

In the mid-20th century, sociology and psychology, new fields of discourse, joined the debate about the doctor–patient relationship. The American sociologist Talcott Parsons in 1951 referred to the 'sick role', in which patients were regarded as passive victims but were expected to want to get better by following the advice of the expert doctor (Parsons 1951). The patient was absolved of responsibility for their illness and allowed to abstain from their usual roles in society until they were better.

Recognising different contexts, the physicians Thomas Szasz and Marc Hollender described three basic models of doctor–patient relationship: activity-passivity, whereby the physician does something to an inert or unresponsive patient; guidance-cooperation, in which the physician tells the patient what to do and the patient complies; and mutual participation, whereby the physician helps the patient to help him- or herself and the patient participates as a partner (Szasz & Hollender 1956). In all situations however, 'compliance', essentially meaning *obeying doctors' orders,* was expected (Stimson 1974). In the name of reducing anxiety, the truth was often withheld from patients, and doctors made decisions about treatment (Freidson 1960). This 'benign paternalism' was the cornerstone of the relationship. Indeed one might characterise it psychodynamically, or in transactional analysis terms, as a parent–child type of relationship (Berne 1961). It was criticised for maintaining doctors' power base at the expense of respecting patient autonomy, and Eliot Freidson called for patients, as consumers, to be actively involved to negotiate effectively for services (Freidson 1986). The nature of the doctor–patient relationship was now up for debate.

Whilst the sociologists were concerned with issues of power, others such as George Engel, Michael Balint and Carl Rogers viewed the relationship through the lens of 'dynamic psychology'. Engel advocated the need for a new medical model that linked science and humanism and used the term 'bio-psychosocial-cultural' (Engel 1977). This integrated information concerning *what was the matter with the patient* and *what mattered to the patient.* Rogers, a humanistic psychologist, maintained that for a person to "grow", he or she needed an environment that provided genuineness, acceptance and empathy. Anyone in a therapeutic relationship, such as a doctor or therapist, needed to demonstrate unconditional positive regard, openness, warmth and a willingness to listen and understand the person (Rogers 1961). The goal was to empower the person to fulfil his or her potential. Rogers' work was hugely important in the 1960s, defining a basis for the doctor–patient relationship, specifying both underlying attitudes and skilled behaviours.

At the same time, the Hungarian psychoanalysts Michael and Enid Balint, working in the UK, recognised the impact on doctors of the limitations of the biomedical model, as they saw doctors struggle with patients where they could find no diagnosis or satisfy the patient. Balint was the first to coin the term 'Patient-centred medicine', to describe the belief that each patient *'has to be understood as a unique human being'* (Balint 1961).

Balint training groups enabled doctors to share situations where they did not know what was going on or what to do for a patient, their frustration when the medical model did not help and the impact of their feelings of helplessness on their behaviour. His book, *The Doctor, His Patient and the Illness* (Balint 1964), was hugely influential on British medicine, and Balint groups spread to the USA and Europe (Salinsky 2003).

The birth of feminism in the 1960s was a significant milestone as a catalyst for social action around the control of women's reproductive rights. The Boston Women's Health Collective publication *Our Bodies, Ourselves* inspired the women's health movement and challenged the pathology/disease approach to normal life events such as giving birth, menopause, aging and death (Boston Women's Health Collective 1970). It maintained that informed health consumers can become their own health experts, and that they have a right to know about controversies surrounding medical practices. Deference was being questioned. Ivan Illich further described how over-medicalization was making people lifelong patients, reducing their capacity to deal with life's problems (Illich 1975a). Doctors, by their classification systems, controlled the definition of illness and tended to see illness and need for treatment rather than normality and health (Foucault 1973). Doctors were neither acknowledging nor explaining risks, and the problem of iatrogenesis (harm caused by medical treatment), both clinical and social, was significant (Illich 1975b).

The two 'realities' in the doctor–patient relationship were defined by Elliot Mishler in the terms 'medicines world' and patients' 'lifeworld'. The world concept and language in each differed (Mishler 1984). The patient is the one who moves in and out of the healthcare setting trying to maintain his or her narrative in the 'lifeworld', and problems arise when the patient is ignored or blocked by doctors' use of the voice of medicine (Kleinman 1988).

The broader context was echoed by the lawyer Ian Kennedy in his book *The Unmasking of Medicine* (Kennedy 1981). He argued that notions of disease, illness and health are not morally neutral and shared decision making was being hindered by protected vested interests and the state-sanctioned power of the medical profession. He advocated a wider debate over values, ethical judgments and the political choices within healthcare, with a moral duty to listen to society at large. He significantly influenced the later introduction of bioethics as a core component of the medical curriculum.

The biopsychosocial concept of health, or 'Whole Person Health', was affirmed in the World Health Organisation's Alma-Ata Declaration in 1978, a major milestone of the 20th century, defining health as *'a state of complete physical, mental, and social well-being, and not merely the absence of disease or infirmity'* (World Health Organisation 1978).

The era of evidence-based medicine: studying the doctor–patient relationship

The seminal research of the American paediatrician Barbara Korsch first demonstrated how outcomes of medical care were affected by doctor–patient communication (Korsch *et al.* 1968). She identified how mothers frequently left the consultation without having expressed their main concerns or questions. Half had not received an explanation of the cause of their child's symptoms and doctors often used jargon that families did not understand.

The concept of 'evidence-based medicine' was beginning to emerge, and in 1972 Archie Cochrane called for evidence as a priority for the NHS (Cochrane 1972). The Cochrane

Collaboration was subsequently established to coordinate and publish systematic reviews. Criticism of evidence-based medicine from within and outside the profession was countered by David Sackett, who argued that evidence-based practice was the integration of individual clinical expertise with the best available external clinical research evidence and judicious application to the care of individual patients (Sackett 1996).

Research on the doctor–patient interaction burgeoned from the 1980s with audio- and videotaping now enabling observation of the process. The ground-breaking work of Patrick Byrne and Barrie Long in the UK identified consultations ranging from heavily doctor-dominated, closed questioning to very open, facilitative listening styles (Byrne & Long 1976). High control styles were common, and interruption of patients only 18 seconds into the consultation, as reported by Howard Beckman and Richard Frankel, led to important information being missed (Beckman & Frankel 1984; Platt & McMath 1979). David Tuckett and colleagues revealed how patients' thoughts and 'expertise', particularly of those from lower socioeconomic groups, remained unknown to doctors (Tuckett et al. 1985).

Howard Waitzkin found that doctors only used about 1 minute of a 20-minute consultation to give advice (Waitzkin 1984). Patient dissatisfaction with information provided was compounded by the finding that doctors did not organise their information to align with patients' thinking, so explanations were less effective, not understood or forgotten (Ley & Spellman 1968). Patients often misinterpreted what doctors were intending to convey, and understanding of terminology, anatomy and disease was poor (Boyle 1970). Aaron Lazare found that despite 99% of patients having treatment preferences, only 37% voiced these spontaneously (Lazare et al. 1975). Moreover Peter Maguire showed how clinicians avoided emotionally challenging situations by using distancing tactics, and in so doing, mental health problems often remained undiagnosed and untreated (Maguire 1985). This highlighted how doctors' own emotions and psychological needs were central in the doctor–patient relationship, as well as the skills they did or did not possess. Hence such studies on the doctor–patient relationship revealed how communication and partnership might be threatened.

Evidence was amassing of correlation between doctor–patient communication and health outcomes and a significant milestone was the publication in 1988 by Judith Hall and colleagues of a meta-analysis study (Hall et al. 1988). Moira Stewart's review found that outcomes associated with doctor–patient communication were, in descending order of frequency, emotional health, symptom resolution, function, physiologic measures (i.e. blood pressure and blood sugar level) and pain control. The key aspects of communication found to enhance patients' cooperation with the management plan were orientation, facilitation of patient's ideas and questions, sharing ideas and humour (Stewart et al. 1999). Ineffective communication was associated with medication errors and malpractice claims (Hulka et al. 1976; Levinson et al. 1997).

During the period 1986–1996, over 40 patient–physician communication instruments were published (Boon & Stewart 1998). Amongst the many, Deborah Roter's Interactional Analysis Scale (Roter 1995) correlated most highly with other instruments and was to become used worldwide with application to more than 45 areas of communication contexts and outcomes.

A significant milestone in 1991 was the evidence-based Toronto consensus statement on doctor–patient communication, with implications for practice and training (Simpson et al. 1991). From their review of research, a strong message emerged; within the relationship, doctors needed to use their power wisely, not to control but to 'find common ground', show care, and guide and empower patients in collaborative relationships and shared decision making to improve outcomes (Brown et al. 1989; Stewart et al. 1999).

Patient-centredness and models of the doctor–patient relationship

The concept of patient-centredness, first mooted by Balint, now increasingly appeared in the literature, and in 1999, the Society of General Internal Medicine in the USA endorsed this approach (Association of American Medical Colleges 1999). The Transformed Clinical Method was proposed by Ian McWhinney and colleagues in Canada to operationalise Engel's biopsychosocial model (McWhinney 1989). The increasingly systematic approach to studying the doctor–patient interaction in practice led to a variety of models of the doctor–patient relationship being developed, which are discussed in Alexia Papageorgiou's chapter on models of the doctor–patient consultation (chapter 4).

The psychodynamic models were highly relevant to the underlying doctor–patient relationship. Notably, Eric Berne's channels of communication identified verbal and nonverbal behaviour embodying 'parent', 'adult' and 'child' (superego, ego and id) states (Berne 1961). The 'parent' relationship maps particularly to the paternalistic approach, whilst the 'adult' relationship embodies respect for patient autonomy and partnership. John Heron described 'authoritative' and 'facilitative' interventions, both of which were appropriate, depending on context (Heron 1976). Additionally he identified inappropriate and potentially 'harmful' interventions that he termed 'perverted'. These arose from conscious or unconscious attitudes and underlying assumptions. The skills-based models have, however, largely dominated in training, and Keith Taylor argues that the change in underlying assumptions about the relationship in the patient-centred model have been more implicit than explicit (Taylor 2009). The concept of patient-centredness has become a dominant paradigm and is discussed in Rosie Illingworth's chapter (chapter 6).

At the end of the 20th century, the concept of 'concordance' was proposed by the Royal Pharmaceutical Society in the UK. This was a radical shift in the consultation dynamic, which traditionally demanded that both parties act to avoid tension or conflict that could jeopardise the encounter in the immediate and long term. It involved honest sharing of ideas and real negotiation *'so that both doctor and patient together can proceed on the basis of reality and not of misunderstanding, distrust or concealment'* (Royal Pharmaceutical Society Great Britain 1997). It was however frequently misunderstood and misrepresented in the literature as 'patient concordance'; in other words a patient behaviour rather than a process in which *'agreement to differ'* could also be legitimate. Kristian Pollock argued that its *true* meaning was not recognised in everyday practice and that professional paternalism with pseudo-concordance prevailed, in which *'informed compliance'* persists (Pollock 2005).

Training on the doctor–patient relationship

Formal training on the doctor–patient relationship and doctor–patient communication emerged in the 1970s. Howard Barrows, a neurologist, introduced standardised patients in 1968 as an educational device to teach history and examination skills (Barrows 1968), whilst Paula Stillman, a paediatrician, trained 'simulated mothers' to teach interviewing skills and assess students' performance (Stillman *et al.* 1976). By the mid-1970s, communication skills training was widespread in the USA, but a third of British medical schools provided no training (Wakefield 1983). In the UK, a group of general practitioners pioneered vocational training on the consultation, and courses for trainers were developed using videotaping of patient consultations (Pendleton *et al.* 1984).

In the USA, the American Association of Medical Colleges established a Task Force on the Doctor and Patient in the 1980s and launched a national facilitator training programme to promote knowledge, attitudes and skills relating to the medical interview across all specialities (Lipkin *et al.* 1995). This prompted the first UK training initiative for senior hospital doctors in 1989, with the founding of the Medical Interview Teaching Association (Bird *et al.* 1993). Postgraduate training was important to promote best practice by clinicians and to develop trainers for the expanding undergraduate and postgraduate teaching. The development of 'clinical communication skills' as a discipline is discussed in Victoria Bates and colleagues' chapter (chapter 27).

National drivers and policy on training about the doctor–patient relationship

The resurgence of neoliberalism worldwide, associated with the ideas of economic theorists such as Milton Friedman, was embraced by the conservative government of Margaret Thatcher in the 1980s (Scott-Samuel *et al.* 2014). It supported extensive economic liberalisation, free trade and reduction in government spending to enhance the private sector in the economy. Within the neoliberal paradigm, healthcare was less a social right and more a market commodity (McGregor 2001). Accordingly, marketization would take care of services, whilst individual personal responsibility and aspirations for healthcare would increase consumer choice and power. Professional power would be tempered. Application of private-sector management principles paved the way for subsequent privatisation of elements of the NHS by Conservative and Labour governments.

The UK government's *Patient's Charter*, published in 1991, called for fuller and greater public and patient involvement in healthcare services at a strategic level to assure accountability for public funds, together with empowerment of patients in their own healthcare decisions (Department of Health 1991). Powerful lobbying charities and independent health policy groups influenced the patient partnership agenda, reflecting wider societal cultural changes towards rights, respect, dignity, openness and partnership (Cayton 2004; Coulter & Collins 2011). Evidence-based medicine also grew at this time with the pressure for public accountability of resources and managerial control over medical practice (Scally & Donaldson 1998). Burgeoning healthcare costs, patient safety issues and recognition that many illnesses and acute exacerbations result from lifestyle factors fuelled the call for a new doctor–patient relationship (Department of Health 1996, 2001, 2010; National Patient Safety Agency 2009).

In the USA, where much of the communication research originated, training and assessment were already widespread in the 1990s (Klass *et al.* 1998). In 1993 the General Medical Council, the registration body in the UK, published *Tomorrow's Doctors*, which recommended that '*communication skills and attitudes that befit a doctor*' be explicitly incorporated into undergraduate medical education (General Medical Council 1993). The doctor–patient relationship could no longer be left to chance or customary practice. The General Medical Council also published *Duties of a Doctor*, which specified honesty as a duty (General Medical Council 1995). Despite scepticism within the profession, these influential documents led to development of curricula, explicit teaching on the doctor–patient relationship and ethics, and the incorporation of communication competences into qualifying examinations across the UK (Doyal & Gillon 1998; Hargie *et al.* 1998).

National consensus documents to foster best practice in communication education established quality criteria (Makoul & Schofield 1999; von Fragstein *et al.* 2008). By 1998 assessment of clinical communication competency was part of licensing examinations for international medical graduates applying for provisional registration to work in the UK (General Medical Council 2013). Compulsory postgraduate advanced communication training for all clinicians working in cancer medicine was introduced as part of the NHS Cancer Plan of 2000 (Department of Health 2000).

The General Medical Council in the UK defined postgraduate communication curriculum outcomes and the Royal Colleges specified the requirement for competency in communication within the new *doctor–patient partnership* and *shared decision-making* model, and assessments of clinical communication became part of membership examinations (Federation of the Royal Colleges of Physician 2006; Academy of Medical Royal Colleges 2009; General Medical Council 2010).

The era of research on training and evidence of its effectiveness

Associations for research into medical education date back to the mid-20th century. However it was not until 1999 that the first Best Evidence Medical Education review of communication skills teaching studies was published (Aspegren 1999). Studies were of low quality with only one long-term follow-up, but key points were that learning methods should be experiential, occur in the 'clinical' (clerkship) years and primarily focus on problem definition. Robert Hulsman and colleagues' review of postgraduate training also found that most of the studies used inadequate research designs (Hulsman *et al.* 1999). Those with the most adequate designs reported the fewest positive training effects, with half or less of the observed behaviours evident. A significant milestone was the publication of the first randomised controlled trial in 2003, showing an enduring effect of communication skills training with transfer to the clinic (Fallowfield *et al.* 2003). However, other research revealed problems with application to clinical settings (Dwamena *et al.* 2012). The issue of transfer of learning to the clinical environment is discussed in John Skelton's chapter (chapter 7).

Public inquiries in the 21st century: Trust in the doctor–patient relationship

At the beginning of this century the doctor–patient relationship came under scrutiny in the UK. A number of high-profile cases of serious failures of care, ranging from Bristol Royal Infirmary Inquiry in 2001 into care of children receiving complex cardiac surgical services (Bristol Royal Infirmary Inquiry 2001), the serial killer Dr Harold Shipman (Home Secretary and the Secretary of State for Health 2007), and the recent Francis Report (Francis 2013) on neglect at the Mid Staffordshire Hospital in 2013, brought trust in the profession into question. The Bristol Inquiry spoke of a 'club culture' with lack of standards for evaluation of performance, quality of care, appraisal and revalidation. These professional failures prompted renewed debate around professionalism and reports on safeguarding patients (Department of Health 2007). Sir Donald Irvine, chairman of the Picker Institute Europe (an international charity), pointed out that *'We know quite a lot about communication and skills and how to teach them but there is not much known about the attitudes that underpin this'* (Royal College of Physicians 2005, p. 33).

In 2005 in the UK, the Royal College of Physicians' report on professionalism restated the values of integrity, compassion, altruism, continuing improvement, excellence, working in partnership with members of the wider healthcare team, personal responsibility and accountability that underpin the science and practice of medicine (Royal College of Physicians 2005). The Kings Fund (an independent charity in the UK) in 2010 included views of lay people, amongst the various stakeholders, to define the basis for a moral contract between the medical profession and society in achieving the goals of best care for both the population as a whole and for the individual (Levenson *et al.* 2010).

In the USA, Matthew Wynia warned about the domination of respect for individual autonomy and loss of the societal aspect of the initial understanding of professionalism. He argued that a contemporary social contract requires retention of commitment to science with negotiation between the patient's expectations, resource distribution, and service to society, artful practice, humility and self-regulation (Wynia 2008).

Whole systems and teamworking

By the turn of the century, healthcare was increasingly complex, with multiprofessional healthcare teams and many traditional duties of a doctor extended to allied professionals. The concept of relationship-centred care had been introduced in the USA in the 1990s and encompassed collaborative relationships within teams, team working and organisational practices impacted on the doctor–patient relationship (Tresolini & the Pew-Fetzer Task Force 1994). The culture and values of an organisation profoundly affected congruence of the workforce. It was recognised that interactions between clinicians and all other staff in the healthcare institution, especially in hierarchical organisations, affected their own well-being in addition to the health of patients. *'When an organisation diverges from core principles of relationship centredness, the practitioner is forced to engage with patients in a manner sometimes quite different from how he or she is treated'* (Beach *et al.* 2006). Stress on healthcare workers had implications for care and risked compromising empathy. In the UK the Francis Report revealed resourcing pressures, stress, attitude and culture as sources of problems (Francis 2013). Increased specialisation in the organisation of care resulted in great benefits of expertise but also weakened continuity of relationships for patients (Cornwall *et al.* 2012). Audits of the patient's experience within the *whole* system became common as one indicator of care quality (Coulter 2005a).

The tension between feeding the data-gathering imperative for financial and management purposes, the needs of research and evidence-based medicine, whilst serving the patient narrative and human experience of care, all within a time-limited consultation, presents a challenge (Iles 2014). The clinician's capacity for self-awareness and integrity, especially the ability to *sustain* these in complex and challenging circumstances, was recognised as a basis for positive relationships with colleagues and patients.

The patient in the patient-doctor relationship: the Internet and democratisation of knowledge

Arguably the most profound effect on the doctor–patient relationship has come from the explosion of information available to the public in the 21st century. The potential for patients themselves to influence the interaction has been supported not only by information from a myriad of websites but also formal training aimed at improving patients' ability to be more skilful in handling the consultation to express their ideas, information and involvement needs. Expert patient programmes evolved to harness the expertise and lay understanding of self-management, to support other patients with long-term conditions, as well as to train health professionals in a collaborative approach to consultations (Department of Health 2001; Wallace *et al.* 2012).

Focus on patients' ability and desire for involvement in their healthcare recognised the importance of 'health literacy', defined as '*the cognitive and social skills which determine the motivation and ability of individuals to gain access to, understand, and use information in ways which promote and maintain good health*' (American Medical Association 1999). Patients with inadequate health literacy experience a complex array of communication difficulties that interact to influence health outcome (Nutbeam 2008). Lack of understanding, feelings of intimidation and associated shame could be reinforced by hospital staff who become frustrated or angry (Parikh *et al.* 1996). Those less able to seek help when needed lack confidence and effectiveness in managing their health and healthcare (Hibbard & Gilbert 2014).

These patient factors affect the doctor–patient encounter. Some authors warned of potential risks of 'victim blaming' in the individual responsibility model, which could damage the doctor–patient relationship (Marantz 1990). Patients' dependency and need for support differ, requiring a flexible approach by clinicians in promoting patient engagement and self-care. Iona Heath argued that if not balanced with unconditional positive regard, nonjudgement and compassion, expectations of patient responsibility could be detrimental and oppressive (Heath 1995).

Globalisation, information technology and consumerism

Increasing global migration in the 21st century brought together doctors and patients from diverse social and cultural backgrounds. In 2009, 58% of new General Medical Council registrants qualified in the UK, 23% were from the European Economic Area and 19% were international medical graduates from outside the European Economic Area (General Medical Council 2010). In addition to sociolinguistic challenges (General Medical Council 2014), doctors and patients hold a range of expectations of the doctor–patient relationship and views on healthcare rights, public accountability and personal responsibility. This requires even greater skill in the doctor–patient interaction to work within a patient-centred model of care.

Information technology revolutionised the collection and storage of patient data, with standards for records recently published by the Royal College of Physicians (Royal College of Physicians 2015). The implications of the electronic patient record on the consultation are emerging, with warnings that bureaucratisation '*risks marginalisation of aspects of quality which lie beyond their focus, in particular attention to patient narrative*' and that doctors need '*to be creative in using templates to avoid privileging "institution-centred" care over patient-centred care*' (Swinglehurst *et al.* 2012). Evidence-based medicine's supremacy, it is argued, has limitations in situations of complex healthcare needs where co-morbidity is so prevalent (Greenhalgh *et al.* 2014).

Are we moving towards a consumerist model in which power relationships are reversed, with the patient taking the active role and the doctor adopting a fairly passive role, acceding to the patient's requests for particular treatments, a second opinion, referral to hospital, a sick note and so on? Picker Institute surveys show that the British public remains strongly in favour of equity and participation, with high-quality services available to all, accountability of providers and independent regulation at arm's length from government (Coulter 2005b).

In the current social, scientific and political climate doctors need to use their expertise wisely in the service of patients and navigate the various demands and constraints within a social contract, whilst at the same time retaining the ability to care, to be trustworthy and share information, decisions, uncertainty and even mistakes openly. The final word must go to Henry Sigerist, who reminds us that "the physician's position in society is never determined by the physician himself, but by the society he is serving" (Sigerist 1933).

References

Academy of Medical Royal Colleges. (2009) *Improving Assessment*. Academy of Medical Royal Colleges, London.

American Medical Association. (1999) Health literacy: Report of the Council on Scientific Affairs. Ad Hoc Committee on Health Literacy for the Council on Scientific Affairs. *JAMA*, 281, 552–557.

Aspegren, K. (1999) BEME guide no. 2: Teaching and learning communication skills in medicine. *Medical Teacher*, 21, 563–570.

Association of American Medical Colleges. (1999) *Contemporary issues in medicine: Communication in medicine*. Medical School Objectives Project 1999 [WWW document]. URL www.aamc.org/meded/msop1.pdf.

Baker, R., Caplan, A., Emanuel, L. & Latham, S. (eds). (1999) *The American Medical Ethics Revolution: How the AMA's Code of Ethics Has Transformed Physicians' Relationships to Patients, Professionals and Society*. John Hopkins University Press, Baltimore, MD.

Balint, M. (1961) The other part of medicine. *Lancet*, 1, 40–42.

Balint, M. (1964) *The Doctor, His Patient and the Illness*. Pitman Medical Publishing, London.

Barrows, H. (1968) Simulated patients in medical teaching. *Canadian Medical Association Journal*, 98, 674–676.

Beach, M., Inui, T. & Relationship-Centred Care Research Network. (2006) Relationship-centered care: A constructive reframing. *Journal of General Internal Medicine*, 21, S3–8.

Beckman, H. & Frankel, R. (1984) The effect of physician behavior on the collection of data. *Annals of Internal Medicine*, 101, 692–696.

Berne, E. (1961) *Transactional Analysis in Psychotherapy: A Systematic Individual and Social Psychiatry*. Grove Press, New York.

Beveridge, W. (1942) *Social Insurance and Allied Services*. Report by Sir William Beveridge. HMSO, London.

Bird, J., Hall, A., Maguire, P. & Heavy, A. (1993) Workshops for consultants on the teaching of clinical communication skills. *Medical Education*, 27, 181–185.

Boon, H. & Stewart, M. (1998) Patient-physician communication assessment instruments: 1986–1996 in review. *Patient Education and Counseling*, 35, 161–176.

Boston Women's Health Collective. (1970) *Our bodies ourselves* [WWW document]. URL http://www.ourbodiesourselves.org/cms/assets/uploads/2014/04/Women-and-Their-Bodies-1970.pdf.

Boyle, C. (1970) Difference between patients' and doctors' interpretation of some common medical terms. *BMJ*, 2, 286–289.

Bristol Royal Infirmary Inquiry. (2001) *Learning from Bristol: The Report of the Public Inquiry into Children's Heart Surgery at the Bristol Royal Infirmary 1984–1995.* HMSO, London.

Brown, J., Weston, W. & Stewart, M. (1989) Patient-centred interviewing. Part II: Finding common ground. *Canadian Family Physician*, 35, 151–158.

Byrne, P. & Long, B. (1976) *Doctors Talking to Patients.* HMSO, London.

Cayton, H. 2004. *Patient Engagement and Patient Decision-Making in England.* The Commonwealth Fund/Nuffield Trust, New York.

Cochrane, A. (1972) *Effectiveness and Efficiency: Random Reflections on Health Services.* The Nuffield Provincial Hospitals Trust, London.

Cornwall, J., Levenson, R., Sonola, L. & Poteliakhoff, E. (2012) *Continuity of Care for Older Hospital Patients: A Call for Action.* The King's Fund, London.

Coulter, A. (2005a) *Trends in patients experience of the NHS.* Picker Institute [WWW document]. URL http://www.pickereurope.org/wp-content/uploads/2014/10/Trends-in-patients-experience-of-the-NHS.pdf.

Coulter, A. (2005b) What do patients and the public want from primary care? *BMJ*, 331, 1199.

Coulter, A. & Collins, A. (2011) *Making Shared Decision-Making a Reality: No Decision about Me, without Me.* The King's Fund, London.

Department of Health. (1991) *The Patient's Charter.* HMSO, London.

Department of Health. (1996) *Patient Partnership: Building a Collaborative Strategy.* HMSO, London.

Department of Health. (2000) *The NHS Cancer Plan: A Plan for Investment, a Plan for Reform.* HMSO, London.

Department of Health. (2001) *The Expert Patient: A New Approach to Chronic Disease Management for the 21st Century.* HMSO, London.

Department of Health. (2007) *Safeguarding Patients: The Government's Response to the Recommendations of the Shipman Inquiry's Fifth Report and to the Recommendations of the Ayling, Neale and Kerr/Haslam Inquiries.* HMSO, London.

Department of Health. (2010) *Equity and Excellence: Liberating the NHS.* Department of Health, London.

Doyal, L. & Gillon, R. (1998) Medical ethics and law as a core subject in medical education. *BMJ*, 316, 1623–1624.

Dwamena, F., Holmes-Rovner, M., Gaulden, C., Jorgenson, S., Sadigh, G., Sikorskii, A., Lewin, S., Smith, R.C., Coffey, J. & Olomu, A. (2012) Interventions for providers to promote a patient-centred approach in clinical consultations. Cochrane Database of Systematic Reviews, 2 (Art. No.: CD003267). doi:10.1002/14651858.CD003267.pub2.

Engel, G. (1977) The need for a new medical model: A challenge for biomedicine. *Science*, 196, 129–136.

European Graduate School: Graduate and Postgraduate Studies. (n.d.) *Sigmund Freud biography* [WWW document]. URL http://www.egs.edu/library/sigmund-freud/biography/.

Fallowfield, L., Jenkins, V., Farewell, V. & Solis-Trapala, I. (2003) Enduring impact of communication skills training: Results of a 12-month follow-up. *British Journal of Cancer*, 89, 1445–1449.

Federation of the Royal Colleges of Physicians. (2006) *Generic Curriculum for the Medical Specialities.* Federation of the Royal Colleges of Physician UK, London.

Foucault, M. 1973. *The Birth of the Clinic: An Archaeology of Medical Perception.* Routledge, London.

Francis, R. (chair). (2013) *Report of the Mid Staffordshire NHS Foundation Trust Public Inquiry.* HMSO, London.

Freidson, E. (1960) Client control and medical practice. *American Journal of Sociology*, 65, 374–382.

Freidson, E. (1986) *Professional Powers: A Study of the Institutionalization of Formal Knowledge.* University of Chicago Press, Chicago.

General Medical Council. (1993) *Tomorrow's Doctors: Recommendations on Undergraduate Medical Education.* General Medical Council, London.

General Medical Council. (1995) *Duties of a Doctor.* General Medical Council, London.

General Medical Council. (2010) *Final Report of the Education and Training Regulation Policy Review: Recommendations and Options for the Future Regulation of Education and Training.* General Medical Council, London.

General Medical Council. (2013) *Response to Freedom of Information request* [WWW document]. URL https://www.whatdotheyknow.com/request/plab_exam_historical_pass_rates.

General Medical Council. (2014) *Making sure all licensed doctors have the necessary knowledge of English to practise safely in the UK* [WWW document]. URL http://www.gmc-uk.org/.

Greenhalgh, T., Howick, J. & Maskrey, N. (2014) Evidence based medicine: a movement in crisis? *BMJ*, 348, G3725. doi:10.1136/bmj.g3725.

Hahn, R. & Kleinman, A. (1983) Biomedical practice and anthropological theory: Frameworks and directions. *Annual Review of Anthropology*, 12, 305–333.

Hall, J., Roter, D. & Katz, N. (1988) Meta-analysis of correlates of provider behaviour in medical encounters. *Medical Care*, 26, 657–675.

Hargie, O., Dickson, D., Boohan, M. & Highes, K. (1998) A survey of communication skills training in UK Schools of Medicine: Present practices and prospective proposals. *Medical Education*, 32, 25–34.

Heath, I. (1995) *The Mystery of General Practice*. The John Fry Trust Fellowship. Nuffield Provincial Hospitals Trust, London.

Heron, J. (1976) A six-category intervention analysis. *British Journal of Guidance and Counseling*, 4, 143–155.

Hibbard, J. & Gilbert, H. (2014) *Supporting people to manage their health: An introduction to patient activation*. Kings Fund [WWW document]. URL http://www.kingsfund.org.uk.

Home Secretary and the Secretary of State for Health. (2007) *Learning from Tragedy, Keeping Patients Safe: Overview of the Government's Action Programme in Response to the Recommendations of the Shipman Inquiry*. HMSO, London.

Hulka, B., Cassel, J., Kupper, L. & Burdette, J. (1976) Communication, compliance, and concordance between physicians and patients with prescribed medications. *American Journal of Public Health*, 66, 847–853.

Hulsman, R., Ros, W., Winnubst, J. & Bensing, J. (1999) Teaching clinically experienced physicians communication skills: A review of evaluation studies. *Medical Education*, 33, 655–668.

Iles, V. (2014) *Why reforming the NHS doesn't work: The importance of understanding how good people offer bad care*. Really Learn [WWW document]. URL http://www.reallylearning.com/.

Illich, I. (1975a) The medicalization of life. *Journal of Medical Ethics*, 1, 73–77.

Illich, I. (1975b) *Medical Nemesis: The Expropriation of Health*. Calder and Boyars, London.

Kennedy, I. (1981) *The Unmasking of Medicine*. Allen and Unwin, London.

Klass, D., DeChamplain, A., Fletcher, E., King, A. & Macmillan, M. (1998) Development of a performance-based test of clinical skills for the United States Medical Licensing Examination. *Federation Bulletin*, 85, 177–185.

Kleinman, A. (1988) *The Illness Narratives: Suffering, Healing, and the Human Condition*. Basic Books, New York.

Korsch, B., Gozzi, E. & Francis, V. (1968) Gaps in doctor–patient communication I: Doctor patient interaction and patient satisfaction. *Pediatrics*, 42, 855–871.

Lazare, A., Eisenthal, S. & Wasserman, L. (1975) The customer approach to patienthood: Attending to patient requests in a walk-in clinic. *Archives of General Psychiatry*, 32, 553–558.

Levenson, R., Atkinson, S. & Shepherd, S. (2010) *The 21st-Century Doctor: Understanding the Doctors of Tomorrow*. The King's Fund, London.

Levinson, W., Roter, D., Mullooly, J., Dull, V. & Frankel, R. (1997) The relationship among malpractice claims among primary care physicians and surgeons. *JAMA*, 277, 553–559.

Ley, P. & Spellman, M. (1968) *Communicating with the Patient*. Staples Press, London.

Lipkin, M.J., Putnam, S. & Lazare, A. (1995) *The Medical Interview: Clinical Care, Education and Research*. Springer-Verlag, New York.

Maguire, P. (1985) Barriers to psychological care of the dying. *BMJ*, 291, 1711–1713.

Makoul, G. & Schofield, T. (1999) Communication teaching and assessment in medical education: An international consensus statement. *Patient Education and Counseling*, 37, 191–195.

Marantz, P. (1990) Blaming the victim: The negative consequences of preventive medicine. *American Journal of Public Health*, 80, 1186–1187.

McGregor, S. (2001) Neoliberalism and health care. *International Journal of Consumer Studies*, 25, 82–89.

McWhinney, I. (1989) The need for a transformed clinical method. In: M. Stewart & D. Roter (eds), *Communicating with Medical Patients*, p. 25. Sage Publications, London.

Mishler, E. (1984) *The Discourse of Medicine: The Dialectics of Medical Interviews*. Ablex, Norwood, NJ.

National Patient Safety Agency. (2009) *Being open framework*. National Reporting and Learning Service [WWW document]. URL http://www.nrls.npsa.nhs.uk/beingopen/.

Nutbeam, D. (2008) The evolving concept of health literacy. *Social Science and Medicine*, 67, 2072–2078.

Osler, S.W. (1914) *Aequinimitas. With Other Addresses to Medical Students, Nurses and Practitioners of Medicine*, second edn. HK Lewis, London.

Parikh, N.S., Parker, R.M., Nurss, J.R., Baker, D.W. & Williams, M.V. (1996) Shame and health literacy: The unspoken connection. *Patient Education and Counseling*, 27, 33–39.

Parsons, T. (1951) Illness and the role of the physician: A sociological perspective. *American Journal of Orthopsychiatry*, 21, 452–460.

Pendleton, D., Schofield, T., Tate, P. & Havelock, P. (1984) *The Consultation: An Approach to Learning and Teaching*. Oxford University Press, Oxford.

Platt, F. & McMath, J. (1979) Clinical hypocompetence: The interview. *Annals of Internal Medicine*, 9, 898–902.

Pollock, K. (2005) *Concordance in Medical Consultations: A Critical Review*. Radcliffe Publishing, Oxford, chaps. 2, 3, and 10.

Porter, R. (1997) *The Greatest Benefit to Mankind: A Medical History of Humanity from Antiquity to the Present*. Harper Collins, London.

Rivett, G. (1998) *From Cradle to Grave, Fifty Years of the NHS*. The Kings Fund, London.

Rogers, C. (1961) The characteristics of a helping relationship. In: *On Becoming a Person: A Therapist's View of Psychotherapy*, pp. 39–58. Houghton Mifflin, Boston, MA.

Roter, D. (1995) *The Roter Method of Interaction Process Analysis*. Department of Health Policy and Management, School of Hygiene and Public Health, Johns Hopkins University, Baltimore, MD.

Royal College of Physicians. (2005) *Doctors in Society: Medical professionalism in a Changing World*. Report of a Working Party of the Royal College of Physicians. London.

Royal College of Physicians. (2015) Healthcare record standards [WWW document]. URL https://www.rcplondon.ac.uk/projects/healthcare-record-standards.

Royal Pharmaceutical Society Great Britain. (1997) *From Compliance to Concordance: Achieving Shared Goals in Medicine Taking*. Royal Pharmaceutical Society Great Britain, London.

Sackett, D.L., Rosenberg, W.M., Gray, J.A., Haynes, R.B. & Richardson, W.S. (1996) Evidence based medicine: What it is and what it isn't. *BMJ*, 312, 71–72.

Salinsky, J. (2003) Balint groups. In: J. Burton & J. Launer (eds), *Supervision and Support in General Practice*. Radcliffe Medical Press, Oxford.

Scally, G. & Donaldson, L. (1998) Clinical governance and the drive for quality improvement in the new NHS in England. *BMJ*, 317, 61–65.

Science Museum. (2014) *Brought to life: Exploring the history of medicine*. Barber-Surgeons [WWW document]. URL http://www.sciencemuseum.org.uk/broughttolife/people/barbersurgeons.aspx.

Scott-Samuel, A., Bambra, C., Collins, C., Hunter, D., McCartney, G. & Smith, K. (2014) Neoliberalism in health care: The impact of Thatcherism on health and well-being in Britain. *International Journal of Health Services*, 44, 53–71.

Sigerist, H. (1933) The physician's profession throughout the ages. *Bulletin of the New York Academy of Medicine*, 12, 661–676.

Simpson, M., Buckman, R., Stewart, M., Maguire, P., Lipkin, M., Novack, D. & Till, J. (1991) Doctor–patient communication: The Toronto consensus statement. *BMJ*, 303, 1385–1387.

Skirry, J. (2006) *Rene Descartes: The mind-body distinction*. Internet Encyclopedia of Philosophy [WWW document]. URL http://www.iep.utm.edu/descmind/.

Stewart, M., Brown, J., Boon, H., Galajda, J., Meredith, L. & Sangster, M. (1999) Evidence on patient-doctor communication. *Cancer Prevention and Control*, 3, 25–30.

Stillman, P., Sabers, D. & Redfield, D. (1976) The use of paraprofessionals to teach interviewing skills. *Pediatrics*, 57, 769–774.

Stimson, G. (1974) Obeying doctors' orders: A view from the other side. *Social Science & Medicine*, 8, 97–104.

Swinglehurst, D., Greenhalgh, T. & Roberts, C. (2012) Computer templates in chronic disease management: Ethnographic case study in general practice. *BMJ Open*, 2 (no. 6). doi:10.1136/bmjopen-2012-001754.

Szasz, T. & Hollender, M. (1956) Contributions to the philosophy: The basic models of the doctor–patient relationship. *Archives of Internal Medicine*, 97, 585–592.

Taylor, K. (2009) Paternalism, participation and partnership – the evolution of patient-centredness in the consultation. *Patient Education and Counseling*, 74, 150–155.

Tresolini, C.P. & Pew-Fetzer Task Force. (1994) *Health Professions Education and Relationship-Centered Care*. Pew Health Professions Commission, San Francisco, CA.

Tuckett, D., Boulton, M., Olsen, C. & Williams, A. (1985) *Meetings between Experts: An Approach to Sharing Ideas in Medical Consultations*. Tavistock, London.

Von Fragstein, M., Silverman, J., Cushing, A., Quilligan, S., Salisbury, H. & Wiskin, C. (2008) UK Council for Clinical Communication Skills Teaching in Undergraduate Medical Education. UK consensus statement on the content of communication curricula in undergraduate medical education. *Medical Education*, 42, 1100–1107.

Waitzkin, H. (1984) Doctor–patient communication: Clinical implications of social scientific research. *JAMA*, 252, 2441–2446.

Wakefield, R. (1983) Communication skills training in United Kingdom medical schools. In: D. Pendleton & J. Hasler (eds), *Doctor–Patient Communication*. Academic Press, London.

Wallace, L., Turner, A., Kosmala-Anderson, J., Sharma, S., Jesuthasan, J., Bourne, C. & Realpe, A. (2012) *Evidence: Co-creating Health: Evaluation of First Phase*. Health Foundation, London.

Warren, M. (2000) *A Chronology of State Medicine, Public Health, Welfare and Related Services in Britain 1066–1999*. Faculty of Public Health Medicine of the Royal College of Physicians of the United Kingdom, London.

World Health Organisation. (1978) Declaration of Alma-Ata 1978.

Wynia, M. (2008) The short history and tenuous future of medical professionalism: The erosion of medicine's social contract. *Perspectives in Biology and Medicine*, 51, 565–578.

CHAPTER 4

Models of the Doctor–Patient Consultation

Alexia Papageorgiou

University of Nicosia Medical School, Nicosia, Cyprus

Historical overview

The models of the doctor–patient consultation that have been developed from ancient times until today have aimed to provide teachers and students with examples of philosophies, skills, processes and behaviours, with the ultimate goal of improving outcomes and satisfaction. They give a framework for learning, teaching and assessing the medical consultation (Silverman *et al.* 2005). The models are based on many different traditions: the reductionist/biomedical, biopsychosocial, patient-centred, relationship-centred, consumerist and systemic (Lussier & Richard 2008).

There is very little evidence of what occurred during the doctor–patient encounter up to the 1850s. Doctors' records, if kept at all, were scant (e.g. noting only fee charged, patient's presenting complaints, physical examinations and prescribed medications). In addition, doctors would spend very little time with their patients. For example, a doctor would see up to 30 patients in an outpatient clinic in 2 hours (equating to around 5 minutes per patient) (Stoeckle & Billings 1987).

Between 1850 and 1950 the content of 'the medical history' was standardized and included the following components (Stoeckle & Billings 1987):
- demographics;
- presenting problem(s);
- history of presenting problem(s);
- past medical history;
- systems enquiry;
- family history;
- medication history and
- social history.

Teaching to medical students would be through observation of the senior doctor questioning the patients at their beds on the hospital ward. Students were assessed by means of a viva at certain points of the medical training. The process of doctor–patient communication resembled interrogation rather than dialogue between equals during that time (Stoeckle & Billings 1987). This process aimed to provide a scientific approach to eliciting and recording health problems and gave clinicians a common language of communication. However, it neglected the effect of the illness on the patient's life and the psychosocial aspects of health and illness, hence it is placed under the reductionistic

Clinical Communication in Medicine, First Edition. Edited by Jo Brown, Lorraine M. Noble, Alexia Papageorgiou and Jane Kidd.

or biomedical philosophical approach (Keller & Carroll 1994; Kurtz *et al.* 1996; see also chapter 3). The traditional medical history performed a number of functions, such as collecting and recording information during clerking, helping doctors to arrive at a diagnosis and recording information in a way that could be shared among members of the team.

The development of psychoanalysis around the end of the 19th century, the two World Wars and the psychological traumas experienced by soldiers brought to light the significance of the psychosocial aspects of illness (Balint 1957; Stoeckle & Billings 1987). Balint and his contemporaries emphasized the importance of psychotherapeutic medical consultations, where doctors viewed the person holistically (physically, psychologically, socially). They encouraged the use of open-ended questions, picking up verbal and nonverbal cues and taking into consideration the importance of transference and counter-transference during the consultations. They introduced weekly group discussions for general practitioners (called Balint Groups) in order to improve the doctors' consultation skills and were the first to use the term 'patient-centred care' (see chapter 6). Still, if we try to answer the question whether Balint provided a consultation model the answer would probably be *no*. He provided a way of practising medicine for general practitioners that was rooted in psychoanalytic theory. The function of this approach was to shift the attention of the doctor away from data collection onto the relationship with the patient and the interaction between two human beings (Balint 1957).

However, the study of helping relationships facilitated the development of models of practitioner–patient interactions. Eric Berne's transactional analysis (1964) contributed an easy-to-follow psychotherapeutic account of human ego states (parent, adult, child) that come into play during consultations. In most medical consultations, for example, the doctor would adopt the parent role while the patient the child one. The model enabled practitioners to become aware of, and hence change, the nature of the relationship.

As mentioned in chapter 3, the 1960s were marked by the birth of feminism and the development of social and communication sciences. Specialized instruments were developed for exploring the patients' experience of illness and their satisfaction with healthcare in general, and the doctor–patient relationship in particular. Consumerism entered healthcare. In the 1970s, the development of clinical, health and social psychology, and the influences from the humanistic, cognitive and behavioural paradigms brought an influx of new ideas into the medical consultation. The Health Belief Model, for example (Becker 1974; Rosenstock *et al.* 1988), provided more insight into human variables that shape health and illness behavior. By considering how people's behaviour is related to their perception of risk, these approaches highlighted the importance of including the patient's perspective of illness and treatment in the doctor–patient consultation.

Some of these influences can be seen in Heron's Six Category Intervention Analysis (Heron 1976). Heron suggested a taxonomy of interaction styles for one-to-one interventions between a practitioner and client. He described six styles, falling under the categories of *authoritative* or *facilitative*.

- Authoritative:
  - prescriptive;
  - informative and
  - confronting.
- Facilitative:
  - cathartic;
  - catalytic and
  - supportive.

Heron emphasised that no one approach was inherently 'better' than another and that practitioners were likely to use a combination of approaches.

Technological advancements enabled medical students and clinicians to audio- or videotape their consultations with either real or simulated patients for training and professional development as well as research purposes. Byrne and Long (1976) tape-recorded over 2,000 doctor–patient consultations in UK general practice and derived a six-stage consultation model. The stages included:

- the doctor's task to establish a relationship with the patient;
- his/her attempt to discover the reasons the patient consulted the doctor;
- the physical examination or the verbal exploration of the problem;
- consideration of the condition by the doctor or the patient or both;
- further treatment or investigations usually suggested by the doctor and
- termination of the consultation, usually by the doctor.

Byrne and Long's study identified that doctors used a range of styles from heavily doctor-dominated, characterised by closed questioning, to very open, facilitative styles where the doctor listened, saying very little. Subsequent research using this approach to observing and quantifying communication found that the successful resolution of the stages was linked to the consultation skills used (Neighbour 2005; Moulton 2009). For example, Beckman and Frankel (1984) discovered that doctors interrupted patients a mean of 18 seconds after the patient started speaking, which had a detrimental effect on the consultation because the patient's agenda was not discovered in full.

So far, we have seen that the main tool that doctors used to consult with patients, the traditional medical history, was enriched by a number of societal changes (e.g. feminism and consumerism) and the development of psychosocial paradigms that added theoretical weight behind simple skills – such as the importance of asking open questions to elicit the patient's concerns or addressing the dynamics in the doctor–patient relationship. The development of psychosocial sciences contributed to both patient and doctor education and changed the focus of the medical consultation from just the treatment of illness to illness prevention and identifying barriers to behaviour change (Kurtz *et al.* 1998). One could say that the function of the models that appeared in the 1960s and 1970s was to pave the way towards patient-centred medicine and emphasize the need for evidence-based practice (Bensing 2000).

Although great progress was achieved, one important aspect that still left a lot to be desired was well-designed research and a coherent and standardized approach to teaching and assessing the medical consultation. During the 1980s, technological advancements made medicine even more complex than before. The need for patients to have more information regarding diagnosis, prognosis and treatment, and more involvement in their care, was recognised. Clinical communication training became widespread in the USA, and the Royal College of General Practitioners led the way in the UK (see chapter 3).

These changes were reflected in new consultation models that operationalised the research findings and the concept of patient-centredness. Pendleton *et al.*'s model of good practice (1984) assigned seven tasks to the medical consultation:

- finding the reasons the patient visits the doctor;
- exploring problems other than the presenting complaint;
- sharing understanding and decision making;
- involving the patient in the consultation;
- empowering him/her to accept responsibility of his/her part in the process of diagnosis, prognosis and treatment;
- efficient and effective management of time and resources and
- building and maintaining a therapeutic relationship.

In order to achieve these tasks, the doctor would have to learn a number of skills and develop the art of reflection and feedback. More on this topic will be found in the last part of the book, which focuses on models of learning and the assessment of clinical communication.

In 1989, McWhinney developed the Disease-Illness Model, which clarified the different aims and goals of the patient and the doctor and the desired outcome. The parts of the traditional medical enquiry were called 'Disease Framework' or 'Doctor's Agenda' while the patient's experience of illness were called 'Illness Framework' or 'Patient's Agenda'. Successful integration of these two agendas was theorised to result in patient-centred consultations, shared decision making and greater patient satisfaction (Stewart *et al.* 1995). Some of the skills that were recommended in order to achieve the tasks above included:
- attentive listening;
- use of open and closed questions;
- clarification;
- summarizing and
- use of verbal and nonverbal behaviours to build and maintain a therapeutic relationship.

Around the same time, Neighbour (1987) developed another approach to the medical consultation, suggesting five main tasks that need to be accomplished:
- connecting;
- summarizing;
- handing over;
- safety netting and
- housekeeping.

Cohen-Cole (1991) developed the three-function approach, focusing on three key tasks:
- building an effective doctor–patient relationship;
- assessing the patient's problems and
- managing the patient's problems.

The authors of both models emphasised the need for doctors to practise the communication skills required to achieve these tasks and to focus on reflecting and evaluating their own skills.

The 1980s started showing a shift from paternalistic and reductionist medical consultations to patient-centred care, at least in the Western world. Teaching and assessing clinical communication with the models mentioned above became part of undergraduate and graduate medical education. Some solid research evidence on the effectiveness of clinical communication training on patient-centredness appeared (Dwamena *et al.* 2012).

Tomorrow's Doctors (General Medical Council 1993; General Medical Council 2003) legitimized the teaching and assessment of clinical communication in the UK, but there was still lack of clarity in the interpretation of what needed to be taught and assessed in both undergraduate and graduate medical education.

The development of the Calgary-Cambridge Guide to the Medical Interview in 1996 gave a framework for overcoming the barriers of implementation in teaching and assessment and has been used extensively in the UK since (Kurtz and Silverman 1996; Silverman *et al.* 2005). This model divided the medical interview into five basic tasks that have to be achieved in order for the consultation to be patient-centred, efficient and effective for both the doctor and the patient. These tasks included information gathering, physical examination, explanation and planning and closing the consultation. Under each task a number of skills had to be mastered in order for the doctor to achieve the task. In addition, the doctor had to use appropriate skills in order to structure the consultation and build and maintain a therapeutic relationship with the patient. All in all, the Calgary-Cambridge model provided about 70 skills and a visual representation of the consultation to be used for both teaching and assessment purposes (Kurtz & Silverman 1996; Kurtz *et al.* 1998; Silverman *et al.* 2005).

While the Calgary-Cambridge model was gaining pace in the UK, in the USA two other models were being developed and used around the same time. One of these was the E4 Model (Keller & Carroll 1994), which suggests that the doctor has two biomedical tasks: *find* what the problem is and *fix* it. In order to do that he/she needs to employ the following communication tasks:

- engage;
- empathise;
- educate and
- enlist.

The other model was the Four Habits Model (Frankel & Stein 1996), which proposes that a doctor needs to learn a family of skills under each of four habits in order to perform efficient and patient-centred medical consultations. These habits, defined as an organised way of thinking and acting in the consultation, are the following:

- invest in the beginning;
- elicit the patient's perspective;
- demonstrate empathy and
- invest in the end.

The majority of the models developed in the eighties and nineties advocated the same principles and families of skills that need to be taught, learned and examined in order to achieve patient-centred consultations. However, as we have seen, these models use different analogies and frameworks upon which to hang the skills that will result in certain behaviours and outcomes of care. There is no research to date to assess whether one model is more effective than another in terms of training and assessing medical students and experienced doctors. But we do have some convincing evidence that training to use medical interviewing skills such as those described by the majority of models is effective in achieving patient-centred care (Dwamena *et al.* 2012).

Current practice

The first decade of the 21st century showed the development of new models such as narrative-based medicine (Launer 2002), which places great emphasis on patients telling their story and the doctor listening and creating a common story between these two people who interact under very specific circumstances.

Warren (2006) advocated the BARD model, which considers the totality of the relationship between a general practitioner, a patient and the roles that are being enacted. Both the doctor's personality and his or her previous experience of the patient will have an impact on the consultation. In order to capture what happens during the consultation and encourage reflection the doctor has four tools at his or her disposal:

1 behaviour (verbal and nonverbal);
2 aims of the consultation;

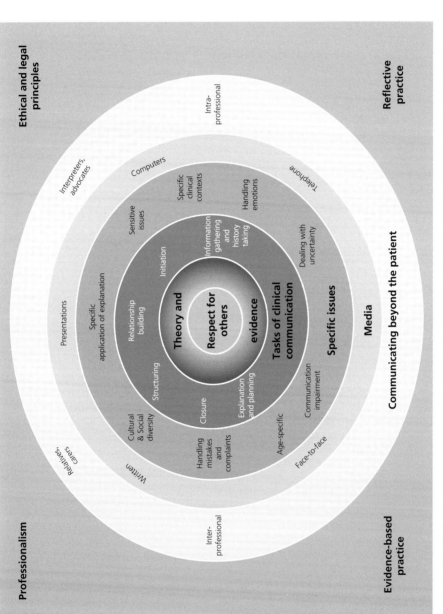

Figure 4.1 The UK Council consensus statement. Source: Von Fragstein 2008. Reproduced with permission of John Wiley and Sons.

3 room (the environment and atmosphere) and
4 dialogue (tone of voice, what you say, language, the ability to confront or challenge).
In addition, models for specific types of consultation were developed; for example, SPIKES for breaking bad news (Baile *et al.* 2000).

To accommodate the growing need for a framework to support patients and doctors making decisions together, Elwyn *et al.* (2012) published Shared Decision Making, a model for clinical practice that involves three steps:
1 introducing choice;
2 describing options, often by integrating the use of patient decision support and
3 helping patients explore preferences and make decisions.
Under each step the authors outline a number of skills clinicians need to master in order to arrive at a shared decision. A tool was also developed to observe and measure these skills: the OPTION grid for shared decision making (Elwyn *et al.* 2005).

Other approaches focused on how to support patients to take up and maintain healthy behaviours. Motivational interviewing, an approach to support patients in achieving long-term behaviour change, was introduced into medical consultations around the first decade of the 21st century (Rollnick *et al.* 2008; see also chapter 16).

Most importantly, during this time the need for consensus and common tools for teaching, assessing and research arose. US experts in the field created the SEGUE Framework during their meeting in Kalamazoo (Makoul 2001a; Makoul 2001b; see also chapter 5).

In 2008, clinical communication skills educators in the UK came together to create their own consensus statement (Figure 4.1) (von Fragstein *et al.* 2008).

Both consensus statements attempted to provide a whole picture of what is important in clinical communication, how to teach and how to assess the subject. They described processes, tasks, professional ideology and skills. Particular emphasis was placed on the 'hidden curriculum', the culture outside the classroom that can undermine modern communication skills teaching, which will be covered more extensively in the last section of this book.

The consensus statements provided a conceptual model and skills that could enable students and doctors to face very complex interactions with their patients, their carers and their colleagues in different healthcare settings and situations. They also provided guidance for doctors' continuous professional development.

As long as these conceptual models are integrated within the continuum of medical education and clinical practice and are evaluated along the way, the medical consultation will continue to evolve and be refined.

Future directions

Patient-centredness has become the cornerstone of the current ideology about conducting effective medical consultations, and the reader will be able to see more on this in chapter 6. As the consensus statements emphasise, medical consultations are very complex interactions and take place in very complex healthcare environments. Consequently, it would be difficult for one model to address that complexity in all situations. Flexibility is paramount. As Lussier and Richard (2008) suggest, the illness and the setting (acute versus chronic and serious versus minor illnesses) all affect the doctor–patient relationship. In the emergency room, when a patient comes with a heart attack, stroke or major trauma, the doctor is the *expert-in-charge*. When a patient comes into hospital with a chronic unstable condition such as diabetes mellitus, arteriosclerotic heart disease or chronic obstructive pulmonary disease, the doctor becomes the *expert-guide*. When this patient's condition is stable the doctor becomes a *partner* in the relationship. Finally, when patients with chronic but minor conditions such as irritable bowel syndrome, osteoarthritis or gastroesophageal reflux disease visit their doctors in primary care or as outpatients, the doctor becomes the *facilitator* (Lussier & Richard 2008).

In this chapter the models that have been briefly described show an important change from the paternalistic medical consultation to patient-centred care, recognising the importance of the patient's illness experience in the consultation. The latter will be illustrated with evidence and from many different angles throughout this book. However, one should not forget the overwhelming evidence of the effect of the sociopolitical systems and the complexity of healthcare environments in the use of different consultation models, which will be a recurring theme throughout the book (see chapter 3; Goold & Lipkin 1999; Bensing 2000; Wirtz *et al.* 2006). In the years to come we may see more consolidation of skills, processes and tasks that promote patient-centredness. We will hopefully see more research on the effectiveness of teaching and assessing clinical communication in undergraduate medical education and in the early years of doctors practising medicine that will strengthen the use of certain models and skills over others. We will also see the effect of the internet and e-learning on the existing models and the development of new medical consultation models.

References

Baile, W.F., Buckman, R., Lenzi, R., Glober, G., Beale, E.A. & Kudelka, A.P. (2000) SPIKES – a six-step protocol for delivering bad news: Application to the patient with cancer. *Oncologist*, 5, 302–311.

Balint, M. (1957) *The Doctor, His Patient and the Illness*. Churchill Livingstone, London.

Becker, M.H. (ed) (1974) The health belief model and personal health behavior. *Health Education Monographs*, 2, 324–508.

Beckman, H.B. & Frankel, R.M. (1984) The effect of physician behavior on the collection of data. *Annals of Internal Medicine*, 101, 692–696.

Bensing, J. (2000) Bridging the gap: The separate worlds of evidence-based medicine and patient-centered medicine. *Patient Education and Counseling*, 39 (no. 1), 17–25.

Berne, E. (1964) *Transactional Analysis: Games People Play*. Ballantine Books, New York.

Byrne, P.S. & Long, B.E. (1976) *Doctors Talking to Patients*. HMSO, London.

Cohen-Cole, S. (1991) *The Medical Interview: The Three Function Approach*. Mosby Year Book, St Louis.

Dwamena, F., Holmes-Rovner, M., Gaulden, C.M., Jorgenson, S., Sadigh, G., Sikorskii, A., Lewin, S., Smith, R.C., Coffey, J. & Olomu, A. (2012) Interventions for providers to promote a patient-centred approach in clinical consultations. Cochrane Database of Systematic Reviews, 2 (Art. No.: CD003267). doi:10.1002/14651858.CD003267.pub2.

Elwyn, G., Hutchings, H., Edwards, A., Rapport, F., Wensing, M., Cheung, W-Y. & Grol, R. (2005) The OPTION scale: Measuring the extent that clinicians involve patients in decision making tasks. *Health Expectations*, 8 (no. 1), 34–42.

Elwyn, G., Frosch, D., Thomson, R., Joseph-Williams, N., Lloyd, A., Kinnersley, P., Cording, E., Tomson, D., Dodd, C., Rollnick, S., Edwards, A. & Barry, M. (2012) Shared decision making: A model for clinical practice. *Journal of General Internal Medicine*, 27 (no. 10), 1361–1367.

Frankel, R.M. & Stein, T.S. (1996) *The Four Habits of Highly Effective Clinicians: A Practical Guide*. Kaiser Permanente Northern California Region: Physician Education & Development, Oakland, CA.

General Medical Council. (1993) *Tomorrow's Doctors*. General Medical Council, London.

General Medical Council. (2003) *Tomorrow's Doctors*. General Medical Council, London.

Goold, S.D. & Lipkin, M. (1999) The doctor–patient relationship: Challenges, opportunities, and strategies. *Journal of General Internal Medicine*, 14 (Supp 1), S26–S33.

Heron, J. (1976) A six-category intervention analysis. *British Journal of Guidance & Counselling*, 4 (no. 2), 143–155.

Keller, V.F. & Carroll, G.J. (1994) A new model for physician-patient communication. *Patient Education and Counseling*, 23, 131–140.

Kurtz, S.M. & Silverman, J.D. (1996) The Calgary – Cambridge Referenced Observation Guides: An aid to defining the curriculum and organizing the teaching in communication training programmes. *Medical Education*, 30 (no. 2), 83–89.

Kurtz, S.M., Silverman, J.D. & Draper, J. (1998) *Teaching and Learning Communication Skills in Medicine*. Radcliffe Medical Press, Oxford.

Launer, J. (2002) *Narrative-Based Primary Care: A Practical Guide*. Radcliffe Medical Press, Oxford.

Lussier, M.T. & Richard, C. (2008) Because one shoe doesn't fit all: A repertoire of doctor–patient relationships. *Canadian Family Physician*, 54, 1089–1092.

Makoul, G. (2001a) The SEGUE Framework for teaching and assessing communication skills. *Patient Education and Counselling*, 45 (no. 1), 23–34.

Makoul, G. (2001b) Essential elements of communication in medical encounters: The Kalamazoo consensus statement. *Academic Medicine*, 76, 390–393.

McWhinney, I. (1989) The need for a transformed clinical method. In: M. Stewart & D. Roter (eds), *Communicating with Medical Patients*, pp. 25–40. Sage Publications, Newbury Park, CA.

Moulton, L. (2009) *The Naked Consultation: A Practical Guide to Primary Care Consultation Skills*. Radcliffe Publishing, Oxford.

Neighbour, R. (1987) *The Inner Consultation: How to Develop an Effective and Intuitive Consulting Style*. MTP Press, Lancaster.

Neighbour, R. (2004) *The Inner Consultation: How to Develop an Effective and Intuitive Consulting Style*, second edn. Radcliffe Publishing, Oxford.

Pendleton, D., Schofield, T., Tate, P. & Havelock, P. (1984) *The Consultation: An Approach to Learning and Teaching*. Oxford University Press, Oxford.

Rollnick, S., Miller, W.R. & Butler, C.C. (2008) *Motivational Interviewing in Health Care: Helping Patients Change Behaviour*. Guilford Press, London.

Rosenstock, I.M., Stretcher, V.J. & Becker, M.H. (1988) Social learning theory and the health belief model. *Health Education Quarterly*, 15, 175–183.

Silverman, J., Kurtz, S. & Draper, J. (2005) *Skills for Communicating with Patients*, second edn. Radcliffe Publishing, Oxford.

Stewart, M., Brown, J.B., Weston, W.W., McWhinney, I.R., McWilliam, C.L. & Freeman, T.R. (1995) *Patient-Centred Medicine: Transforming the Clinical Method*. Sage Publications, Newbury Park, CA.

Stoeckle, J.D. & Billings, A.J. (1987) A history of history-taking. *Journal of General Internal Medicine*, 2, 119–127.

von Fragstein, M., Silverman, J., Cushing, A., Quilligan, S., Salisbury, H., Wiskin, C. & on behalf of the UK Council of Clinical Communication in Undergraduate Medical Education. (2008). UK consensus statement on the content of communication curricula in undergraduate medical education. *Medical Education*, 42, 1100–1107.

Warren, E. (2006) *B.A.R.D. in the Practice: A Guide for Family Doctors to Consult Efficiently, Effectively and Happily*. Radcliffe Publishing, Oxford.

Wirtz, V., Cribb, A. & Barber, N. (2006) Patient-doctor decision-making about treatment within the consultation – a critical analysis of models. *Social Science and Medicine*, 62, 116–124.

CHAPTER 5

What Is Effective Doctor–Patient Communication? Review of the Evidence

Gregory Makoul[1,2,3] and Sandra van Dulmen[4,5,6]

[1]PatientWisdom, Chicago, IL, USA
[2]Connecticut Institute for Primary Care Innovation, Hartford, CT, USA
[3]University of Connecticut School of Medicine, Farmington, CT, USA
[4]Netherlands Institute for Health Services Research (NIVEL), Utrecht, the Netherlands
[5]Radboud University Medical Center, Nijmegen, the Netherlands
[6]Buskerud and Vestfold University College, Drammen, Norway

Over the past 50 years, a confluence of research evidence and teaching practice has positioned effective communication as the linchpin of doctor–patient relationships, highlighting the impact on patient outcomes such as information recall, adherence to treatment plans and likelihood to sue for malpractice (e.g. Levinson *et al.* 1997; Zolnierek & DiMatteo 2009; Dillon 2012). More recent work has also pointed to communication as the key to prevent burnout and increase job satisfaction among doctors (Bensing *et al.* 2013). This chapter focuses on doctor–patient communication and takes a step back, examining the fundamental question underlying the connection between communication and outcomes: what is effective communication? Put even more simply: what works, and how do we know? The answer to these questions can help guide communication teaching, assessment, research and clinical practice.

Models for teaching and assessing communication skills

As described in previous chapters within this section (chapters 3 and 4), the literature is replete with models of medicine, models of the doctor–patient relationship and models of communication skills. The major models – or frameworks – for teaching and assessing communication skills offer a useful lens for addressing the question of effective doctor–patient communication. Established models include:
• Calgary-Cambridge Guide (Silverman *et al.* 1998; Silverman *et al.* 2013);
• E4 Model (Keller & Carroll 1994);
• Essential Elements (Makoul 2001a);

- Four Habits (Frankel & Stein 2001);
- Patient-Centered Clinical Method (Brown *et al.* 1986);
- Patient-Centered Interviewing (Smith *et al.* 2000; Fortin *et al.* 2012);
- SEGUE Framework (Makoul 2001b) and
- Three-Function Model (Bird & Cohen-Cole 1990).

Sources of evidence for the components of these models vary. For instance, groups that developed the Calgary-Cambridge Guide and the Patient-Centered Interviewing model undertook extensive reviews of the published literature to support and illuminate their recommendations, while the SEGUE Framework was derived from primary research evidence gained through physician surveys, patient surveys and video analysis of doctor–patient encounters.

Although generated in different ways, at different times and in different countries, all of these models are consistent, differentiated primarily by level of abstraction (e.g. focusing on tasks to be accomplished versus particular skills and strategies for accomplishing them). The Essential Elements of Communication in Medical Encounters (Makoul 2001a) represent a consensus based upon expert review of five major models for teaching and assessing communication skills. More specifically, 21 leaders from prominent medical education and professional organizations worked together to synthesize the models. The group reviewed the research base, overarching views of the medical encounter and current applications of the Calgary-Cambridge Guide, E4 Model, Patient-Centered Clinical Method, SEGUE Framework and Three-Function Model. Analysis focused on identifying similarities and differences across the models, which yielded the Essential Elements. This model offers an evidence-based, educator-endorsed touchstone (see Box 5.1). As discussed later in this chapter, the essence of these Essential Elements has also been endorsed by patients (Makoul *et al.* 2007).

The Essential Elements favor the 'task approach', acknowledging that multiple skills and strategies can be used to accomplish communication tasks and that trainees and doctors will employ those that work best for their patient, for them and for the situation (i.e. they may approach the same patient differently in different clinical contexts). Moreover, the task approach reflects communication behavior that serves specific functions and goals, as articulated by de Haes and Bensing (2009), in relation to immediate, intermediate and long-term outcomes of communication. While all of the tasks are considered essential, the one that requires further explication in the context of this chapter is Build a Relationship. As noted in the original article (Makoul 2001a):

> A strong, therapeutic, and effective relationship is the sine qua non of physician-patient communication. The group endorses a patient-centered approach to care, which emphasizes both the patient's disease and his or her illness experience. This requires eliciting the patient's story of illness while guiding the interview through a process of diagnostic reasoning. It also requires an awareness that the ideas, feelings, and values of both the patient and the physician influence the relationship. Further, this approach regards the physician-patient relationship as a partnership, and respects patients' active participation in decision-making. The task of building a relationship is also relevant for work with patients' families and support networks. In essence, building a relationship is an ongoing task within and across encounters.

A patient-centered approach that puts emphasis on building and maintaining a therapeutic relationship between patient, doctor and care team is also referred to as a

Box 5.1 Essential Elements (Makoul 2001a).

Build a Relationship

- Elicit the patient's story of illness.
- Be aware that ideas, feelings and values of patient and doctor influence the relationship.
- Respect patient's active participation.

Open the Discussion

- Allow the patient to complete his or her opening statement.
- Elicit the patient's full set of concerns.
- Establish/maintain a personal connection.

Gather Information

- Use open-ended and closed-ended questions appropriately.
- Structure, clarify and summarize information.
- Actively listen.

Understand the Patient's Perspective

- Explore contextual factors (e.g. family, culture, gender, age, socioeconomic status, spirituality).
- Explore beliefs, concerns and expectations about health and illness.
- Acknowledge and respond to the patient's ideas, feelings and values.

Share Information

- Use language the patient can understand.
- Check for understanding.
- Encourage questions.

Reach Agreement on Problems and Plans

- Encourage the patient to participate in decisions to the extent he or she desires.
- Check the patient's willingness and ability to follow the plan.
- Identify and enlist resources and supports.

Provide Closure

- Ask whether the patient has other issues or concerns.
- Summarize and affirm agreement with the plan of action.
- Discuss follow-up (e.g. next visit, plan for unexpected outcomes).

---

relationship-centered approach. According to Beach *et al.* (2006), relationship-centered care is founded upon four principles:

1 that relationships in health care ought to include the personhood of the participants;
2 that affect and emotion are important components of these relationships;
3 that all healthcare relationships occur in the context of reciprocal influence and
4 that the formation and maintenance of genuine relationships in healthcare is morally valuable.

Clearly, a central component of such an approach is for doctors to convey that they see their patients as people (i.e. not simply cases with biomedical defects). This is reflected in the excerpt above and part of Open the Discussion, another of the Essential Elements: making a personal connection with patients, in the sense of going beyond the medical issue at hand.

Making a personal connection can be done by expressing genuine interest in a patient's life world; it does not require reciprocal self-disclosure on the part of the doctor (Beach *et al.* 2004). In a study of initial clinical encounters (i.e. the doctor and patient were meeting for the very first time), patients who had encounters that included a brief personal connection reported, on a postconsultation survey, that their doctor knew them significantly better than did patients in encounters that never went beyond the medical issue at hand (Makoul & Strauss 2003). Video analysis documented that these personal connections tended to be about rather mundane topics such as work or school. Others too found that making a personal connection by expressing only seconds of compassion and attention can make a huge difference to patients; study participants reported better information recall, less anxiety and fewer concerns after having seen an empathic doctor (Fogarty *et al.* 1999; Van Vliet *et al.* 2013; Sep *et al.* 2014; Van Osch *et al.* 2014). These findings support the positioning of Build a Relationship as "the fundamental communication task" in the Essential Elements consensus statement (Makoul 2001a), particularly in light of the notion that perceived familiarity engenders trust, which increases the likelihood of mediators critical to patient care such as open and honest communication, adherence to treatment plans and commitment to follow-up.

Patient perspectives on essential communication skills

As patient views offer an equally important type of evidence for determining what constitutes effective doctor–patient communication, we now examine the Communication Assessment Tool (CAT), which was developed to gauge patient perspectives on doctor communication and has been established as a reliable and valid instrument (Makoul *et al.* 2007). Indeed, the instrument development process, and outcome, are directly relevant to the question of what works. More specifically, the CAT is based on a literature review as well as focus groups with a diverse group of patients and, importantly, a random-digit-dial, representative survey of more than 1,000 Americans to determine the importance people attach to the communication tasks considered for inclusion. This process yielded a 14-item instrument to be answered on a five-rating scale (from 1 'poor' to 5 'excellent') that represents patient views of effective communication in medical encounters (see Box 5.2).

It is interesting and instructive to compare the CAT items to the Essential Elements, as there is considerable overlap in specific tasks, with one framework often providing useful explication for the other. For instance, the CAT includes four clear instantiations of relationship building: Greeted me in a way that makes me feel comfortable; Treated me with respect; Showed interest in my ideas about my health; and Showed care and concern. The Essential Elements tend to be more mechanistic. Some guide doctor behavior in ways that are entirely consistent with the CAT items. For instance, the Essential Elements task of exploring patient beliefs, concerns and expectations about health and illness was the substrate for the CAT task of showing interest in patients' ideas about their health. Others highlight communication tasks that focus either on the process of communication (e.g. use open-ended and closed-ended

Box 5.2 CAT items.

- Greeted me in a way that makes me feel comfortable.
- Treated me with respect.
- Showed interest in my ideas about my health.
- Understood my main health concerns.
- Paid attention to me (looked at me, listened carefully).
- Let me talk without interruptions.
- Gave me as much information as I want.
- Talked in terms I can understand.
- Checked to be sure I understand everything.
- Encouraged me to ask questions.
- Involved me in decisions as much as I want.
- Discussed next steps, including any follow-up plans.
- Showed care and concern.
- Spent the right amount of time with me.

questions appropriately; structure, clarify and summarize information) or key processes of the clinical encounter (e.g. check the patient's willingness and ability to follow the plan; identify and enlist resources and supports).

In several published studies conducted across a broad range of clinical settings, medical specialties, stages of training and levels of seniority, we have detected a striking pattern of results. Patients consistently report that two CAT tasks are lacking in clinical encounters, both of which are also integral to the Essential Elements:
1 encouraging patients to ask questions and
2 involving patients in decisions to the extent they want.
This discrepancy is further highlighted by a recent study among patients in the Netherlands, Italy, the UK and Belgium that indicates that what they give foremost value to is to be given space to talk (Mazzi *et al.* 2013). Moreover, while the CAT was developed in the United States, it has been pilot tested with nearly 20,000 patients across 20 countries. Results of the large-scale CAT pilot test (Makoul *et al.* 2010) indicate that patients in all 20 countries find their doctors least effective in accomplishing these same two tasks of encouraging questions and involving the patient in decisions.

These results send a clear, consistent and compelling message about discrete aspects of effective communication that need attention. Moreover, they are consistent with other evidence demonstrating that patient perceptions of the quality of communication in different countries are strikingly similar (Van den Brink-Muinen *et al.* 2003). We are in the process of a more in-depth investigation designed to examine cultural differences, including the importance attached to each CAT task in different countries.

How communication heals

The relevance of encouraging patients' views and involvement in decision making becomes clear when we consider the pathways along which communication heals. Street *et al.* (2009) make clear that some pathways through which doctor–patient communication influences health outcomes are direct. However, in most cases, communication affects health more indirectly through immediate, or proximal, outcomes of the interaction (e.g. satisfaction with care, motivation to adhere, trust in the clinician, self-efficacy, shared understanding) that affect health or that contribute to intermediate outcomes (e.g. adherence, self-management skills, social support) that lead to better health. Indeed, Street *et al.* (2009) describe seven pathways through which communication can lead to better health:

- increased access to care;
- greater patient knowledge and shared understanding;
- higher quality medical decisions;
- enhanced therapeutic alliances;
- increased social support;
- patient agency and empowerment and
- better management of emotions.

The pathway of patient agency and empowerment most clearly illustrates the clinical relevance of encouraging patients' contribution to the conversation and involvement in decision making. According to Street *et al.* (2009), patient 'agency' ranges from active participation in medical encounters and decision making to self-care skills for managing everyday health-related activities. Clinicians can facilitate involvement in the decision-making process by helping patients actively seek information, clarify treatment goals and express concerns and feelings.

A seemingly simple premise

A book published 30 years ago – *Meetings between Experts* (Tuckett *et al.* 1985) – was based on a seemingly simple premise: doctors are experts on clinical medicine; patients are experts on their lives and values. The expertise of doctors is earned through intensive clinical training and subsequent practice. The expertise of patients is equally compelling and hard earned, given the fact most have nearly 6,000 waking hours a year (16 hours/day × 7 days/week × 52 weeks/year) to deal with their health. Only a fraction of that time is spent with a doctor (see also Asch *et al.* 2012). Clearly, the most effective encounters will be those in which the doctor and patient work together to acknowledge, access and act upon the expertise of one another. This interdependent interaction is central to shared decision making.

However, despite a tremendous amount of excellent research and dedicated teaching over the past 30 years, the state of affairs described in *Meetings between Experts* and replicated by other researchers has not changed radically (Makoul *et al.* 1995; Van Dulmen & Bensing 2002; Kramer *et al.* 2004; Cheraghi-Sohi & Bower 2008; Fernandez-Olano *et al.* 2008; Ho *et al.* 2010). Studies continue to indicate that patient views are rarely solicited during clinical encounters and that patients are often interrupted prematurely, leaving major complaints or concerns unnoticed (Marvel *et al.* 1999; Langewitz *et al.* 2002). These results are echoed by the CAT studies mentioned above. Persistent reports that there is a relative lack of patient-centered exchange in most clinical encounters suggest that we need to change our approach to teaching, assessment and research.

While there are always opportunities for improvement in the formal curriculum, there may be more value in directly addressing the 'hidden curriculum' (i.e. the culture and behavior of everyday clinical practice), as comments or role modeling in the 'real world' can contravene points and progress made in the classroom or simulation center (Hafferty 1998; Francis 2013). In other words, there are deeply rooted, insidious obstacles to true transformative learning in the sense of transferring communication skills from classroom to consulting room (Van den Eertwegh *et al.* 2013). Strategies for addressing the hidden curriculum include communication training, ideally with observation and feedback, for faculty and staff as well as making the hidden curriculum more visible to learners and providing them with a safe way to alert communication faculty of counter-models in the clinical environment. A nice example of how to accomplish this is can be seen in Zagreb, Croatia (Cikes *et al.* 2014). As part of the new medical curriculum, faculty members in Zagreb were invited to refresh their communication skills and to each become communication supervisor of a fixed group of medical students throughout their 6-year medical curriculum. Many medical specialists volunteered and became enthusiastic, motivating models for students. This approach helped students more readily acknowledge the importance of effective communication as one of the core competencies of becoming a doctor – why else would medical specialists invest in these skills?

Meeting the challenges of contemporary practice

Time and doctor capacity to adapt to patient language, culture and health literacy have long been recognized as significant barriers to effective communication. With the advent and expanding use of the electronic health record (EHR), the Internet, telemedicine and team-based care, the clinical encounter has become markedly more complex. The EHR has been likened to a third person in the room, one that often draws the doctor's attention – both literally and figuratively – away from the patient; fortunately, the doctor gradually seems to adapt to this intruder (Noordman *et al.* 2010). While there is no quality control on the Internet, it is now relatively common for patients to have tried diagnosing and/or treating themselves based on what they find on websites. Still, most patients, especially those who are older and/or chronically ill, continue to rely foremost on their doctor for reassurance and information (Muusses *et al.* 2012). And, while care delivered by multidisciplinary teams holds promise in terms of extending the doctor's reach, many patients still expect to have unfettered access to their doctor. That said, innovations in care delivery (e.g. health coaches, access to care settings with an emphasis on convenience instead of continuity) offer alternatives to the traditional doctor–patient relationship.

On the whole, the conceptualization of communication in medicine – as well as the approach to teaching and assessment – have only begun to incorporate these developments. For instance, Wald and colleagues actively advocate communication training that highlights the role of EHRs in the doctor–patient encounter, and they offer an evidence-based approach on this front (Wald *et al.* 2014). Bridging the traditional gap between communication teaching and clinical practice is critical (Makoul & Schofield 1999; Malhotra *et al.* 2009; Van den Eertwegh *et al.* 2013; Van den Eertwegh *et al.* 2014). Approaches for strengthening that bridge must include attention to communication in the real world of contemporary practice (Van Weel-Baumgarten *et al.* 2013).

Future directions

In sum, most models of effective doctor–patient communication – whether derived by medical educators or patients – overlap considerably and offer a coherent sense of what works. Rather than creating additional models for teaching, assessment, research and clinical practice, it may be wise to choose one of the prominent tools already available and tailor it as needed. This approach would provide a solid foundation for embedding knowledge of what works throughout the continuum of medical education, in terms of both learning stages and real-world training sites. Perhaps the most important point regarding effective communication is that it is only effective if genuinely incorporated into everyday clinical practice, not just in educational or exam settings. Otherwise, we run the risk of passing the test but failing the patient.

References

Asch, D.A., Muller, R.W. & Volpp, K.G. (2012) Automated hovering in health care – watching over the 5000 hours. *New England Journal of Medicine*, 367, 1–3.

Beach, M.C., Inui, T. & Relationship-Centered Care Research Network. (2006) Relationship-centered care: A constructive reframing. *Journal of General Internal Medicine*, 21 (Suppl. 1), S3–S8.

Beach, M.C., Roter, D., Rubin, H., Frankel, R., Levinson, W. & Ford, D.E. (2004) Is physician self-disclosure related to patient evaluation of office visits? *Journal of General Internal Medicine*, 19, 905–910.

Bensing, J.M., van Den Brink-Muinen, A., Boerma, W. & van Dulmen, S. (2013) The manifestation of job satisfaction in doctor–patient communication: A ten-country European study. *International Journal of Person Centered Medicine*, 3, 44–52.

Bird, J. & Cohen-Cole, S.A. (1990) The three-function model of the medical interview: An educational device. *Advances in Psychosomatic Medicine*, 20, 65–88.

Brown, J., Stewart, M., McCracken, E., McWhinney, I.R. & Levenstein, J. (1986) The patient-centred clinical method. 2. Definition and application. *Family Practice*, 3, 75–79.

Cheraghi-Sohi, S. & Bower, P. (2008) Can the feedback of patient assessments, brief training, or their combination, improve the interpersonal skills of primary care physicians? A systematic review. *BMC Health Services Research*, 8, 179.

Cikes, N., Pavlekovic., G, Kujundzic Tiljak, M., Bras, M. & Matijevic, R. (2014) *Teaching generic competencies in the continuum of medical education (abstract)*. AMEE conference, 2014 [WWW document]. URL http://www.amee.org/getattachment/Conferences/AMEE-2014/AMEE-2014-APP-Data/7E-SHORT-COMMUNICATIONS.pdf.

Dillon, P.J. (2012) Assessing the influence of patient participation in primary care medical interviews on recall of treatment recommendations. *Health Communication*, 27, 58–65.

Fernandez-Olano, C., Montoya-Fernandez, J. & Salinas-Sanchez, A.S. (2008) Impact of clinical interview training on the empathy level of medical students and medical residents. *Medical Teacher*, 30, 322–324.

Fogarty, L.A., Curbow, B.A., Wingard, J.R., McDonnell, K. & Somerfield, M.R. (1999) Can 40 seconds of compassion reduce patient anxiety? *Journal of Clinical Oncology*, 17, 371–379.

Fortin, A.H., Dwamena, F.C., Frankel, R.M. & Smith, R.C. (2012) *Smith's Patient-Centered Interviewing: An Evidence-Based Method*, third edn. McGraw-Hill Global Education, Columbus, OH.

Francis, R. (2013) *Report of the Mid Staffordshire NHS Foundation Trust Public Inquiry (HC 947)*. The Stationery Office, London.

Frankel, R.M. & Stein, T. (2001) Getting the most out of the clinical encounter: The Four Habits Model. *Journal of Medical Practice Management*, 16, 184–191.

Haes, H. de & Bensing, J. (2009) Endpoints in medical communication research, proposing a framework of functions and outcomes. *Patient Education and Counseling*, 74, 287–294.

Hafferty, F.W. (1998) Beyond curriculum reform: Confronting medicine's hidden curriculum. *Academic Medicine*, 73, 403–407.

Ho, M.J., Yao, G., Lee, K.L., Hwang, T.J. & Beach, M.C. (2010) Long-term effectiveness of patient-centered training in cultural competence: What is retained? What is lost? *Academic Medicine*, 85, 660–664.

Keller, V.F. & Carroll, J.G. (1994) A new model for physician-patient communication. *Patient Education and Counseling*, 23, 131–140.

Kramer, A., Duesman, H., Tan, L. & van der Vleuten, C. (2004) Acquisition of communication skills in postgraduate training for General Practice. *Medical Education*, 38, 158–167.

Langewitz, W., Denz, M., Keller, A., Kiss, A., Rüttimann, S. & Wössmer, B. (2002) Spontaneous talking time at start of consultation in outpatient clinic: Cohort study. *BMJ*, 325, 682–683.

Levinson, W., Roter, D.L., Mullooly, J.P., Dull, V.T. & Frankel, R.M. (1997) Physician-patient communication: The relationship with malpractice claims among primary care physicians and surgeons. *JAMA*, 277, 553–559.

Makoul, G. (2001a) Essential elements of communication in medical encounters: The Kalamazoo consensus statement. *Academic Medicine*, 76, 390–393.

Makoul, G. (2001b) The SEGUE Framework for teaching and assessing communication skills. *Patient Education and Counseling*, 45, 23–34.

Makoul, G. & Schofield, T. (1999). Communication teaching and assessment in medical education: An international consensus statement. Netherlands Institute of Primary Health Care. *Patient Education and Counseling*, 37, 191–195.

Makoul, G. & Strauss, A. (2003) Building therapeutic relationships during patient visits. *Journal of General Internal Medicine*, 18, 275.

Makoul, G., Arntson, P. & Schofield, T. (1995) Health promotion in primary care: Physician–patient communication and decision making about prescription medications. *Social Science & Medicine*, 41, 1241–1254.

Makoul, G., Krupat, E. & Chang, C.H. (2007) Measuring patient views of physician communication skills: Development and testing of the Communication Assessment Tool. *Patient Education and Counseling*, 67, 333–342.

Makoul, G., Myerholtz, L., Williams, M. & Wolf, S. (2010) Priorities for effective communication: Patterns emerging from Communication Assessment Tool (CAT) data. Presented at the International Conference on Communication in Healthcare, Verona.

Malhotra, A., Gregory, I., Darvill, E., Goble, E., Pryce-Roberts, A., Lundberg, K., Konradsen, S. & Hafstad, H. (2009) Mind the gap: Learners' perspectives on what they learn in communication compared to how they and others behave in the real world. *Patient Education and Counseling*, 76, 385–390.

Marvel, M.K., Epstein, R.M., Flowers, K. & Beckman, H.B. (1999) Soliciting the patient's agenda. Have we improved? *JAMA*, 281, 283–287.

Mazzi, M.A., Bensing, J., Rimondini, M., Fletcher, I., van Vliet, L., Zimmermann, C. & Deveugele, M. (2013) How do lay people assess the quality of physicians' communicative responses to patients' emotional cues and concerns? An international multicentre study based on video-taped medical consultations. *Patient Education and Counseling*, 90, 347–353.

Muusses, L., van Weert, J., Jansen, J. & van Dulmen, S. (2012) Chemotherapy and information-seeking behaviour: Predicting mass media information source usage. *Psycho-Oncology*, 9, 993–1002.

Noordman, J., Verhaak, P., van Beljouw, I. & van Dulmen, S. (2010) Consultation-room computers and the effect on general practitioner-patient communication: Comparing two periods of computer use. *Family Practice*, 27, 644–651.

Sep, M.S., van Osch, M., van Vliet, L.M., Smets, E.M. & Bensing, J.M. (2014) The power of clinicians' affective communication: How reassurance about non-abandonment can reduce patients' physiological arousal and increase information recall in bad news consultations. An experimental study using analogue patients. *Patient Education and Counseling*, 95, 45–52.

Silverman, J.D., Kurtz, S.M. & Draper, J. (1998) *Skills for Communicating with Patients*. Radcliffe Medical Press, Oxford.

Silverman, J.D., Kurtz, S.M. & Draper, J. (2013) *Skills for Communicating with Patients*, third edn. Radcliffe Medical Press, Oxford.

Smith, R.C., Marshall-Dorsey, A.A., Osborn, G.G., Shebroe, V., Lyles, J.S., Stoffelmayr, B.E., van Egeren, L.F., Mettler, J., Maduschke, K., Stanley, J.M. & Gardiner, J.C. (2000)

Evidence-based guidelines for teaching patient-centered interviewing. *Patient Education and Counseling*, 39, 27–36.

Street, R.L., Jr, Makoul, G., Arora, N.K. & Epstein, R.M. (2009) How does communication heal? Pathways linking clinician-patient communication to health outcomes. *Patient Education and Counseling*, 74, 295–301.

Tuckett, D., Boulton, M., Olson, C. & Williams, A. (1985) *Meetings between Experts*. Tavistock Publications, London.

Van den Brink-Muinen, A., van Dulmen, A.M., Bensing, J.M., Maaroos, H.-I., Tähepöld, H., Krol, Z.J., Plawecka, L., Oana, S.C., Boros, M., Satterlund-Larsson, U. & Bengtsson, B.-M. (2003) *Eurocommunication II: A Comparative Study between Countries in Central- and Western Europe on Doctor–Patient Communication in General Practice*. NIVEL, Utrecht.

Van den Eertwegh, V., van Dulmen, S., van Dalen, J., Scherpbier, A.J.J.A. & van der Vleuten, C.P.M. (2013) Learning in context; Identifying gaps in research on the transfer of medical communication skills to the clinical workplace. *Patient Education and Counseling*, 90, 184–192.

Van den Eertwegh, V., van Dalen, J., van Dulmen, S., van der Vleuten, C.P.M. & Scherpbier, A.J.J.A. (2014) Barriers to transformative communication skills learning: contrasting two medical working contexts in postgraduate training. *Patient Education and Counseling*, 95, 91–97.

Van Dulmen, A.M. & Bensing, J.M. (2002) Health promoting effects of the physician–patient encounter. *Psychology, Health & Medicine*, 7, 289–300.

Van Osch, M., Sep, M., van Vliet, L.M., van Dulmen, S. & Bensing, J.M. (2014) Reducing patients' anxiety and uncertainty, and improving recall in bad news consultations. *Health Psychology*, 33, 1382–1390.

Van Vliet, L.M., van der Wall, E., Plum, N.M. & Bensing, J.M. (2013) Explicit prognostic information and reassurance about nonabandonment when entering palliative breast cancer care: Findings from a scripted video-vignette study. *Journal of Clinical Oncology*, 31, 3242–3249.

Van Weel-Baumgarten, E., Bolhuis, S., Rosenbaum, M. & Silverman, J. (2013) Bridging the gap: How is integrating communication skills with medical content throughout the curriculum valued by students? *Patient Education and Counseling*, 90, 177–183.

Wald, H.S., George, P., Reis, S.P. & Taylor, J.S. (2014) Electronic health record training in undergraduate medical education: Bridging theory to practice with curricula for empowering patient- and relationship-centered care in the computerized setting. *Academic Medicine*, 89, 380–386.

Zolnierek, K.B. & Dimatteo, M.R. (2009) Physician communication and patient adherence to treatment: A meta-analysis. *Medical Care*, 47, 826–834.

CHAPTER 6

Patient-Centredness

Rosie Illingworth

Manchester Medical School, University of Manchester, Manchester, UK

The term 'patient-centredness' appears with regularity in the healthcare literature (Scholl *et al.* 2014). Where has this term come from? What does it mean in practice? Is there evidence of the effect on healthcare outcomes? Patient-centredness is taught and promoted to medical students, but what is absorbed? This chapter explores and addresses these questions, focusing on the doctor–patient relationship, though there is an increasing literature on the concept of 'patient-centred healthcare' from a health policy perspective, for example (Dulmen *et al.* 2013).

Evolution of the term 'patient-centred'

Prior to the 19th century, the only sources of information available to doctors were the individual's account of his or her illness, external observation and examination. Hence in the early days of medicine the patient's account was absolutely at the centre and there was no need to conceptualise 'patient-centred'; it was simply the norm.

Scientific and technological developments allowed diseases and disorders to be identified, understood, classified and treated. In this context the individual's account became less significant. Medicine became 'doctor-centred' and 'disease-centred' with less regard to the illness experience of the patient (Jewson 1976).

In the 21st century the 'digital age' is here, with exponential development of diagnostic testing, keyhole surgery and robotic applications, further distancing healthcare from the human experience. The dominant paradigm is an evidence-based, scientific model. However, a patient may suffer the same disease as another patient, but his or her experience of living with the illness may be different (Stewart 2001).

It was Enid Balint, in the UK, who appears to have first used the term 'patient-centred' to conceptualise the idea of 'the whole person' needing to be taken into account to make an 'overall diagnosis' (Balint 1969). In 1976, Byrne and Long used the phrase in their analysis of doctors' verbal consultation styles. They discovered a spectrum from a 'doctor-centred' heavily doctor-dominated consultation, with minimal contribution from the patient, to a 'patient-centred' consultation; the latter meaning that the consultation was driven by the agenda of the patient, with the doctor encouraging and facilitating the patient, particularly in regard to the diagnosis (Byrne & Long 1976).

Clinical Communication in Medicine, First Edition. Edited by Jo Brown, Lorraine M. Noble, Alexia Papageorgiou and Jane Kidd.
© 2016 John Wiley & Sons, Ltd. Published 2016 by John Wiley & Sons, Ltd.

In 1995 the phrase 'patient-centered medicine' appeared as the title of a model of the consultation (Stewart 1995). Stewart identified six interactive components of the patient-centred approach:
- exploring both the disease and the individual's illness experience;
- understanding the whole person within his or her social context;
- finding common ground;
- incorporating prevention and health promotion;
- enhancing the patient–doctor relationship through sharing and caring;
- being realistic and working within the constraints of time and resources.

The broad scope of this term has posed challenges for its definition, and it has become apparent that the term 'patient-centred' means different things to different authors (Mead & Bower 2000). On the one hand it has been described as a 'key philosophy' (Bower & Mead 2007), whilst on the other it has been called a 'fuzzy concept' (Bensing 2000). Since the concept is hard to encapsulate, assumptions are made about its meaning. A global meaning is taken to be that *the patient is at the centre of his or her own healthcare*. However, this does not convey the subtlety of the concept. I propose to select three definitions. The first as the most often cited, the second for its simplicity and the third as the most contemporary.

Mead and Bower (2000) undertook a literature review to examine the various meanings of the term and categorised five dimensions that they initially described as 'distinct':
- biopsychosocial perspective;
- patient as person;
- sharing power and responsibility;
- therapeutic alliance and
- doctor as person.

However, in their 2007 paper, they referred to these as 'a number of interconnecting components from a theoretical perspective' (Bower & Mead 2007).

A simpler definition of patient-centredness from the Department of Health (2004) gives two dimensions to the concept:

> Patient-centred is a philosophy of care that encourages:
> (a) a focus in the consultation on the patient as a whole person who has individual preferences situated within social contexts, and/or
> (b) shared control of the consultation, decisions about interventions or management of health problems with the patient.

It is indicative of the problems concerning the concept that there is an 'and/or' included in their definition.

The most recent contribution to the field comes from Scholl *et al.* (2014), who undertook a systematic review and concept analysis of 'patient-centredness'. These investigators found that many studies that included the term in their title or abstract failed to include a definition. From the studies that did include a definition, Scholl *et al.* identified 15 dimensions of patient-centredness, which they grouped into three categories:
- principles: essential characteristics of the clinician, clinician–patient relationship, patient as a unique person, biopsychosocial perspective;
- enablers: clinician–patient communication, integration of medical and nonmedical care, teamwork and teambuilding, access to care, coordination and continuity of care; and

- activities: patient information, patient involvement in care, involvement of family and friends, patient empowerment, physical support, emotional support.

This conceptualisation explicitly relates clinical communication to patient-centredness. However, I would argue that it is implicit in the various definitions of patient-centredness: you cannot have patient-centredness without effective clinical communication; they are entwined. The dimensions identified are incorporated into the two-way exchange between doctor and patient through the medium of communication. This view was also taken by Bensing, who used the phrase 'Communication: the royal pathway to patient-centered medicine' (Bensing *et al.* 2000).

What is the evidence of the effect of patient-centred care on healthcare outcomes?

This question has been examined and reexamined many times. The answer continues to be problematic whilst the terminology of patient-centredness is heterogenous. In essence studies lack comparability. As I write now, in 2014, this problem remains unresolved. The evidence is mixed. This in turn makes it hard to summarise such complex information with any succinctness.

The three most recent studies each take a slightly different but related outlook at health outcomes.

Rathert *et al.* (2012) conducted a systematic review of the patient-centred care literature to examine the evidence for the concept and for its outcomes. They categorised patient-centred care using the Institute of Medicine definition (Institute of Medicine 2001). Their results, with a detailed examination of 40 studies, found contradictory evidence. Whilst some studies demonstrated a significant relationship between specific elements of patient-centred care and outcomes, other studies found no relationship. There was evidence that *patient satisfaction and self-management were positively influenced* by patient-centred care.

McMillan *et al.* (2013) specifically evaluated the efficacy of patient-centred care interventions for people with chronic conditions and, via a systematic review, identified 30 randomised controlled trials. They took a robust study approach by categorising aspects of patient-centred care using the Morgan and Yoder categorization (Morgan & Yoder 2012). In doing so, they identified that most interventions used the aspect of 'empowering care', alongside educating patients; an aspect that encourages patient autonomy and self-confidence. They classified outcomes under three headings: patient satisfaction, perceived quality of care and health outcomes, with the latter further broken down into clinical, functional, personal and system outcomes. For future researchers it is worth looking at the detail of their findings. However, overall McMillan *et al.* could conclude no more than there '*appeared to be benefits associated*' with patient-centred care in terms of patient satisfaction and the perceived quality of care.

Dwamena and colleagues (2012) examined the effects of interventions for providers to promote a patient-centred approach in clinical consultations. Hence it is of direct relevance to readers here as an evidence base for clinical communication. The definition of patient-centredness they used was akin to the Department of Health definition (Department of Health 2004). They concluded that training interventions were largely successful in transferring new skills to providers and that, interestingly, short-term training of less than 10 hours was as effective as longer training. This conclusion was drawn from studies across numerous high-income countries and several clinical settings.

What was less clear was the effect on healthcare outcomes for patients. A proportion of the studies were found to include interventions to educate patients as well as the providers. In these cases they reported 'modest support' for an effect on health status. Overall, however, they report mixed effects on patient satisfaction, health behaviour and health status. Their tentative conclusion was that in complex interventions involving providers and patients that include condition-specific educational materials, there is *some indication of beneficial effects*.

Note my italicized text in each summary indicating that researchers are cautious about their claims. Whilst the current research provides positive support for the continuance of training staff in patient-centredness, more robust research is needed to examine the effect on health outcomes. In my opinion this will only be possible once more homogenous terminology is adopted.

Is the concept of *patient-centred care* justified?

It could be argued that patient-centredness is such an amorphous concept, with such mixed evidence of its effects, that it is unjustifiable to use it as a basis for healthcare. Perhaps it is merely a fashion. Few authors stop to pose this as a question, let alone address it. It is as if it has become a 'sacred cow' (Illingworth 2008).

Others propose a moral justification. McWhinney stated, 'Some things are good in themselves' (McWhinney 1995). Similarly Dwamena *et al.*'s Cochrane Review concluded that patient-centredness is justified if it is 'seen as worthy in its own right' (Dwamena *et al.* 2012). From the patient's point of view, the International Alliance of Patients' Organizations states that patients and carers have a 'fundamental right to patient-centred healthcare' (International Alliance of Patients' Organizations 2007).

But the question remains to be asked and answered. Is there sufficient justification for this concept? What would happen if doctors were not, in any sense, patient-centred?

Teaching and learning of patient-centredness with medical students

The current standard for medical graduates in the UK (General Medical Council 2009) states that a doctor should be able to:

> Demonstrate awareness of the clinical responsibilities and role of the doctor, making the care of the patient the first concern. Recognise the principles of patient-centred care, including self-care, and deal with the patients' healthcare needs in consultation with them and, where appropriate, their relatives or carers.
>
> *(Outcome 3: 20 b)*

However, the General Medical Council fail to define what they mean by 'patient-centred'.

The use of patient-centred frameworks to teach consultation skills, such as the Calgary-Cambridge Guide, are widespread (Kurtz *et al.* 2005). Such frameworks include features of patient-centredness, such as exploring the 'patient's perspective' and engaging in 'shared decision-making', as essential components.

However, there is a growing body of research that records the *decline of various aspects of medical students' skills and attitudes that are related to patient-centredness* as they progress through medical school. Paradoxically, Bombeke *et al.* demonstrated that students are more patient-centred, using the Mead and Bower definitions, when they enter than when they leave medical school (Bombeke *et al.* 2010).

Krupat *et al.* (2009) noted that 'Students have been found to become less idealistic, less empathic, less patient-centred, less attuned to the needs of special populations, and less sensitive to ethical issues'; and that this has been found in accounts across the years and internationally. Some of these areas will be examined in more detail.

Empathy

A working definition of empathy (a term that of itself has generated multiple meanings) is:

> a cognitive attribute that involves an understanding of the inner experiences and perspectives of the patient as a separate individual, combined with a capability to communicate this understanding to the patient.
>
> *(Hojat et al. 2004)*

There have been many studies providing empirical evidence that empathy declines as a student/resident progresses through medical school. These were brought together in a systematic review undertaken by Neumann and colleagues, where 18 studies met the inclusion criteria; specifically, that the studies did not include interventions to enhance empathy (Neumann *et al.* 2011). Of the 11 studies of medical students, 9 (3 longitudinal and 6 cross-sectional studies) showed a decrease in empathy during medical school that was significant. It was the clinical practice phase of training that particularly showed the downward trend.

Interviewing to gather information

In a longitudinal study, Pfeiffer and colleagues noted a rise, followed by a fall, of students' skill in obtaining a medical history (Pfeiffer *et al.* 1998). The decline in skill in taking a social history was of particular note.

A later cohort study, following a curriculum review, showed earlier acquisition and a less steep decline in interviewing and interpersonal skills during students' time in medical school (Hook & Pfeiffer 2007). However, the decline remained and seemed to be linked with the clinical years.

Patient-centred attitudes

In the 1980s Mizrahi found that medical students saw patients as an annoyance and that part of their focus was to 'get rid of the patient' – colloquially known as GROP (Mizrahi 1986). Her work also showed that the students' main aim was survival and that they were immersed in a culture in which patients were 'turfed' (transferred to another department) and referred to as 'gomers' (get out of my emergency room). The jargon was not perceived to be derogatory by students.

Haidet and colleagues set out to describe and quantify student attitudes towards the doctor–patient relationship in the first, third and fourth years of a large medical school in the USA (Haidet *et al.* 2002). The validated instrument they used was the Patient–Practitioner Orientation Scale, which measures an individual's attitudes along two dimensions termed 'sharing' and 'caring' (Krupat *et al.* 1996). They produced direct evidence of the decline of students' patient-centred attitudes over time whilst at medical school.

Another study of students' patient-centred attitudes, using the same measure, was undertaken in Greece (Tsimtsiou *et al.* 2007). By contrast, this was a longitudinal study testing a student cohort at year 4 and then again at the end of year 6. Their findings again suggested that medical students' attitudes became more doctor-centred. In this study, the sharing dimension showed decline, whereas the caring dimension remained constant. Tsimtsiou and colleagues noted that previous studies had also suggested that students developed a more paternalistic idea of the doctor's role during their progress through medical school (de Monchy *et al.* 1988; Trovato *et al.* 2004). A Canadian longitudinal study reported a persistent decline in several attitude scores as students progressed through medical school and commented that this was counter to the intention of the school (Woloschuk *et al.* 2004). It included decline in the students' attitude towards recognising the importance of doctor–patient relations interpersonally and emotionally.

A UK study from Noble and colleagues demonstrated that a teaching intervention, which included professional skills training in years 1 and 2 of the curriculum, led to increasing patient-centred attitudes in students (measured on the scale devised by de Monchy *et al.* 1988) relative to a traditional curriculum (Noble *et al.* 2007). However, this study is again of the preclinical years.

The effect of culture and curriculum

Pfeiffer *et al.* proposed potential explanations for their findings (Pfeiffer *et al.* 1998). One was that the very culture of medicine de-emphasizes the need for interpersonal skills. The focus was on 'hard' facts and scientific data. Their clinical clerkships started in year 3, when the decline became particularly noticeable. Another reason they put forward was that the fourth-year students might be so preoccupied with establishing differential diagnoses that they ignored the patient's social history and considered rapport as irrelevant. The final hypothesis was that students learned to regard patients as an annoyance in their clerkships and aimed to 'get rid of patients' (Mizrahi 1986). In my opinion these findings (Pfeiffer *et al.* 1998; Hook & Pfeiffer 2007) link with what is known about the socialisation of medical students and how they learn to 'discount the social stuff' (Conrad 1988).

Others comment similarly: 'Medical sociologists and anthropologists suggest that methods for managing work, mistakes and emotions, in addition to the language and manner of presentation that students acquire during their training, direct students away from patient-centred patterns of interactions in both peer groups and with patients' (Haidet *et al.* 2002).

Within the structure of medical education, formal teaching of patient-centred aspects, however defined, often occurs in the preclinical years. It is when medical students are in their clinical attachment years that the decline is more visible. Hence Woloschuk *et al.* (2004) proposed that the 'unintentional or null curriculum' (whereby teaching on communication and doctor–patient relations ceases at the end of the preclinical phase) may transmit that these areas are unimportant.

A major influence on medical students comes from the unplanned, informal, hidden curriculum (Hafferty 1998; Cribb & Bignold 1999). If students see things done differently in the 'real' world that is what they will follow, rather than what is taught in the training room. Poor role modelling and 'rolelessness' of the medical student (having no role other than that of learner) may be major factors leading to the decline of patient-centredness (Illingworth 2008).

Bombeke and colleagues identified a 'huge gap between education and practice' (Bombeke *et al.* 2012). They found that the 'reality shock' of clinical practice was such that many students concluded that the communication skills they had been taught were not feasible or realistic in the workplace. Students reported that they felt they were marked down if they 'lost time practising patient-centred communication', thus giving students a clear incentive to stop using a patient-centred approach.

Interventions to foster patient-centredness

As the decline of patient-centredness, in its various guises, occurs particularly in the clinical years, interventions must occur during these years to counter-balance this trend. As a practitioner, it seems to me that active learning approaches should be used, in context, to nurture patient-centred attitudes and skills. Branch and colleagues recommended a move from the unconscious ('hidden curriculum') to the conscious use of role modelling humanism with patients, in the presence of students (Branch *et al.* 2001). Students learn from the role models they see, and to nurture patient-centredness in the doctor–patient relationship, positive role modelling is essential (Illingworth 2008).

Some interventions have reported a maintenance and/or improvement in patient-centredness. Krupat *et al.* (2009) set out to prevent the erosion of students' patient-centred beliefs with a group of third-year students and demonstrated that students in an intervention group showed no decline in attitudes, compared to a control group. Whilst it was a small pilot study it is interesting to note that the intervention was to place students with a team on one hospital site, giving them continuity with faculty and patients, hence increasing their sense of having a 'role' and working in a team (Illingworth 2008).

Hojat and colleagues reported 10 approaches to enhancing empathy in healthcare staff, such as experiencing hospitalization and positive role models (Hojat *et al.* 2009). Oswald *et al.* reported an intervention using patient-educators with second-year students and demonstrated gains in the students' insights into the lives of patients living with chronic conditions (Oswald *et al.* 2014). Perhaps this intervention translates to clinical years and could assist the student to continue to see the patient as a person.

Future directions

In this chapter the evolution of patient-centredness has been explored and the various attempts at defining the concept have been examined. With such heterogeneity of terms in use it has been difficult to demonstrate the healthcare outcomes of patient-centred behaviours, including clinical communication.

Since the health systems of the 21st century require a patient-centred approach this needs to be nurtured in the doctors of tomorrow. The evidence of the effect of medical school on students demonstrates that, far from fostering patient-centred attitudes and behaviours, students often leave with a measurable decline in patient-centredness. Further research is needed once definitive terminology has been agreed and is in use. A few ideas from the researchers in the field have been proposed to foster the patient-centredness of medical students, which will also need to be evaluated robustly.

References

Balint, E. (1969) The possibilities of patient-centred medicine. *Journal of the Royal College of General Practice*, 17, 269–276.

Bensing, J. (2000) Bridging the gap: The separate worlds of evidence-based medicine and patient-centred medicine. *Patient Education and Counseling*, 39 (no. 1), 17–25.

Bensing, J.M., Verhaak, P.F., van Dulmen, A.M. & Visser, A.P. (2000) Communication: The royal pathway to patient-centered medicine. *Patient Education and Counseling*, 39 (no. 1), 1–3.

Bombeke, K., Symons, L., Debaene, L., De Winter, B. Schol, S. & Van Royen, P. (2010) Help, I'm losing patient-centredness! Experiences of medical students and their teachers. *Medical Education*, 44 (no. 7), 662–673.

Bombeke, K., Symons, L., Vermeire, E., Debaene, L., Schol, S., De Winter, B. & Van Royen, P. (2012) Patient-centredness from education to practice: The 'lived' impact of communication skills training. *Medical Teacher*, 34 (no. 5), E338–E348.

Bower, P. & Mead, N. (2007) Patient-centred healthcare. In: S. Ayers, A. Baum, C. McManus *et al.*, *Cambridge Handbook of Psychology, Health and Medicine*, p. 968. Cambridge University Press, Cambridge.

Branch, W.T., Jr, Kern, D.E., Haidet, P., Weissman, P., Gracey, C.F., Mitchell, G. & Inui, T.S. (2001) Teaching the human dimensions of care in clinical settings. *JAMA*, 286, 1067–1074.

Byrne, P.S. & Long, B.E.L. (1976) *Doctors Talking to Patients: A Study of the Verbal Behaviours of Doctors in the Consultation*. HMSO, London.

Conrad, P. (1988) Learning to doctor: Reflections on recent accounts of the medical school years. *Journal of Health and Social Behavior*, 29 (no. 4), 323–332.

Cribb, A. & Bignold, S. (1999) Towards the reflexive medical school: The hidden curriculum and medical education research. *Studies in Higher Education*, 24 (no. 2), 195–209.

de Monchy, C., Richardson, R., Brown, R.A. & Harden, R.M. (1988) Measuring attitudes of doctors: The doctor–patient (DP) rating. *Medical Education*, 22, 231–239.

Department of Health. (2004) *Patient and Public Involvement in Health: The Evidence for Policy Implementation*. Department of Health, London.

Dulmen, S.A., Lukersmith, S., Muxlow, J., Santa Mina, E., Nijhuis-van der Sanden, M.W. & Wees, P.J. (2013) *Supporting a Person-Centred Approach in Clinical Guidelines: A Position Paper of the Allied Health Community–Guidelines International Network (G-I-N)*. Health Expectations. doi:10.1111/hex.12144.

Dwamena, F., Holmes-Rovner, M., Gaulden, C., Jorgenson, S., Sadigh, G., Sikorskii, A., Lewin, S., Smith, R.C., Coffey, J. & Olomu, A. (2012) Interventions for providers to promote a patient-centred approach in clinical consultations. Cochrane Database of Systematic Reviews, 2 (Art. No.: CD003267). doi:10.1002/14651858.CD003267.pub2.

General Medical Council. (2009) *Tomorrow's Doctors: Outcomes and Standards for Medical Education*. General Medical Council, London.

Hafferty, F.W. (1998) Beyond curriculum reform: Confronting medicine's hidden curriculum. *Academic Medicine*, 73 (no. 4), 403–407.

Haidet, P., Dains, J.E., Paterniti, D.A., Hechtel, L., Chang, T., Tseng, E. & Rogers, J.C. (2002) Medical student attitudes toward the doctor–patient relationship. *Medical Education*, 36 (no. 6), 568–574.

Hojat, M., Mangione, S., Nasca, T.J., Rattner, S., Erdmann, J.B., Gonnella, J.S. & Magee, M. (2004) An empirical study of decline in empathy in medical school. *Medical Education*, 38 (no. 9), 934–941.

Hojat, M., Vergare, M.J., Maxwell, K., Brainard, G., Herrine, S.K., Isenberg, G.A., Veloski, J. & Gonnella, J.S. (2009) The devil is in the third year: A longitudinal study of erosion of empathy in medical school. *Academic Medicine*, 84 (no. 9), 1182–1191.

Hook, K.M. & Pfeiffer, C.A. (2007) Impact of a new curriculum on medical students' interpersonal and interviewing skills. *Medical Education*, 41, 154–159.

Illingworth, R.E. (2008) Teaching and learning of patient-centred medicine: A study of medical students' accounts. PhD Thesis, University of Manchester, Manchester.

Institute of Medicine. (2001) *Crossing the Quality Chasm: A New Health System for the 21st Century*. National Academies Press, Washington, DC.

International Alliance of Patients' Organizations. (2007) *What Is Patient-Centred Health Care? A Review of Definitions and Principles*. International Alliance of Patients' Organizations, London.

Jewson, N.D. (1976) The disappearance of the sick-man from medical cosmology, 1770–1870. *Sociology*, 10 (no. 2), 225–244.

Krupat, E., Putnam, S.M. & Yeager, C. (1996) The fit between doctors and patients: Can it be measured? *Journal of General Internal Medicine* 1 (Suppl), 134.

Krupat, E., Pelletier, S., Alexander, E.K., Hirsh, D., Ogur, B. & Schwartzstein, R. (2009) Can changes in the principal clinical year prevent the erosion of students' patient-centered beliefs? *Academic Medicine*, 84 (no. 5), 582–586.

Kurtz, S.M., Silverman, J. & Draper, J. (2005) *Teaching and Learning Communication Skills in Medicine*. Radcliffe Publishing, Oxford.

McMillan, S.S., Kendall, E., Sav, A., King, M.A., Whitty, J.A., Kelly, F. & Wheeler, A.J. (2013) Patient-centered approaches to health care: A systematic review of randomized controlled trials. *Medical Care Research and Review*, 70 (no. 7), 567–596. doi:10.1177/1077558713496318.

McWhinney, I.R. (1995) Why we need a new clinical method. In: M. Stewart, J. B. Brown, W. W. Weston *et al.*, *Patient-Centred Medicine: Transforming the Clinical Method*. London, Sage.

Mead, N. & Bower, P. (2000) Patient-centredness: A conceptual framework and review of the empirical literature. *Social Science & Medicine* 51 (no. 7), 1087–1110.

Mizrahi, T. (1986) *Getting Rid of Patients: Contradictions in the Socialization of Physicians*. Rutgers University Press, New Brunswick, NJ.

Morgan, S. & Yoder, L.H. (2012) A concept analysis of person-centered care. *Journal of Holistic Nursing*, 30 (no. 1), 6–15.

Neumann, M., Edelhäuser, F., Tauschel, D., Fischer, M.R., Wirtz, M., Woopen, C., Haramati, A. & Scheffer, C. (2011) Empathy decline and its reasons: A systematic review of studies with medical students and residents. *Academic Medicine*, 86 (no. 8), 996–1009. doi:1010.1097/ACM.1000b1013e318221e318615.

Noble, L.M., Kubacki, A., Martin, J. & Lloyd, M. (2007) The effect of professional skills training on patient-centredness and confidence in communicating with patients. *Medical Education* 41, 432–440.

Oswald, A., Czupryn, J., Wiseman, J. & Snell, L. (2014) Patient-centred education: What do students think? *Medical Education*, 48 (no. 2), 170–180.

Pfeiffer, C., Madray, H., Ardolino, A. & Willms, J. (1998) The rise and fall of students' skill in obtaining a medical history. *Medical Education*, 32 (no. 3), 283–288.

Rathert, C., Wyrwich, M.D. & Boren, S.A. (2012) Patient-centered care and outcomes: A systematic review of the literature. *Medical Care Research and Review*, 70 (no. 4), 351–379.

Scholl, I., Zill, J.M., Harter, M. & Dirmaier, J. (2014) An integrative model of patient-centeredness – a systematic review and concept analysis. *PLoS One*, 9 (no. 9), e107828.

Stewart, M. (1995) Effective physician-patient communication and health outcomes: A review. *Canadian Medical Association Journal*, 152, 1423–1433.

Stewart, M. (2001) Towards a global definition of patient centred care. *BMJ*, 322, 444–445.

Trovato, G., Catalano, D., Di Nuovo, S. & Di Corrado, D. (2004) Perception of cultural correlates of medicine: A comparison between medical and non-medical students – the authoritarian health. *European Review for Medical and Pharmacological Sciences*, 8, 59–68.

Tsimtsiou, Z., Kerasidou, O., Efstathiou, N., Papaharitou, S., Hatzimouratidis, K. & Hatzichristou, D. (2007) Medical students' attitudes toward patient-centred care: A longitudinal survey. *Medical Education*, 41 (no. 2), 146–153.

Woloschuk, W., Harasym, P.H. & Temple, W. (2004) Attitude change during medical school: A cohort study. *Medical Education* 38, 522–534.

CHAPTER 7

The Impact of Training

John Skelton

University of Birmingham, Birmingham, UK

The impact of training is essentially concerned with two things. First, there is the question of how, if at all, training changes practice in the workplace. Second, there is the impact on the learner of what is taught and assessed. I shall look at both of these issues.

A fundamental difficulty in all education is separating out the effect of a particular educational intervention from the myriad other influences at play in the learner's life. What one does in the classroom – the way a tutor teaches a particular clinical skill at the bedside, the ethical principles discussed in a seminar, the lecture on the sociology of health-seeking behaviour - may be undermined, enhanced or distorted by later exposure to the workplace, by the learner's prior learning or simply by his or her experience of life. Indeed, the areas where it is possible to isolate the effect of teaching with some confidence tend to be those that are simpler.

The problem is spelled out in a much-cited review from the late 1980s (Baldwin & Ford 1988):

> The tasks used [in the existing research] limit generalizability of the results to short-term simple motor tasks and memory skills training. The use of such tasks is problematic, given that organizational training is often conducted to enhance individual competence on long-term complex skills such as interpersonal communication and managerial problem solving.

The authors conclude that the effect of applying 'learning principles' is unknown when it comes to these more complex issues. The quandary detailed here is one that is still a common one in education: the smaller the element being evaluated, the easier it is to measure change, but it becomes less likely that you will be measuring anything meaningful. Equally, if small elements are what get tested (say, "Does the doctor greet the patient?") the more likely it is that the teaching will emphasise just those bits and pieces of behaviour. Picking up Baldwin and Ford's use of the word, I shall call such things 'simple' changes.

Transfer and clinical communication

As regards clinical communication, a major tradition over many years has been to concentrate on identifying bits of communication behaviour that are easy to isolate and teach as good practice (e.g. greeting the patient, maintaining eye contact, asking open questions). However, just as the medical student who can successfully demonstrate a particular clinical skill may do so without understanding the principles, and may therefore be unsafe, so we may assume a student who demonstrated the desired communication behaviour may do so mechanically, and their values may not match the skills. There have been doubts expressed about whether the learning of communication skills in a simulated environment transfers into improved clinical practice.

Thus van den Eertwegh *et al.* (2013), in a narrative review, talk of the "inconsistencies of findings and the apparent low transfer of communication skills from training to medical practice". Uitterhoeve (2009), looking at the effects of training on patient outcome – which might imply a transfer of training – identified just seven studies, of which five were randomised, and given the 'inconclusive' nature of the evidence in key areas, call for "more high quality studies". Barth and Lannen (2011) similarly looked at 13 trials and concluded that there is "a potential gap between training and clinical impact." And Liénard *et al.* (2010) found that "transfer was directly related to training attendance but remained limited" following a 40-hour programme.

Yet there have been important indications to the contrary, that long-term transfer can be identified through the traditional method of a randomised controlled trial. Fallowfield *et al.* (2003), reporting on their 3-day course, found that, 3 months after the end of the course, participants showed significantly better results than a control group with reference to focused and open questions, expressions of empathy, appropriate responses to patient cues and a decrease in the number of leading questions. More interestingly, most of these skills were retained "approximately 15 months post-course" (Fallowfield *et al.* 2003). In addition, the participants were "exhibiting additional, important and effective skills" – thus, there was less evidence of doctors interrupting patients. This is intriguing evidence for participants taking responsibility for future learning and for identifying ways in which the principles of what they have been taught – not the behavioural elements, but the underlying ethos – can be enacted.

Fallowfield *et al.* raise the issue of self-efficacy as a means of accounting for the maintenance and development of the skills over time. This concept, first developed by Bandura (e.g. Bandura 1977), refers to the way individuals who believe they are capable of doing something successfully are more likely to attempt it and more likely to persevere with it. Bandura (1982) argues that "the self-efficacy mechanism may have wide explanatory power"; certainly it is often very easy to account for educational success by reference to it.

The central implication of the construct is that learning is associated not merely with the enactment of simple behaviours but with what Baldwin and Ford call "personal characteristics". A great deal of recent medical education, as I shall suggest, has dealt essentially with versions of this switch away from simple behaviours to the people who use them.

What factors improve the chance of transfer?

There are three areas that might affect training transfer – or, more broadly, the success or failure of an educational intervention. These are, unsurprisingly (using Baldwin and Ford's terms): 'trainee characteristics', 'training design' and 'work environment'. Self-efficacy is, clearly, a 'personal characteristic', and one that has been widely explored. Thus within clinical education, Parle *et al.* (1997) report a training intervention designed to improve self-efficacy, amongst other things, and Ammentorp *et al.* (2007) report on a randomised controlled trial designed to see whether 'self-efficacy' could be improved for nurses and doctors as a result of a 30-hour course. They make the point that communication courses should (of course) 'promote introspection and self-awareness as a necessary condition for self-reflection'. Gulbrandsen *et al.* (2013) found that their 'communication skills course led to improved communication skills self-efficacy more than 3 years later' (note the timescale). This was a crossover randomised trial, over 20 hours, and it is worth noting, therefore, that – as with the programmes described by Liénard *et al.*, Fallowfield *et al.* and Ammentorp *et al.*, there is a substantial amount of small group work involved.

Other personal characteristics which seem to affect successful transfer are reviewed by Burke and Hutchins (2007). These are 'cognitive ability', 'pre-training motivation', 'anxiety' (i.e. a lack of anxiety), 'openness to experience', 'perceived utility', 'career planning', 'self-efficacy' (again) and 'organizational commitment'. For other characteristics that one might expect to have a role to play, such as having an internal locus of control, the authors say the evidence is uncertain. Similarly, Salas and Cannon-Bowers (2001) suggest there are three over-arching 'individual characteristics': 'cognitive ability', 'self-efficacy' and 'goal orientation' (i.e. a desire to succeed).

As regards training design, the evidence is not unexpected, and it is well summed up by Berkhof *et al.* (2011) in their overview of systematic reviews: 'Training programmes were effective if they lasted for at least one day, were learner-centred, and focused on practising skills. The best training strategies within the programmes included role-play, feedback and small group discussions.'

Berkhof *et al.* are referring here to doctors, and it is worth recalling that medical students normally have more than the 1 day of training specified, and because the interventions are spread over a period of years, there is plenty of time for reflection. Finally, there is the work environment and its role in ensuring transfer. At its simplest level, this is self-evident. Training that cannot be used is likely to atrophy. If one studies French in a classroom setting, then goes to live in France, transfer will take place. Indeed, under normal circumstances (assuming one is not living in isolation), one's competence at French will improve out of all recognition, and for that matter to such an extent that the effect of training rather than practice *in situ* will become unmeasurable. This is the fundamental difficulty implicit in Miller's pyramid of assessing clinical skills competence (Miller 1990), that full integration often means that formal teaching becomes invisible. Miller argued that there are four 'levels' of learning, leading through *knowledge, competence* and *performance* to *action.* These terms are often presented as 'knows', 'knows how', 'shows how' and 'does'. Thus, people learning to drive are likely to know, prior to lesson one, what the pedals are called (they 'know' this); that they are operated by pushing down on them with their feet ('knows how'); can work them successfully, to the satisfaction of their instructor ('shows how'); and then, on a year in year out basis, put everything into action ('does'). It is important to be aware here also that, underpinning the concept of 'does' is the concept of successful enactment. For a doctor this will mean not merely an appropriate level of clinical competence but with the appropriate values and attitudes, just as successful enactment behind the wheel of the car implies 'does safely'.

Go and live in Germany, however, and there will be no transfer because there is no point. And in fact, training of which the learner 'sees the point' is likely to work. This is one of the principal themes of Brown's (2010) study of how medical students perceived communication teaching when they were in a clinical setting. Thus: 'I thought it [clinical communication skills] was a load of tosh…Only when I got into my clinical years did I realize oh my gosh, I'm so grateful that I did have the opportunity.'

Where the need is self-evident, transfer will happen. In this sense, one of the areas that training should emphasise is the need to raise awareness, so that what is self-evident to the trainer will become so to the learner.

How else can the workplace support the learning?

Some readers will recall that, 20 years ago, there was a government report ('The Kennedy Report', Bristol Royal Infirmary Inquiry 2001) into poor standards of care in neonatal cardiology at the Bristol Royal Infirmary. The inquiry's chairman, Professor Ian Kennedy, spoke of the need to 'broaden the notion of clinical competence', specifying in particular that 'greater priority than at present should be given to non-clinical aspects of care…in the education, training and continuing professional development of health care professionals'. The relevant areas were: 'skills in communicating with patients and colleagues', 'education about the principles and organisation of the NHS', 'skills required for management', 'the development of teamwork', 'shared learning across professional boundaries', 'clinical audit and reflective practice' and 'leadership'.

The contextualisation of clinical communication offered here is important. It helps us to recognise the importance of seeing communication not as something isolated but as something that happens as part of the daily routine of medicine and of being a doctor. The recent Francis Report into problems in Mid Staffordshire, with its emphasis on the importance of NHS 'culture' (a word used 69 times in the executive summary alone), offers a not dissimilar reminder (Mid Staffordshire NHS Foundation Trust Public Inquiry 2013). We should recognise that attention to communication is a part of the creation of a good workplace culture. The Kennedy Report is, interestingly, echoed in a recent systematic review of the assessment of professionalism (Wilkinson *et al*. 2009). Five 'clusters of professionalism' were identified: 'adherence to ethical principles; effective interactions with patients and…people…important to [them]; effective interactions with people working within the health system; reliability; and a commitment to…improvement of competence in oneself, others and systems'.

The various ideas that have been suggested to support workplace training in this respect run from those things that ought to happen anyway – senior doctors should role model good practice, simply because they themselves undertake good practice. Thus Russ-Eft (2002) identifies 'supervisor support', 'opportunity to use', 'workload' (i.e. having the time to practise as necessary) and 'peer support' as relevant. She also, perhaps less comfortably, mentions 'supervisor sanction', that is, the anxiety that the trainee will have to conform to what is required or get into trouble. Heaven *et al*. (2006) make the case for 'the potential of clinical supervision in enhancing the transfer process', something that is, perhaps, obvious, but often does not happen properly. Other suggestions (from multiple sources) include follow-up training to ensure retention, identifying 'buddies' to support and exchange ideas, and so forth.

The learners medical schools create

The great achievement of the communication skills movement is that every doctor in the UK and in many other countries under the age of, say, 40 knows that communication skills matter. In the UK, all medical schools teach and assess communication, and a large number of postgraduate specialties assess it during examinations that determine career progression.

But this probably means, in effect, that *some* doctors typically now graduate with an understanding that good communication is the exercise of a range of simple behavioural entities like 'asking open questions' to enact patient-centredness. But this is a very restricted view. One unintended effect of training has been that 'communication' has tended to become synonymous with 'empathy' and a kind of counselling style, and for that matter, has come to mean almost exclusively spoken communication. What Hafferty (2000) was calling an 'artificial dichotomy' at the turn of the century – the question of whether we want doctors who are competently boorish or incompetently sensitive – is not without resonance even today. Hafferty concludes: 'The object of medical education is not emotional sensitivity. It is professionalism.'

In this respect, it is worth observing that there are many areas where language and communication have central roles, and that doctors undertake, but that recent graduates, and their trainers, are rather unlikely to think of as 'communication skills tasks'. For example, despite the highly conventionalised language features of scientific writing (there is a major research tradition of relevance; e.g. see Swales & Feak 2004 as a starting point), it is not normally considered part of the 'communication' remit. Nor is the developing genre of writing a reflective log. Nor is the widely used 'SBAR' technique for communicating information between members of a team (Institute for Healthcare Improvement 2015). Equally, the concept of 'respectful challenging' (when a senior colleague has made a mistake) may not particularly be seen as 'communication'.

But with the shift of focus towards a better understanding of how to help learners become reflective practitioners and take responsibility for their professional development, it seems likely that aspects of communication training will be repositioned within the preoccupations this suggests. Communication, in this light, is a 'manifestation' (Stern 2006) of professionalism. Thus, what will seem to matter increasingly may be an awareness of the role of communication in a much wider range of contexts, echoed still to some extent by the areas mentioned by Kennedy, Wilkinson *et al.*, and with the impact of Francis, as a means of modelling and upholding the appropriate 'culture'. 'Communication' in this sense is a more fully integrated concept, and one likely to be taught (though perhaps with attention to the caveats mentioned above) in a more fully integrated context, alongside other training, and folded within it. Bradley (2006) sketches aspects of a possible framework for this, in which a mix of elements coexists under the broad heading of 'simulation'. Of particular relevance is the possibility of 'routine learning and rehearsal of clinical and communication skills at all levels', with all this implies in terms of, for instance, interprofessional learning and teamwork.

A further unintended consequence of communication skills training has been, precisely, to promote a certain set of simple skills as having inherent rather than contextual value. But it is evident that the relentless pursuit of any skill – for example, *only* asking open questions – is a bad idea. What matters is the ability to choose intelligently, 'creatively' (Salmon & Young 2011) from a range of communication resources; to know when it's fine to say to a patient 'You'll live' and when it isn't; when you can laughingly say 'Oh, don't be a dope' to a colleague, and so on. The ability to choose judiciously is known as 'communicative competence' (Hymes 1972). Communication is a highly flexible resource that thoughtful individuals use to achieve particular professional, ethical ends. Communication teaching will be subsumed into such things as professional development (e.g. Stern 2006). This suggests a move away from teaching, testing and researching 'communication skills' in itself. Checklists have always had their place in teaching, as pegs to hang discussion on. But the discussion should not get stuck here.

This leaves the issue of evidence, as a means of both testing students and doctors and of assessing change. There are efforts now to demonstrate the psychometric appropriateness of measuring, for example (and using both these terms in the narrowest sense), *clinical skills* (say, undertaking a pelvic examination) and *communication skills* (communicating appropriately with the lady being examined) together. For example, see Moulton *et al.* (2009), who found that 'technical' and 'communication' skills could be tested together but could be separated out successfully – indeed, the finding was that the two components did not correlate. (For an overview of the difficulties and complexities involved in assessing relevant areas together, see Stern 2006.) From a different angle, in a study of considerable importance, van der Vleuten & Schuwirth (2005) discuss how testing theory and practice can enable both 'integration' and 'authenticity'. They argue that 'selecting an assessment method involves context-dependent compromises', and that 'we need more methods that rely on qualitative information and thus require professional judgement.' The authors stress that 'reliability can also be achieved with less standardised assessment situations and more subjective evaluations, provided the sampling is appropriate.' With judicious, repeated sampling, high levels of reliability can be achieved without compromising too much on validity.

Future directions

All of this, then, offers validation for the current shift towards hi-tech, rich context simulations *and* for reflective logs. However, preparing oneself or one's trainee for an examination can be a reductive process, and it remains to be seen whether there is a drift back to a formulaic approach (witness the number of people who think you demonstrate reflection by beginning lots of sentences with 'I reflected that…'). Just at the moment, however, there is optimism: essentially, a hope that the humanisation of medical education, to pick up a phrase much used at present, is possible. The best medical students and doctors have, we might reasonably hope, always seen beyond the simple skills – have always, in effect, transferred more than their training, have reflected on the hidden as well as the overt curriculum and have explored the way one uses language to represent oneself in the world and to be a decent human being in the workplace.

References

Ammentorp, J., Sabroe, S., Kofoed, P.-E. & Mainz, J. (2007) The effect of training on medical doctors' and nurses' self-efficacy: A randomized controlled trial. *Patient Education and Counselling*, 66 (no. 3), 270–277.

Baldwin, T.T. & Ford J.K. (1988) Transfer of training: A review and directions for future research. *Personnel Psychology*, 41, 63–105.

Bandura, A. (1977) Self-efficacy: Toward a unifying theory of behavioural change. *Psychological Review*, 84 (no. 2), 184–195.

Bandura, A. (1982) Self-efficacy mechanism in human agency. *American Psychologist*, 37 (no. 2), 122–147.

Barth, J. & Lannen, P. (2011) Efficacy of communication skills training courses in oncology: A systematic review and meta-analysis. *Annals of Oncology*, 22 (no. 5), 1030–1040.

Berkhof, M., van Rijssen, H.J., Schellart, A.J.M., Anema, J.R. & van der Beek, A.J. (2011) Effective training strategies for teaching communication skills to physicians: An overview of systematic reviews. *Patient Education and Counselling*, 84, 152–162.

Bradley, P. (2006) The history of simulation in medical education and possible future directions. *Medical Education*, 40, 254–262.

Bristol Royal Infirmary Inquiry. (2001) *The Report of the Public Enquiry into Children's Heart Surgery at the Bristol Royal Infirmary 1984–1995: Learning from Bristol ("The Kennedy Report")* [WWW document]. URL http://webarchive.nationalarchives.gov.uk/+/www.dh.gov.uk/en/Publicationsandstatistics/Publications/PublicationsPolicyAndGuidance/DH_4005620 [accessed on 18 February 2014].

Brown, J. (2010) Transferring clinical communication skills from the classroom to the clinical environment: Perceptions of a group of medical students in the United Kingdom. *Academic Medicine*, 85 (no. 6), 1052–1059.

Burke, L. & Hutchins, H. (2007) Training transfer: An integrative literature review. *Human Resource Development Review*, 6 (no. 3), 263–296.

Fallowfield, L., Jenkins, V., Farewell, V. & Solis-Trapala, I. (2003) Enduring impact of communication skills training: Results of a 12-month follow-up. *British Journal of Cancer*, 89 (no. 8), 1445–1449.

Gulbrandsen, P., Jensen, B.F., Finset, A. & Blanch-Hartigan, D. (2013) Long-term effect of communication training on the relationship between physicians' self-efficacy and performance. *Patient Education and Counselling*, 91, 180–185.

Hafferty, F.W. (2000) In search of a lost cord: Professionalism and medical education's hidden curriculum. In: D. Wear & J. Bickel, J (eds), *Educating for Professionalism: Creating a Culture of Humanism in Medical Education*, pp. 11–34. University of Iowa Press, Iowa City.

Heaven, C., Clegg, J. & Maguire, P. (2006) Transfer of communication skills training from workshop to workplace: The impact of clinical supervision. *Patient Education and Counselling*, 60, 313–325.

Hymes, D. (1972) On communicative competence. In: J.B. Pride & J. Holmes J. (eds), *Sociolinguistics: Selected Readings*, pp. 269–293. Penguin, Harmondsworth.

Institute for Healthcare Improvement. (2015) *SBAR Technique for Communication: A Situational Briefing Model* [WWW document]. URL http://www.ihi.org/resources/Pages/Tools/SBARTechniqueforCommunicationAsituationalBriefingModel.aspx.

Liénard, A., Merckaert, I., Libert, Y., Bragard, I., *et al.* (2010) Transfer of communication skills to the workplace during clinical rounds: Impact of a programme for residents. *PLoS One*, 5 (no. 8), e12426. DOI:10.1371/journal.pone.0012426.

Mid Staffordshire NHS Foundation Trust Public Inquiry. (2013) *Report of the Mid Staffordshire NHS Foundation Trust Public Inquiry ("The Francis Report")* http://www.midstaffspublicinquiry.com/report (Accessed 18th February 2014).

Miller, G.E. (1990) The assessment of clinical skills/competence/performance. *Academic Medicine*, 65, S63–S67.

Moulton, C.-A., Tabak, D., Kneebone, R., Nestel, D., Macrae, H. & LeBlanc, V.R (2009) Teaching communication skills using the integrated procedural performance instrument (IPPI): A randomized controlled trial. *American Journal of Surgery*, 197, 113–118.

Parle, M., Maguire, P. & Heaven, C. (1997) The development of a training model to improve health professionals' skills, self-efficacy and outcome expectancies when communicating with cancer patients. *Social Science and Medicine*, 44 (no. 2), 231–240.

Russ-Eft, D. (2002) A typology of training design and work environment factors affecting workplace learning and transfer. *Human Resource Development Review*, 1 (no. 1), 45–65.

Saks, A.M. (2002) So what is a good transfer of training estimate? A reply to Fitzpatrick. *Industrial-Organizational Psychologist*, 39, 29–30.

Salas, E. & Cannon-Bowers, J.A. (2001) The science of training: A decade of progress. *Annual Review of Psychology*, 52, 471–499.

Salmon, P. & Young, B. (2011) Creativity in clinical communication: From communication skills to skilled communication. *Medical Education*, 45, 217–226.

Stern, D.T. (2006) A framework for measuring professionalism. In: D.T. Stern (ed), *Measuring Medical Professionalism*, pp. 3–13. Oxford University Press, New York.

Swales, J.M. & Feak, C. (2004) *Academic Writing for Graduate Students: Essential Tasks and Skills.* University of Michigan Press, Ann Arbor.

Uitterhoeve, R.J. (2009) The effect of communication skills training on patient outcomes in cancer care: A systematic review of the literature. *European Journal of Cancer Care*, 19, 442–457.

van den Eertwegh, V., van Dulmen, S., van Dalen, J., Scherpbier, A.J. & van der Vleuten, C.P. (2013). Learning in context: Identifying gaps in research on the transfer of medical communication skills to the clinical workplace. *Patient Education and Counselling*, 90, 184–192.

van der Vleuten, C.P.M. & Schuwirth, L.W.T. (2005) Assessing professional competence: From methods to programmes. *Medical Education*, 39 (no. 3), 309–317.

Wilkinson, T.J., Wade, W.B. & Knock, D.L. (2009) A blueprint to assess professionalism: Results of a systematic review. *Academic Medicine*, 84 (no. 5), 551–558.

CHAPTER 8

The Future of the Doctor–Patient Relationship

Lorraine M. Noble

University College London Medical School, London, UK

This is the century of the patient.

(Gray 2014)

Current practice

We have seen in the preceding chapters that the conceptualisation of the doctor–patient relationship is related to the perceived role of the doctor – as a tradesman, keeper of expert knowledge, accountable professional or public servant – which in turn reflects the broader societal context (see chapters 3 and 4). The rise of approaches such as 'patient-centred care' and 'shared decision making' owe much to expert commentary (e.g. Engel 1977) and the evidence base (e.g. Hall *et al.* 1988; Stewart 1995). But equally important have been society's changing expectations about the rights of the individual (e.g. the 1950 European Convention on Human Rights and the Human Rights Act 1998). The increased focus on the *perspective* of the persons whose health is at issue, their *role* in their own healthcare and their *rights* is central to current approaches to clinical communication. But this change is not exclusive to *clinical communication:* it is fundamental to recent developments in healthcare policy and quality standards that apply across all aspects of healthcare (e.g. Department of Health 2010; NICE 2012).

Whilst the doctor–patient relationship is complex and has been formulated in numerous ways, there is consensus about the features of a professional and caring approach (Makoul 2001; von Fragstein *et al.* 2008; General Medical Council 2013; Silverman *et al.* 2013; see also chapter 5). Nonetheless, it would be a mistake to assume that there is at present a single, universally agreed conceptualisation of the doctor–patient relationship. Practising doctors may have received their basic training decades ago, and many were taught almost exclusively using the biomedical model, although it would have been unlikely to have been labelled as such. More recent graduates will have been provided – either explicitly or implicitly – with a variety of models of the professional–patient relationship. This results in the common complaint that there is a discrepancy between classroom-based teaching and experience on clinical clerkships, which is difficult for learners to resolve (Malhotra *et al.* 2009).

Clinical Communication in Medicine, First Edition. Edited by Jo Brown, Lorraine M. Noble, Alexia Papageorgiou and Jane Kidd.

The dominance of the biomedical model – not just in medical training but in the fabric of healthcare itself – and its continuing impact on the professional–patient relationship cannot be underestimated. The biomedical approach to the consultation was initially modified to incorporate 'the patient's perspective' by *adding* an additional, parallel stream of activity, for example, the Patient-Centred Clinical Method (Levenstein *et al.* 1986) or the 4Es Model (Keller & Carroll 1994). Subsequent formulations of the consultation *integrated* both biomedical tasks and the patient's perspective in a single chronological stream, for example, Calgary-Cambridge (Kurtz *et al.* 2003) or shared decision making (Coulter & Collins 2011). Integrating the anticipated 'goals' of the patient and the doctor theoretically achieves a unified model of care and eliminates the potential for one perspective to dominate, or for the perspectives to be set in opposition to each other. But whilst current frameworks promote the doctor–patient relationship as a *partnership* where the patient is actively involved in decisions about his or her own healthcare (Department of Health 2010; General Medical Council 2013), observed practice shows a more complex picture. For example, recent studies have found:
• doctors actively directing the discussion away from patients' concerns, emotions or accounts of their illness, whilst emphasising biomedical aspects (Agledahl *et al.* 2011);
• doctors prescribing placebo interventions (Howick *et al.* 2013) and
• marked discrepancies in the opinions of patients and doctors about whether patients should have access to their consultation notes (Delbanco *et al.* 2012).

The persisting confusion about the concept of 'patient-centredness' (Mead & Bower 2000; see also chapter 6) is understandable when considered from the perspective of clinicians immersed in a 'fug' of simultaneously coexisting formulations of the doctor–patient relationship. In theory, patient-centredness is the natural successor to the biopsychosocial approach. In practice, the rate of change is much slower. According to the 'diffusion of innovations' theory, when a new idea is introduced into a population, people can be categorised as innovators, early adopters, the early majority, the late majority and laggards (Rogers 1962; Berwick 2003). At any given time, therefore, there will be those who have embraced the new idea and those who have not. Current, sophisticated approaches to the consultation (e.g. Silverman *et al.* 2011; Elwyn *et al.* 2013) are predicated on a modern, partnership model of the doctor–patient relationship. These approaches contribute to the *process* of change, whilst not necessarily reflecting current practice (Leape *et al.* 2012). Medical students swiftly pick up on this confusion and face the ongoing dilemma of which approach to adopt under which circumstances. Unfortunately, in healthcare, as in the corporate world, 'culture eats strategy for breakfast' (Wynia 2012).

Future directions

Healthcare faces the increasing demands of an ageing population with complex, long-term needs, conditions related to health-related 'lifestyle' behaviours and serious conditions requiring difficult and intensive treatment (Select Committee on Public Service and Demographic Change 2013). In the UK, one-third of babies born in 2013 are expected to live to 100 (Office for National Statistics 2013), but about two-thirds of adults and 3 out of 10 children in England are overweight or obese (Health and Social Care Information Centre 2013). More than a third of people develop cancer in their

lifetime, with the risk increasing with age (Office for National Statistics 2014). Healthcare professionals can expect to spend increasing amounts of consultation time:
- identifying the healthcare priorities of patients with multiple morbidities;
- navigating complex, high-stakes decisions (often with a delicate balance of benefit versus harm);
- treating conditions with uncertain outcome and
- supporting patients in establishing long-term behavioural change.

In the traditional model of the doctor–patient relationship, there is an implicit 'contract' defining the roles of both parties. At its simplest level, the patient's role is to present with clearly specified signs and symptoms (ideally corresponding to an identifiable diagnosis), and the doctor's role is to name and treat the illness (where 'treat' in this context means 'cure'). Deviations from this optimal enactment of roles are difficult for both parties and result in inherently unsatisfactory consultations, for example, when:
- a patient is not subjectively experiencing symptoms, and the patient and doctor disagree about whether the patient is 'ill' and requires treatment;
- a patient reports chronic symptoms for which no identifiable cause is found from biomedical testing;
- a doctor has to break the news that there is no cure and the patient's condition will inevitably worsen.

The responsibility *felt* by the doctor to 'make it better', and *invested in* the doctor by the patient, is an undercurrent in the consultation, placing the onus on the doctor to effect change. This occurs even as the direction of travel is towards a doctor–patient partnership (e.g. General Medical Council 2013), and with patients showing an increasing preference for involvement in decision making over time (Chewning *et al.* 2012). The changing demands on healthcare will require doctors to have, as standard, a sophisticated repertoire of consultation skills, incorporating elements of:
- motivational interviewing;
- risk communication;
- shared decision making;
- managing uncertainty;
- negotiation;
- conflict resolution and
- breaking bad news.

Changes to the healthcare infrastructure and working patterns have resulted in patients experiencing less continuity with a single doctor. Continuity of care itself comprises several dimensions (Haggerty *et al.* 2003; Parker *et al.* 2011), including continuity of information, management and relationships. Studies of patient preferences have found that continuity of relationship is regarded as particularly important in managing long-term, complex and emotional problems, particularly in primary care and mental health settings (Haggerty *et al.* 2003; Ridd *et al.* 2009). Staff mobility, such as turnover of junior doctors, is not necessarily regarded as a disadvantage, providing staff work well as a team; rather, patients appreciate the benefits (such as 'young hotshots' keeping senior staff 'on their toes') (Brown *et al.* 1997). Haggerty *et al.* (2003) emphasised that continuity of care is not the same as the structural *processes* designed to improve continuity. Rather, continuity is the *experience* that care is 'connected and coherent' and can be experienced (or not) by both patients and professionals.

The implications of lack of 'relational continuity' (seeing the same doctor over time) in current practice for the doctor–patient relationship have yet to be fully explored, given the underpinning assumption that there is one doctor who has a central role in the patient's care. However, many patients increasingly experience a '*doctors*–patient relationship' or 'multidisciplinary team members–patient relationship'. The importance of considering the broader network of relationships beyond the central doctor–patient dyad has been highlighted by the 'relationship-centred care' framework (Tresolini & the Pew Fetzer Task Force 1994; Beach & Inui 2006), which emphasises that the moral foundation and emotional impact of doctors' working relationships applies also to doctor–doctor and doctor–community relations. However, research considering this broader context has tended to focus on interprofessional relationships from the perspective of the professionals, rather than the conceptualisation of these multiple relationships, experienced over time, from the perspective of the patient. How *patients* conceptualise the doctor–patient relationship in this changing landscape remains to be seen. For example, whether patients, who may experience healthcare as a series of encounters with a different professional every time, would describe themselves as having experienced a doctor–patient relationship at all (Vanderminden & Potter 2009).

The increasing use of technology for healthcare delivery inevitably plays a part in this. Telemedicine, defined as the use of telecommunications to diagnose and treat disease and ill health (World Health Organization 2014), has been dated back to the 1850s (Bashshur 2009); essentially, as soon as technological developments (such as the telephone and telegraph) became available, they were put to use for communicating about patient care. E-health, defined more broadly as the use of electronic means to deliver health resources and health care (World Health Organization 2014), often assumes a specifically designed, technological infrastructure, such as systems for recording and monitoring patient data. However, the pervasiveness of sophisticated gadgets in the pockets of the general population has given rise to the concept of 'u-health' (ubiquitous health service), which assumes that – at least in theory – healthcare can be delivered to anyone, anywhere, at any time (Jeong *et al.* 2009).

Studies of the impact of telemedicine on doctor–patient communication and the doctor–patient relationship have found both positive and negative effects – with neither dominating – and some evidence that the conventional pattern of the consultation is simply maintained (i.e. doctor-dominated conversation focusing on tasks rather than socio-emotional exchange), but no compelling evidence of an impact on patient-centredness (Miller 2001; 2003; 2011). In contrast to conventional telemedicine services – where, by definition, communication between the doctor and patient is conducted remotely – health services have also been designed to use a combination of approaches, irrespective of geographical distance between the patient and the health service. One aim of these services is to use technology to reduce the number of face-to-face appointments, for example, by gathering information about a new problem by taking an online history or teleconferencing over the patient's mobile phone (Bachman 2003; Adamson and Bachman 2010; Stephens 2014). However, the aim is not to *eliminate* face-to-face interaction but to reduce the amount of time spent on face-to-face appointments where tasks can be accomplished equally well by other means. The result, in theory, is an improvement in the *quality* of time that the patient and doctor do spend in face-to-face consultations. For example, gathering detailed information in advance of the consultation theoretically frees up more time during the consultation to review the implications of the information and perform other tasks, such as physical examination and planning a course of action (Bachman 2003). Studies of what patients want from the doctor–patient relationship have highlighted that the quality and depth of the relationship and specific consultation skills are more important to patients than the quantity of consultations (Ridd *et al.* 2009).

The use of technology *within* the consultation has had a mixed reception. Optimism about the potential uses to which computers can be put (Ball & Lillis 2001) has been tempered by the reality of having 'a third person in the room' presenting 'a dilemma of attention'. This results in a triadic, rather than dyadic, consultation, where there is a third agency with its own agenda (Swinglehurst *et al.* 2010; Pearce *et al.* 2011). This creates, in effect, a 'triadic relationship' (doctor–computer–patient relationship). It could be argued, however, that this simply mirrors the increasingly social role played by technological gadgets in everyday interpersonal interactions (Srivastava 2005), and that it is unrealistic to expect the doctor–patient consultation to be unaffected by this cultural change.

A more recent development is patient-initiated recording of consultations, which has had an equally mixed reception among clinicians, with strong views on both sides (Gainor 2012; Eden 2013; Zack 2014). In fact, interventions to provide patients with a recording of their consultation have been studied for nearly four decades (Butt 1977). When patients are given a record of their consultation (either as an audiorecording or written summary), they consistently value and use it, and there is a positive impact, for example, on information recall (Pitkethly *et al.* 2008). Patients also value having *access* to a record of their consultation, whether or not they use it (Delbanco *et al.* 2012). The debate about patients having access to their own healthcare records in many respects mirrors the state of flux of the doctor–patient relationship, caught between the culturally embedded paternalistic model and the move to a more equal partnership.

The concept of working in partnership (General Medical Council 2013) assumes that both the patient and the doctor have active roles. Both are experts in their own way (Tuckett *et al.* 1985), and both have the ability to effect change. The importance of fostering patient self-efficacy is integral to the patient-centred approach. Evidence supports the notion that patients who are 'activated' and 'engaged' are more able and willing to manage their health and healthcare and have better outcomes (Hibbard & Greene 2013). There are dissenting voices, however; initiatives to promote an active patient role (such as the concept of the 'expert patient' and patient 'self-management' interventions) have been challenged as originating from, and potentially reinforcing, the dominant biomedical paradigm rather than service users' own perspectives on health and illness (Wilson 2001; Wilson *et al.* 2007). Nonetheless, such initiatives contribute to the overall direction of travel (Wilson *et al.* 2007; Richards *et al.* 2013).

Conclusion

The doctor–patient relationship has never been static, reflecting changing societal expectations as much as the needs of the individuals in the doctor–patient dyad. Current drivers for change include changing demands on healthcare services, the organisation of healthcare delivery, use of technology and a focus on the rights of the individual. However, at any given time, there are multiple formulations of the doctor–patient relationship at play, even as the direction of travel is towards a doctor–patient partnership.

References

Adamson, S.C. & Bachman, J.W. (2010) Pilot study of providing online care in a primary care setting. *Mayo Clinic Proceedings*, 85 (no. 8), 704–710.

Agledahl, K.M., Gulbrandsen, P., Førde, R.R. & Wifstad, A. (2011) Courteous but not curious: How doctors' politeness masks their existential neglect: A qualitative study of video-recorded patient consultations. *Journal of Medical Ethics*, 37 (no. 11), 650–654.

Bachman, J.W. (2003) The patient–computer interview: A neglected tool that can aid the clinician. *Mayo Clinic Proceedings*, 78 (no. 1), 67–78.

Ball, M.J. & Lillis, J. (2001) E-health: Transforming the physician/patient relationship. *International Journal of Medical Informatics*, 61 (no. 1), 1–10.

Bashshur, R. (2009) The genesis of telemedicine: 1870 to 1955. In: R. Bashshur & G. Shannon, *History of Telemedicine: Evolution, Context and Transformation*, pp. 131–153. Mary-Ann Liebert, New York.

Beach, M.C. & Inui, T. (2006) Relationship-centered care. *Journal of General Internal Medicine*, 21 (Suppl. 1), S3–S8.

Berwick, D.M. (2003) Disseminating innovations in health care. *JAMA*, 289 (no. 15), 1969–1975.

Brown, J.B., Dickie, I., Brown, L., & Biehn, J. (1997) Long-term attendance at a family practice teaching unit: Qualitative study of patients' views. *Canadian Family Physician*, 43, 901–906.

Butt, H.R. (1977) A method for better physician–patient communication. *Annals of Internal Medicine*, 86 (no. 4), 478–480.

Chewning, B., Bylund, C.L., Shah, B., Arora, N.K., Gueguen, J.A. & Makoul, G. (2012) Patient preferences for shared decisions: A systematic review. *Patient Education and Counseling*, 86 (no. 1), 9–18.

Coulter, A. & Collins, A. (2011) *Making Shared Decision-Making a Reality: No Decision about Me, without Me*. The King's Fund, London.

Delbanco, T., Walker, J., Bell, S.K., *et al.* (2012) Inviting patients to read their doctors' notes: A quasi-experimental study and a look ahead. *Annals of Internal Medicine*, 157 (no. 7), 461–470.

Department of Health. (2010) *Equity and Excellence: Liberating the NHS (White Paper)*. The Stationery Office, London.

Eden, C. (2013) *Good health viewpoint: Why I believe patients should film consultants on their phones* [WWW document]. URL http://www.dailymail.co.uk/health/article-2358576/Good-Health-Viewpoint-Why-I-believe-patients-film-consultants-phones.html [accessed on 10 November 2014].

Elwyn, G., Lloyd, A., Joseph-Williams, N. Cording, E., Thomson, R., Durand, M.A. & Edwards A. (2013) Option grids: Shared decision making made easier. *Patient Education and Counseling*, 90 (no. 2), 207–212.

Engel, G.L. (1977) The need for a new medical model: A challenge for biomedicine. *Science*, 196 (no. 4286), 129–136.

Gainor, J.F. (2012) Is there an app for that? *Oncologist*, 17 (no. 12), e58–e59.

General Medical Council. (2013) *Good Medical Practice*. General Medical Council, London.

Gray, M. (2014) *Evidence-based medicine: An oral history*. Chapter 3: The future [WWW document]. URL ebm.jamanetwork.com/index.html [accessed on 10 November 2014].

Haggerty, J.L., Reid, R.J., Freeman, G.K. Starfield, B.H., Adair, C.E. & McKendry, R. (2003) Continuity of care: A multidisciplinary review. *BMJ*, 327 (no. 7425), 1219–1221.

Hall, J.A., Roter, D.L. & Katz, N.R. (1988) Meta-analysis of correlates of provider behaviour in medical encounters. *Medical Care*, 26 (no. 7), 657–675.

Health and Social Care Information Centre. (2013) *Statistics on obesity, physical activity and diet: England 2013* [WWW document]. URL http://www.hscic.gov.uk/catalogue/PUB10364/obes-phys-acti-diet-eng-2013-rep.pdf [accessed on 10 November 2014].

Hibbard, J.H. & Greene, J. (2013) What the evidence shows about patient activation: Better health outcomes and care experiences; fewer data on costs. *Health Affairs*, 32 (no. 2), 207–214.

Howick, J., Bishop, F.L., Heneghan, C., Wolstenholme, J. Stevens, S., Hobbs, F.D. & Lewith, G. (2013) Placebo use in the United Kingdom: Results from a national survey of primary care practitioners. *PloS One*, 8 (no. 3), e58247.

Jeong, K., Jung, E.Y. & Park, D.K. (2009) Trend of wireless u-health. In: *9th International Symposium on Communications and Information Technology*, ISCIT 2009, pp. 829–833.

Keller, V.F. & Carroll, J.G. (1994) A new model for physician–patient communication. *Patient Education and Counseling*, 23 (no. 2), 131–140.

Kurtz, S., Silverman, J., Benson, J. & Draper, J. (2003) Marrying content and process in clinical method teaching: Enhancing the Calgary-Cambridge guides. *Academic Medicine*, 78 (no. 8), 802–809.

Leape, L.L., Shore, M.F., Dienstag, J.L., *et al.* (2012) Perspective: A culture of respect, part 1: The nature and causes of disrespectful behavior by physicians. *Academic Medicine*, 87 (no. 7), 845–852.

Levenstein, J.H., McCracken, E.C., McWhinney, I.R. Stewart, M.A. & Brown, J.B. (1986) The patient-centred clinical method. 1. A model for the doctor–patient interaction in family medicine. *Family Practice*, 3 (no. 1), 24–30.

Makoul, G. (2001) Essential elements of communication in medical encounters: The Kalamazoo consensus statement. *Academic Medicine*, 76 (no. 4), 390–393.

Malhotra, A., Gregory, I., Darvill, A. Goble, E., Pryce-Roberts, A., Lundberg, K., Konradsen, S. & Hafstad, H. (2009) Mind the gap: Learners' perspectives on what they learn in communication compared to how they and others behave in the real world. *Patient Education and Counseling*, 76 (no. 3), 385–390.

Mead, N. & Bower, P. (2000) Patient-centredness: A conceptual framework and review of the empirical literature. *Social Science & Medicine*, 51 (no. 7), 1087–1110.

Miller, E.A. (2001) Telemedicine and doctor–patient communication: An analytical survey of the literature. *Journal of Telemedicine and Telecare*, 7 (no. 1), 1–17.

Miller, E.A. (2003) The technical and interpersonal aspects of telemedicine: Effects on doctor–patient communication. *Journal of Telemedicine and Telecare*, 9 (no. 1), 1–7.

Miller, E.A. (2011) The continuing need to investigate the nature and content of teleconsultation communication using interaction analysis techniques. *Journal of Telemedicine and Telecare*, 17 (no. 2), 55–64.

NICE (National Institute for Health and Care Excellence). (2012) *Quality standard for patient experience in adult NHS services*. NICE quality standards QS15 [WWW document]. URL http://www.nice.org.uk/Guidance/QS15 [accessed on 10 November 2014].

Office for National Statistics. (2013) *One third of babies born in 2013 are expected to live to 100: Part of historic and projected data from the period and cohort life tables, 2012-based release* [WWW document]. URL http://www.ons.gov.uk/ons/rel/lifetables/historic-and-projected-data-from-the-period-and-cohort-life-tables/2012-based/sty-babies-living-to-100.html [accessed on 10 November 2014].

Office for National Statistics. (2014) *National cancer statistics for England, 2013* [video]. URL http://www.ons.gov.uk/ons/rel/vsob1/cancer-statistics-registrations--england--series-mb1-/no--42--2011/vid-cancer-statistics.html [accessed on 10 November 2014].

Parker, G., Corden, A. & Heaton, J. (2011) Experiences of and influences on continuity of care for service users and carers: Synthesis of evidence from a research programme. *Health and Social Care in the Community*, 19 (no. 6), 576–601.

Pearce, C., Arnold, M., Phillips, C., Trumble, S. & Dwan, K. (2011) The patient and the computer in the primary care consultation. *Journal of the American Medical Informatics Association*, 18 (no. 2), 138–142.

Pitkethly, M., MacGillivray, S. & Ryan, R. (2008) Recordings or summaries of consultations for people with cancer. Cochrane Database Systematic Reviews, 3 (Art. No. CD001539).

Richards, T., Montori, V.M., Godlee, F. & Paul, D. (2013) Let the patient revolution begin. *BMJ*, 346, f2614.

Ridd, M., Shaw, A., Lewis, G. & Salisbury, C. (2009) The patient–doctor relationship: A synthesis of the qualitative literature on patients' perspectives. *British Journal of General Practice*, 59 (no. 561), e116–e133.

Rogers, E. (1962) *Diffusion of Innovations*. Free Press, New York.

Select Committee on Public Service and Demographic Change. (2013) *First report: Ready for ageing?* [WWW document]. URL http://www.publications.parliament.uk/pa/ld201213/ldselect/ldpublic/140/14002.htm [accessed on 10 November 2014].

Silverman, J., Archer, J., Gillard, S., Howells, R. & Benson, J. (2011) Initial evaluation of EPSCALE, a rating scale that assesses the process of explanation and planning in the medical interview. *Patient Education and Counseling*, 82 (no. 1), 89–93.

Silverman, J., Kurtz, S. & Draper, J. (2013) *Skills for Communicating with Patients*, third edn. Radcliffe, Oxford.

Srivastava, L. (2005) Mobile phones and the evolution of social behaviour. *Behaviour and Information Technology*, 24 (no. 2), 111–129.

Stephens, P. (2014) *AI, robots, pocket doctors: Patient-centred health tech* [WWW document]. URL http://www.bbc.co.uk/news/business-29259571 [accessed on 10 November 2014].

Stewart, M.A. (1995) Effective physician-patient communication and health outcomes: A review. *Canadian Medical Association Journal*, 152 (no. 9), 1423–1433.

Swinglehurst, D., Roberts, C. & Greenhalgh, T. (2010) Opening up the 'black box' of the electronic patient record: A linguistic ethnographic study in general practice. *Communication and Medicine*, 8 (no. 1), 3–15.

Tresolini, C.P. & the Pew-Fetzer Task Force (1994) *Health Professions Education and Relationship-Centered Care*. Pew Health Professions Commission, San Francisco, CA.

Tuckett, D., Boulton, M., Olson, C. & Williams, A. (1985) *Meetings between Experts: An Approach to Sharing Ideas in Medical Consultations*. Tavistock, London.

Vanderminden, J. & Potter, S.J. (2009) Challenges to the doctor patient relationship in the twenty-first century. In: W.C. Cockerham (ed), *The New Blackwell Companion to Medical Sociology*, pp. 355–372. Wiley-Blackwell, Oxford.

von Fragstein, M., Silverman, J., Cushing, A., et al. (2008) UK consensus statement on the content of communication curricula in undergraduate medical education. *Medical Education*, 42 (no. 11), 1100–1107.

Wilson, P.M. (2001) A policy analysis of the Expert Patient in the United Kingdom: Self-care as an expression of pastoral power? *Health and Social Care in the Community*, 9 (no. 3), 134–142.

Wilson, P.M., Kendall, S. & Brooks, F. (2007) The Expert Patients Programme: A paradox of patient empowerment and medical dominance. *Health and Social Care in the Community*, 15 (no. 5), 426–438.

World Health Organization. (2014) *E-health* [WWW document]. URL http://www.who.int/trade/glossary/story021/en/ [accessed on 10 November 2014].

Wynia, M.K. (2012) Making it easier to do the right thing: A modern communication QI agenda. *Patient Education and Counseling*, 88 (no. 3), 364–366.

Zack, P. (2014) *Medio-legal: Patients who record their consultations* [WWW document]. URL http://www.gponline.com/medico-legal-patients-record-consultations/article/122722 [accessed on 10 November 2014].

PART 2
Components of Communication

Section Lead Editor: Alexia Papageorgiou

PART 2A

Core Tasks in Clinical Communication

CHAPTER 9

Overview of Core Tasks in Clinical Communication

Jonathan Silverman

University of Cambridge School of Clinical Medicine, Cambridge; European Association for Communication in Healthcare, Salisbury, UK

The importance of structure

Practitioners, learners, teachers and assessors of healthcare communication all require a way of conceptualising the complex process of clinical communication, of organising what is inherently a highly dynamic process into manageable elements. Without structure, it is all too easy for consultations to be unsystematic or unproductive and for experiential communication teaching to appear random and opportunistic. Paradoxically, structure sets us free – it provides us with an awareness of the distinct phases of the interview as we consult and the flexibility to move away from a fixed path when appropriate, with the security of understanding how to return to our structure in due course. It enables teachers to be learner-centred during experiential teaching yet able to piece together the learning lessons into a conceptual framework for learners to take away.

Core tasks, core skills and specific issues

In order to provide this degree of organisation, the healthcare interview can be conceptualised as a set of core tasks, broadly applicable to all healthcare interactions. These tasks can then be further subdivided into a number of discrete, observable, specific behavioural skills relevant to the execution of each task. These core tasks and skills provide the foundations for effective practitioner–patient communication in a variety of different clinical contexts, providing a secure platform for approaching many specific communication issues (Kurtz *et al.* 2003; Kurtz *et al.* 2005).

Core tasks and skills are of fundamental importance: once they have been mastered, specific communication challenges such as anger, addiction, breaking bad news or diversity issues are much more readily tackled. This platform of core tasks and skills serves as the primary resource for dealing with all challenges. Rather than inventing a new set of skills for each issue, we need to consider how to use particular subsets of skills with greater intention, intensity and awareness. This interrelationship between tasks, skills and issues is well represented in the curriculum wheel developed by the UK Council of Clinical Communication in Undergraduate Medical Education

Clinical Communication in Medicine, First Edition. Edited by Jo Brown, Lorraine M. Noble, Alexia Papageorgiou and Jane Kidd.
© 2016 John Wiley & Sons, Ltd. Published 2016 by John Wiley & Sons, Ltd.

(von Fragstein *et al.* 2008). As mentioned in previous chapters of this book, a number of widely used consultation models and frameworks have been developed by teachers and researchers that list these skills and tasks in a variety of ways (van Thiel & van Dalen 1995; Frankel & Stein 1999; Cole & Bird 2000; Makoul 2001; Participants in the Bayer-Fetzer Conference on Physician–Patient Communication in Medical Education 2001; Kalet *et al.* 2004; de Haes and Bensing, 2009; Silverman *et al.* 2013).

Going beyond specific skills into individuality is the real challenge of experiential learning (Kurtz *et al.* 2005; Skelton 2005). Indeed a potential conflict between skills teaching and creativity has been highlighted by Salmon and Young (2011). However, although we must recognise that there are considerable variables that influence what is best for any individual in any given situation, we can also advocate certain behaviourally specific skills that are proven to be more effective than others (Silverman *et al.* 2011). The specific skills of effective communication provide a toolkit of evidence-based approaches to enable clinicians to put intentions into practice.

Content, process and clinical reasoning

So far we have concentrated on communication process tasks and skills. However, communication process is inextricably linked with the content of the clinical interview and the clinician's thought processes. Healthcare communication is purposeful and not an end in itself. For instance, the communication task of gathering information, achieved via a set of specific process skills, enables the practitioner to obtain the content of the medical history. These two elements of content and process are inextricably linked. Rather than seeing communication as a separate endeavour, it is important for learners to appreciate what they are trying to achieve and how the various tasks within the consultation contribute to achieving that overall goal. This dictates an integrated approach to communication process and content in the healthcare curriculum. We shall explore this fundamental issue in health care communication and its teaching in more depth in chapter 11 when we explore the relationship between effective clinical communication and clinical reasoning

Over the next three chapters, we shall look at three specific core tasks of clinical communication: relationship building, information gathering, information sharing and shared decision making.

References

Cole, S. & Bird, J. (2000) *The Medical Interview: The Three Function Approach*. Mosby, St. Louis, MO.
de Haes, H. & Bensing, J. (2009) Endpoints in medical communication research, proposing a framework of functions and outcomes. *Patient Education and Counseling*, 74, 287–294.
Frankel, R. & Stein, T. (1999) Getting the most out of the clinical encounter: The Four Habits Model. *Permanente Journal*, 3, 79–88.
Kalet, A., Pugnaire, M. P., Cole-Kelly, K., Janicik, R., Ferrara, E., Schwartz, M.D., Lipkin, M., Jr. & Lazare, A. (2004) Teaching communication in clinical clerkships: Models from the Macy Initiative in Health Communication. *Academic Medicine*, 76, 511–520.
Kurtz, S., Silverman, J., Benson, J. & Draper, J. (2003) Marrying content and process in clinical method teaching: Enhancing the Calgary-Cambridge guides. *Academic Medicine*, 78, 802–809.
Kurtz, S.M., Silverman, J. & Draper, J. (2005) *Teaching and Learning Communication Skills in Medicine*. Radcliffe Medical, Oxford.

Makoul, G. (2001) The SEGUE Framework for teaching and assessing communication skills. *Patient Education and Counseling*, 45, 23–34.

Participants in the Bayer-Fetzer Conference on Physician–Patient Communication in Medical Education. (2001) Essential elements of communication in medical encounters: The Kalamazoo consensus statement. *Academic Medicine*, 76, 390–393.

Salmon, P. & Young, B. (2011) Creativity in clinical communication: From communication skills to skilled communication. *Medical Education*, 45, 217–226.

Silverman, J., Deveugele, M., de Haes, H. & Rosenbaum, M. (2011) Unskilled creativity is counterproductive. *Medical Education*, 45, 959–960; author reply 961–962.

Silverman, J., Kurtz, S.M. & Draper, J. (2013) *Skills for Communicating with Patients*. Radcliffe Publishing, Oxford.

Skelton, J.R. (2005) Everything you were afraid to ask about communication skills. *British Journal of General Practice*, 55, 40–46.

van Thiel, J. & van Dalen, J. (1995) MAAS-Globaal criterialijst, versie voor de vaardigheidstoets Medisch Basiscurriculum. Universiteit Maastricht, the Netherlands.

von Fragstein, M., Silverman, J., Cushing, A., Quilligan, S., Salisbury, H. & Wiskin, C. (2008) UK consensus statement on the content of communication curricula in undergraduate medical education. *Medical Education*, 42, 1100–1107.

CHAPTER 10

Relationship Building

Jonathan Silverman

University of Cambridge School of Clinical Medicine, Cambridge; European Association for Communication in Healthcare, Salisbury, UK

Not surprisingly the task of relationship building takes centre stage in many models of clinical communication. Relationship makes a difference to communication in healthcare, to the people involved and to healthcare outcomes. Forging a relationship with the patient is central to the success of every consultation, whatever the context.

Building the relationship is a task easily taken for granted by healthcare practitioners. The sequential components of the interview such as information gathering often dominate as the clinician moves through the consultation making sense of the patient's illness and disease. Yet without paying specific attention to the skills of relationship building, these more 'concrete' tasks become much more difficult to achieve.

Paradoxically, communication teaching is often thought to be only about relationship-building skills. Communication teaching is often criticised by clinicians for overemphasising empathy and concern at the expense of medical problem solving. Communication skills teachers need to emphasise that relationship building is one of several tasks we promote, albeit an essential enabler of all other tasks.

Historical context

As documented earlier in this book, there has been a gradual historical progression from biomedical consultations, through a biopsychosocial paradigm, to patient-centred medicine. Although an imbalance of power is inherent in medical interviewing, there has been a subtle change towards a more equal relationship. This shift away from paternalism requires an increased emphasis on learning relationship-building skills.

From the very earliest research into medical communication, relationship problems have featured highly as predictors of poor outcome. In Korsch *et al.*'s seminal study of 800 visits to paediatric outpatients (Korsch *et al.* 1968), physician lack of warmth and friendliness was one of the most important variables related to poor levels of patient satisfaction and compliance.

Poole and Sanson-Fisher demonstrated significant problems in medical education in the development of relationship-building skills (Poole & Sanson-Fisher 1979). They demonstrated poor skills in empathy in both first- and final-year medical students. They also showed that psychiatric residents who might be thought to develop these skills in their training also demonstrated low empathy skills.

Clinical Communication in Medicine, First Edition. Edited by Jo Brown, Lorraine M. Noble, Alexia Papageorgiou and Jane Kidd.
© 2016 John Wiley & Sons, Ltd. Published 2016 by John Wiley & Sons, Ltd.

More recently, Morse *et al.* found that doctors missed 90% of opportunities to express empathy in a study in cancer care (Morse *et al.* 2008), and Hsu *et al.* found that providers missed most opportunities to respond empathically to their HIV patient's emotions (Hsu *et al.* 2012).

Institutional factors have a major part to play in this historical context. Suchman and Williamson discussed how medical schools affect the development of students' relationship skills (Suchman & Williamson, pers. comm. 2003). They stated that if students 'see powerful figures in medicine routinely entering into non-healing or even negative relationships with one another and their patients; if they see their mentors emphasizing the importance of expert technical knowledge above all else, especially above knowledge of self and other; and if they experience hazing or humiliation as standard techniques of medical pedagogy', this will have a powerful impact on their lifelong practice.

Current practice – the skills of relationship building

So what can teachers of communication skills recommend to learners to enable them to achieve more effective relationship building in the clinical interview? All modern consultation models and frameworks advocate specific relationship-building skills. Typical examples would be:
- the use of appropriate nonverbal behaviour (Hall *et al.* 1981; Ambady *et al.* 2002a; Ambady *et al.* 2002b; Hannawa 2012; Swayden *et al.* 2012; Duke *et al.* 2013);
- rapport-building skills (including respectfulness, acceptance, empathy, acknowledgement, sensitivity and supportiveness) (Williamson 2011) and
- patient involvement skills such as sharing thinking and explaining rationale (Heritage & Stivers 1999; Robins *et al.* 2011).

The evidence base for the use of these skills is critical to teaching practice. We must know both whether these skills are important in clinical practice and whether they are learnable. Space in this chapter does not allow a detailed exploration of the evidence for all these skills, but instead we explore one particular skill, empathy, as an example of the importance of critically analysing communication curricula.

One of the key skills in building the doctor–patient relationship is the use of empathy (Spiro 1992; Garden 2009). Neumann *et al.* suggest that clinical empathy is a fundamental determinant of quality in medical care, enabling the clinician to fulfill key medical tasks more accurately and thereby leading to enhanced health outcomes (Neumann *et al.* 2009).

Of all consultation skills, empathy is the one most often thought to be a matter of personality and therefore inherently not teachable. Certainly, a first step in empathy is the internal motivation to understand the patient's perspective, and this must be present, as well as appropriate communication skills (Norfolk *et al.* 2007). However, although some may naturally be better at demonstrating empathy than others, the skills of empathy can be learned. Over the course of a medical undergraduate curriculum, empathy significantly declines if not taught (Newton *et al.* 2008; Hojat *et al.* 2009).

Poole and Sanson-Fisher demonstrated that empathy is a construct that can be learned (Poole & Sanson-Fisher 1979). Medical students' ability to empathise did not improve over their curriculum without specific training. Bonvicini *et al.* demonstrated that communication training with practising physicians made a significant difference in empathic expression with patients 6 months after training (Bonvicini *et al.* 2009).

The challenge in teaching is to identify the building blocks of the empathic response and enable learners to integrate the elements of empathy into their natural style (Bellet & Maloney 1991; Platt & Keller 1994; Gazda *et al.* 1995; Coulehan *et al.* 2001; Buckman 2002; Frankel 2009). Empathy is a two-stage process:

1 the understanding and sensitive appreciation of another person's predicament or feelings and
2 the communication of that understanding back to the patient in a supportive way.

Many core skills of communication such as attentive listening, facilitation and picking up cues demonstrate to patients a genuine interest in hearing about their thoughts. Together they provide an atmosphere that facilitates disclosure and enables the first step of empathy – understanding the patient's predicament – to take place. Further nonverbal and verbal skills are required to complete the second step of empathy, communicating understanding back to the patient. Effective nonverbal communication can clearly signal to the patient that we are sensitive to his or her predicament. Empathic statements such as 'I can see that your husband's memory loss has been very difficult for you to cope with' more directly name and appreciate the patient's affect or predicament (Platt & Keller 1994).

Future directions

There has been debate about whether skills-based training and assessment of empathy trivialises the very qualities we are trying to instil by reducing them to surface behaviours. Others believe that surface manifestations of behavioural empathy should be assessed and taught because these are essential skills for the compassionate and effective care of patients. A learner who is unable to display these basic communication skills is likely to be deficient in the other, deeper components of empathy as well. Clearly skills-based training should be complemented by other approaches that enhance students' capacities for compassion and authentic presence and enable students to more readily identify with patients' feelings (Teherani *et al.* 2008; Wear & Varley 2008; Blatt *et al.* 2010; Sibley *et al.* 2011). Simultaneously, institutional barriers that create time pressure and unsupportive working environments and inhibit relationship building need to be addressed.

References

Ambady, N., Koo, J., Rosenthal, R. & Winograd, C.H. (2002a) Physical therapists' nonverbal communication predicts geriatric patients' health outcomes. *Psychology and Aging*, 17, 443–452.

Ambady, N., Laplante, D., Nguyen, T., Rosenthal, R., Chaumeton, N. & Levinson, W. (2002b) Surgeons' tone of voice: A clue to malpractice history. *Surgery*, 132, 5–9.

Bellet, P.S. & Maloney, M.J. (1991) The importance of empathy as an interviewing skill in medicine. *JAMA*, 266, 1831–1832.

Blatt, B., Lelacheur, S.F., Galinsky, A.D., Simmens, S.J. & Greenberg, L. (2010) Does perspective-taking increase patient satisfaction in medical encounters? *Academic Medicine*, 85, 1445–1452.

Bonvicini, K.A., Perlin, M.J., Bylund, C.L., Carroll, G., Rouse, R.A. & Goldstein, M.G. (2009) Impact of communication training on physician expression of empathy in patient encounters. *Patient Education and Counseling*, 75, 3–10.

Buckman, R. (2002) Communications and emotions. *BMJ*, 325, 672.

Coulehan, J.L., Platt, F.W., Egener, B., Frankel, R., Lin, C.T., Lown, B. & Salazar, W.H. (2001) 'Let me see if I have this right…': words that help build empathy. *Annals of Internal Medicine*, 135, 221–227.

Duke, P., Frankel, R.M. & Reis, S. (2013) How to integrate the electronic health record and patient-centered communication into the medical visit: A skills-based approach. *Teaching and Learning in Medicine*, 25, 358–365.

Frankel, R.M. (2009) Empathy research: A complex challenge. *Patient Education and Counseling*, 75, 1–2.

Garden, R. (2009) Expanding clinical empathy: An activist perspective. *Journal of General Internal Medicine*, 24, 122–125.

Gazda, G.M., Asbury, F.R., Balzer, F.J., Childers, W.C., Phelps, R.E. & Walters, R.P. (1995) *Human Relations Development, A Manual for Educators*, Allyn and Bacon, Boston, MA.

Hall, J.A., Roter, D.L. & Rand, C.S. (1981) Communication of affect between patient and physician. *Journal of Health and Social Behaviour*, 22, 18–30.

Hannawa, A.F. (2012) 'Explicitly implicit': Examining the importance of physician nonverbal involvement during error disclosures. *Swiss Medical Weekly*, 142, w13576.

Heritage, J. & Stivers, T. (1999) Online commentary in acute medical visits: A method of shaping patient expectations. *Social Science & Medicine*, 49, 1501–1517.

Hojat, M., Vergare, M.J., Maxwell, K., Brainard, G., Herrine, S.K., Isenberg, G.A., Veloski, J. & Gonnella, J.S. (2009) The devil is in the third year: A longitudinal study of erosion of empathy in medical school. *Academic Medicine*, 84, 1182–1191.

Hsu, I., Saha, S., Korthuis, P.T., Sharp, V., Cohn, J., Moore, R.D. & Beach, M.C. (2012) Providing support to patients in emotional encounters: A new perspective on missed empathic opportunities. *Patient Education and Counseling*, 88, 436–442.

Korsch, B.M., Gozzi, E.K. & Francis, V. (1968) Gaps in doctor–patient communication. *Pediatrics*, 42, 855–871.

Morse, D.S., Edwardsen, E.A. & Gordon, H.S. (2008) Missed opportunities for interval empathy in lung cancer communication. *Archives of Internal Medicine*, 168, 1853–1858.

Neumann, M., Bensing, J., Mercer, S., Ernstmann, N., Ommen, O. & Pfaff, H. (2009) Analyzing the 'nature' and 'specific effectiveness' of clinical empathy: A theoretical overview and contribution towards a theory-based research agenda. *Patient Education and Counseling*, 74, 339–346.

Newton, B.W., Barber, L., Clardy, J., Cleveland, E. & O'Sullivan, P. (2008) Is there hardening of the heart during medical school? *Academic Medicine*, 83, 244–249.

Norfolk, T., Birdi, K. & Walsh, D. (2007) The role of empathy in establishing rapport in the consultation: A new model. *Medical Education*, 41, 690–697.

Platt, F.W. & Keller, V.F. (1994) Empathic communication: A teachable and learnable skill. *Journal of General Internal Medicine*, 9, 222–226.

Poole, A.D. & Sanson-Fisher, R.W. (1979) Understanding the patient: A neglected aspect of medical eduction. *Social Science & Medicine*, 13A, 37–43.

Robins, L., Witteborn, S., Miner, L., Mauksch, L., Edwards, K. & Brock, D. (2011) Identifying transparency in physician communication. *Patient Education and Counseling*, 83, 73–79.

Sibley, A., Latter, S., Richard, C., Lussier, M.T., Roberge, D., Skinner, T.C., Cradock, S. & Zinken, K.M. (2011) Medication discussion between nurse prescribers and people with diabetes: An analysis of content and participation using MEDICODE. *Journal of Advanced Nursing*, 67, 2323–2336.

Spiro, H. (1992) What is empathy and can it be taught? *Annals of Internal Medicine*, 16, 843–846.

Swayden, K.J., Anderson, K K., Connelly, L.M., Moran, J.S., McMahon, J.K. & Arnold, P.M. (2012) Effect of sitting vs. standing on perception of provider time at bedside: A pilot study. *Patient Education and Counseling*, 86, 166–171.

Teherani, A., Hauer, K.E. & O'Sullivan, P. (2008) Can simulations measure empathy? Considerations on how to assess behavioral empathy via simulations. *Patient Education and Counseling*, 71, 148–152.

Wear, D. & Varley, J.D. (2008) Rituals of verification: The role of simulation in developing and evaluating empathic communication. *Patient Education and Counseling*, 71, 153–156.

Williamson, P.R. (2011) Appendix 1: A 4-step model of relationship-centered communication. *In:* A. Suchman, D.M. Sluyter & P.R. Williamson (eds), *Leading Change in Healthcare: Transforming Organizations Using Complexity Positive Psychology and Relationship-Centered Care*. Radcliffe Publishing, Oxford.

CHAPTER 11

Information Gathering and Clinical Reasoning

Jonathan Silverman

University of Cambridge School of Clinical Medicine, Cambridge; European Association for Communication in Healthcare, Salisbury, UK

Information gathering has always been a key task in the communication curriculum. Learners need to discover accurate, efficient and supportive ways of exploring the biomedical and patient's perspective of his or her illness. Yet the way that many health professionals have been previously taught to "take a history" can lead to inaccuracy and inefficiency. Traditional questioning methods do not encourage comprehensive history taking or effective hypothesis generation. Fortunately, developments in communication theory and research have greatly improved our understanding of the communication process skills to enable effective information gathering.

The evidence base for ineffective information gathering spreads over many years. Platt and McMath observed hospital physicians and showed that both a "high control style" and premature focus on medical problems lead to an over-narrow approach to hypothesis generation and to limitation of the patients' ability to communicate their concerns (Platt & McMath 1979). More recently, Agledahl *et al.* observed a consistent pattern in hospital clinicians who were primarily concerned with their patients' biomedical health: doctors actively directed the focus away from their patients' concerns (Agledahl *et al.* 2011). Mjaaland *et al.* demonstrated the lack of exploration by hospital physicians of negative emotions expressed as cues and concerns (Mjaaland *et al.* 2011).

Historical context

As communication curricula have become more prominent over the last 30 years, a tension has become apparent between the teaching of history taking and clinical communication. Towards the end of the 19th century, a structured method of recording the encounter was established, forging an ordered approach to history taking. This method still dominates medicine today. While this standardised approach has many advantages, it has also led to considerable problems:

1 It has unwittingly led many health professionals towards a closed approach to question asking, as they mistake the template for recording clinical information (content) with the methodology for obtaining that information (process). Similarly, because learners are still rarely observed taking histories in clinical practice, they are rewarded predominantly for the content of their presentations, and they

Clinical Communication in Medicine, First Edition. Edited by Jo Brown, Lorraine M. Noble, Alexia Papageorgiou and Jane Kidd.

mistakenly conclude that the presentation content schema also represents the process of obtaining the history.

2 The traditional standard history only covers the biomedical perspective, the symptoms and signs that are expected to lead the clinician to a differential diagnosis. It omits the illness framework as conceptualised by McWhinney's team in Western Ontario in the 1980s (McWhinney 1989; Stewart *et al.* 2003). This illness framework relates to the individual patient's unique experience of sickness, his or her ideas, concerns, expectations and feelings. Discovering the patient's perspective is not only an entry into more supportive medical care but also a vital component in enabling the elucidation of the biomedical story. Studies of patient satisfaction, adherence, recall and physiological outcome all validate the need for a broader view of history taking that encompasses the patient's life-world as well as the doctor's more focused biological perspective (Silverman *et al.* 2013).

Unfortunately, it is commonplace for two different groups of educators from separate clinical backgrounds and in different courses to teach history taking (mainly hospital specialists) and clinical communication (mainly general practitioners, psychiatrists, palliative care physicians and psychologists). Learners potentially get the impression that those teaching history taking are only interested in the following:

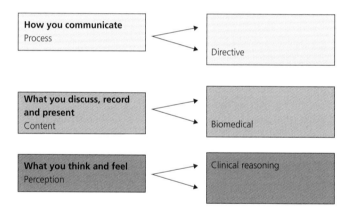

whilst those teaching communication skills are only interested in:

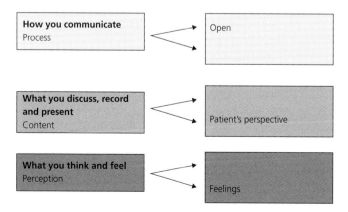

This can lead learners to choose one model over another or alternatively perceive that the history-taking model is more suited to hospital medicine and the communication model to general practice. In fact, there should be only one combined model; effective process, content and perceptual skills need to be taught together by the same teachers in an integrated fashion, producing an effective comprehensive clinical method:

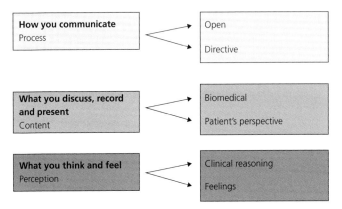

Current teaching practice – the skills of Information gathering

So what can teachers of communication skills recommend to learners to enable them to achieve more effective information gathering in the clinical interview? The information-gathering communication skills advocated in modern consultation models include:
- the narrative thread (Mishler 1984);
- open and closed questioning techniques (Takemura *et al.* 2007);
- attentive listening (Marvel *et al.* 1999; Ruiz Moral *et al.* 2006);
- facilitation skills (Levinson *et al.* 1997);
- picking up cues;
- summary (Takemura *et al.* 2007; Quilligan & Silverman 2012) and
- specific skills related to exploring the patient's ideas, concerns, expectations and feelings.

The evidence base for the use of these skills is critical to teaching practice. Space in this chapter does not allow a detailed exploration of the evidence for all these skills, but instead we explore one particular skill, picking up and exploring cues, as an example of the importance of understanding the literature for teaching.

Communication teaching is only perceived as beneficial if it enables practitioners to work efficiently within their time constraints. One particularly important skill in this regard is picking up cues. Patients are keen to tell us about their own thoughts and feelings but often do so covertly in cues rather than direct comments. In Tuckett *et al.*'s research, 26% of patients spontaneously offered an explanation of their symptoms. However, when patients did express their views, only 7% of doctors actively encouraged their patients to elaborate, and 81% made no effort to listen or deliberately interrupted. Half of patients' views were expressed covertly rather than overtly (Tuckett *et al.* 1985). Butow *et al.* demonstrated that doctors effectively identify and respond to the majority of informational cues; however, they are less observant of and able to address cues for emotional support (Butow *et al.* 2002). Zimmerman *et al.* undertook a systematic review of patient expressions of cues and concerns and concluded that physicians missed most cues and concerns and adopted behaviours that discouraged disclosure – communication training improved the detection of cues and concerns (Zimmermann *et al.* 2007). Del Piccolo *et al.* concluded that listening, together with supporting and emotion-centred expressions, activate cue emission, whereas physician closed questions tend to suppress cue expressions (Del Piccolo *et al.* 2007). On the other hand, soliciting a patient's expression of personal needs by open enquiry and active listening will satisfy the patient's needs and lower cue offers. Levinson *et al.* showed that consultations that were cue based were shorter that those in which cues were missed by 12% in general practice and 10.7% in surgery (Levinson *et al.* 2000). In oncology consultations, addressing cues reduced consultation times by 10–12% (Butow *et al.* 2002).

Future directions

A key area for development in the teaching of information gathering will be the integration of communication with effective clinical reasoning. Without integrating communication back into the larger medical curriculum, communication will be perceived as a separate entity divorced from "real medicine" – an inessential frill rather than a basic skill relevant to all encounters with patients. It is important therefore for communication teachers to understand the influence of clinical reasoning on the process of gathering information and vice versa.

Clinicians use a variety of approaches to clinical reasoning as subject expertise increases, from hypothetico-deductive reasoning, through schema-driven approaches and finally pattern recognition (Elstein and Schwarz 2002; Dornan & Carroll, 2003). All of these different approaches to clinical reasoning necessitate doctors starting the process of problem solving early on as the interview proceeds. At first sight, this might suggest that clinicians employing such techniques should move more quickly to closed questioning as they test out their clinical reasoning. In fact, the opposite is true. All these approaches are critically dependent on adopting the same open-to-closed approach to the process of information gathering. The potential danger of all three approaches is starting down a path of clinical reasoning prematurely. Early closed questioning can quickly lead to the exploration of one particular avenue that may well prove inappropriate and lead inexorably to a dead end. The doctor may have to start again and generate a different problem-solving strategy; inefficient and inaccurate information gathering ensues.

All approaches to clinical reasoning in fact depend on a clear and careful listening phase through which the clinician can obtain enough of the picture first to apply the right schema or increase the chance of the right pattern being recognized. Wise use of the process skills of screening, open questioning, attentive listening and discovering the patient's narrative in the opening minutes of the interview allows clinicians more time to generate their problem-solving strategies and provides them with more information on which to base their theories and hypotheses.

Here we see how perceptual, content and process skills in communication are inextricably linked and cannot be considered in isolation. Future teaching practice needs to follow suit so that learners can see the importance of effective communication to clinical problem solving.

References

Agledahl, K.M., Gulbrandsen, P., Forde, R. & Wifstad, A. (2011) Courteous but not curious: How doctors' politeness masks their existential neglect. A qualitative study of video-recorded patient consultations. *Journal of Medical Ethics*, 37, 650–654.

Butow, P.N., Brown, R.F., Cogar, S., Tattersall, M.H. & Dunn, S.M. (2002) Oncologists' reactions to cancer patients' verbal cues. *Psycho-Oncology*, 11, 47–58.

Del Piccolo, L., Mazzi, M.A., Dunn, G., Sandri, M. & Zimmermann, C. (2007) Sequence analysis in multilevel models: A study on different sources of patient cues in medical consultations. *Social Science & Medicine*, 65, 2357–2370.

Dornan, T. & Carroll, C. (2003) Medical communication and diabetes. *Diabetic Medicine*, 20, 85–87.

Elstein, A.S. & Schwarz, A. (2002) Clinical problem solving and diagnostic decision making: Selective review of the cognitive literature. *BMJ*, 324, 729–732.

Levinson, W., Roter, D.L., Mullooly, J.P., Dull, V.T. & Frankel, R.M. (1997) The relationship with malpractice claims among primary care physicians and surgeons. *JAMA*, 277, 553–559.

Levinson, W., Gorawara-Bhat, R. & Lamb, J. (2000) A study of patient clues and physician responses in primary care and surgical settings. *JAMA*, 284, 1021–1027.

Marvel, M.K., Epstein, R.M., Flowers, K. & Beckman, H.B. (1999) Soliciting the patient's agenda: Have we improved? *JAMA*, 281, 283–287.

McWhinney, I. (1989) The need for a transformed clinical method. In: M. Stewart & D. Roter (eds), *Communicating with Medical Patients*. Sage Publications, Newbury Park, CA.

Mishler, E.G. (1984) *The Discourse of Medicine: Dialectics of Medical Interviews*. Ablex, Norwood, NJ.

Mjaaland, T.A., Finset, A., Jensen, B.F. & Gulbrandsen, P. (2011) Physicians' responses to patients' expressions of negative emotions in hospital consultations: A video-based observational study. *Patient Education and Counseling*, 84, 332–337.

Platt, F.W. & McMath, J.C. (1979) Clinical hypocompetence: The interview. *Annals of Internal Medicine*, 91, 898–902.

Quilligan, S. & Silverman, J. (2012) The skill of summary in clinician–patient communication: A case study. *Patient Education and Counseling*, 86, 354–359.

Ruiz Moral, R., Parras Rejano, J.M. & Perula De Torres, L.A. (2006) Is the expression 'Oh, by the way...' a problem that arises in the early moments of a consultation? *European Journal of General Practice*, 12, 40–41.

Silverman, J., Kurtz, S.M. & Draper, J. (2013) *Skills for Communicating with Patients*. Radcliffe Medical, Oxford.

Stewart, M.A., Brown, J.B., Weston, W.W., McWhinney, I.R. & McWilliam, C.L. (2003) *Patient-Centered Medicine: Transforming the Clinical Method*. Radcliffe Medical, Oxford.

Takemura, Y., Atsumi, R. & Tsuda, T. (2007) Identifying medical interview behaviors that best elicit information from patients in clinical practice. *Tohoku Journal of Experimental Medicine*, 213, 121–127.

Tuckett, D., Boulton, M., Olson, C. & Williams, A. (1985) *Meetings between Experts: An Approach to Sharing Ideas in Medical Consultations*. Tavistock, London.

Zimmermann, C., Del Piccolo, L. & Finset, A. (2007) Cues and concerns by patients in medical consultations: A literature review. *Psychological Bulletin*, 133, 438–463.

CHAPTER 12

Information Sharing and Shared Decision Making

Jonathan Silverman

University of Cambridge School of Clinical Medicine, Cambridge; European Association for Communication in Healthcare, Salisbury, UK

Most communication teaching programmes concentrate on the first half of the interview and neglect or underplay information sharing and shared decision making (Sanson-Fisher *et al.* 1991; Elwyn *et al.* 1999). Yet there are problems in current practice that suggest the need for considerable efforts in our communication teaching of this component of the interview:

1 not enough information given by doctors to match their patients' needs (Richard & Lussier 2003; Richard & Lussier, 2007; Sibley *et al.* 2011);
2 omission of key elements of information (Jenkins *et al.* 2011);
3 use of language that patients cannot understand (Castro *et al.* 2007; Koch-Weser *et al.* 2009);
4 underusing techniques to enable patient recall and understanding (Dunn *et al.* 1993; Murphy *et al.* 2004) and
5 lack of involvement of patients in decision making to the level they wish (Degner *et al.* 1997; Beach *et al.* 2007; Audrey *et al.* 2008, Chewning *et al.* 2012).

Unfortunately these difficulties do not appear to be resolving with time, possibly accentuated by the recent emphasis in medical practice on 'protocolized' care and the effect of computerisation, both of which have had the unintended consequences of leading doctors away from attempts to forge an active partnership with patients (Bensing *et al.* 2006).

Historical context

Many of these problems originally emanated from a traditional view of the doctor–patient relationship between a paternalistic doctor and passive patient, as discussed in Annie Cushing's chapter in this book (chapter 3). However, over several decades, there has been a gradual shift towards a more collaborative approach (Quill 1983; Roter & Hall 1992; Stewart *et al.* 1997) and towards the concept of shared decision making as formulated by Charles *et al.* (1997). In shared decision making, there is a genuine two-way exchange of information including the technical information brought to the interview (mostly but not always by the doctor) and the patient's information concerning his or her unique ideas, concerns and expectations. Both

Clinical Communication in Medicine, First Edition. Edited by Jo Brown, Lorraine M. Noble, Alexia Papageorgiou and Jane Kidd.
© 2016 John Wiley & Sons, Ltd. Published 2016 by John Wiley & Sons, Ltd.

parties reveal their preferences and come to a collaborative decision (Coulter 1999; Elwyn *et al.* 1999; Holmes-Rovner *et al.* 2000; Elwyn *et al.* 2001; Schofield *et al.* 2003).

Current teaching practice – the skills of Information sharing and shared decision making

So what can teachers of communication skills recommend to learners to enable them to achieve more effective information sharing and shared decision making in the clinical interview? Consultation models tend to emphasise the following tasks and skills:
* *providing the correct amount and type of information* (Jenkins *et al.* 2001; Hagerty *et al.* 2004; Claramita *et al.* 2011)
  - assessing the patient's starting point;
  - chunking and checking and
  - eliciting patient's questions
* *aiding accurate recall and understanding* (Kemp *et al.* 2008; van der Meulen *et al.* 2008; Shaw *et al.* 2009; Fink *et al.* 2010)
  - explicit organisation and signposting;
  - repetition and summary;
  - clarity of language;
  - visual methods of communication and
  - checking patient's understanding
* *achieving a shared understanding* (Tuckett *et al.* 1985; Hudak *et al.* 2008; Slade *et al.* 2008)
  - relating explanations to the patient's perspective;
  - providing opportunities to contribute;
  - picking up cues and
  - eliciting reactions and feelings
* *shared decision making* (Kaplan *et al.* 1996; Brown *et al.* 2001; Dimoska *et al.* 2008; Coulter 2012; Langseth *et al.* 2012)
  - sharing thinking;
  - involving the patient;
  - exploring options;
  - ascertaining level of involvement patient wishes and
  - negotiating a mutually acceptable plan, checking.

Again, the evidence base for the use of these skills is critical to teaching practice. Here, we explore one particular skill, ascertaining the level of involvement the patient wishes to make in decisions, as an example of the importance of understanding the literature for truly effective teaching.

In their systematic review of studies on patient preferences for shared decisions, Chewning *et al.* demonstrated that the number of patients who prefer participation in decision making has increased over the past three decades to 71% (Chewning *et al.* 2012). However, all of the studies in the review identified a subset of patients who want to delegate decisions.

In Degner *et al.*'s study of women with a confirmed diagnosis of breast cancer attending hospital oncology clinics, 22% wanted to select their own cancer treatment, 44% wanted to select their treatment collaboratively with their doctors, and 34% wanted to delegate this decision making to their doctors. Only 42% of women believed they actually achieved their preferred level of control in decision making (Degner *et al.*

1997). In Gattellari *et al.*'s study of cancer patients, mismatch between patients' preferred roles in decision making and what they perceived happened led to increased patient anxiety (Gattellari *et al.* 2001). However, whatever the preference of the patient prior to the interview, satisfaction with the consultation and the amount of information and emotional support received were significantly greater in those who reported a shared role. This gives support to the concept that as well as respecting individual differences in patient preference, part of the doctor's role might include gentle encouragement of patients over time to take part in shared decision making.

Beach *et al.* looked further at the relationship between shared decision making and patient outcomes in patients with HIV (Beach *et al.* 2007). They found that patients who preferred to share decisions with their HIV provider had better outcomes than both those who wanted their HIV provider to make decisions and those who wanted to make decisions alone. They suggest that practising clinicians ought to encourage patients toward a shared decision-making role.

It is difficult to guess each patient's desire for involvement in making decisions without enquiring directly. Rather than guess or force all patients to adopt a collaborative role, it is the doctor's task to ascertain individual patient's preferences for participation and to tailor the approach accordingly. Even if the patient does not wish to be involved in decision making at the moment, such a discussion will alert the patient that this is an option that he or she can return to in the future without criticism from the doctor. Since a patient's preferences for participation and information may vary on the nature or stage of the illness (Beaver *et al.* 1996; Chewning *et al.* 2012), preferences need to be discussed periodically over time and from situation to situation. Thus discovering a patient's preference for participation in decision making should be conceptualised as an on-going task. An article by Mulley *et al.* called 'Stop the Silent Misdiagnosis: Patient Preferences Matter' summarises the evidence for the importance of patient preferences in decision making (Mulley *et al.* 2012).

Future directions

The world of doctor–patient information sharing and shared decision making is changing rapidly with the digital age and the ever-increasing availability of information through the Internet. The challenge will be how to enhance patients' decision making in this new era of mushrooming information. And the cutting edge of future development will be how to enable patients to not only understand the information but to help them to understand the scientific uncertainty and clarify their own personal preferences and values and how these impact on their eventual decisions (O'Connor *et al.* 1999; Robinson & Thomson 2001; Sepucha & Mulley 2003; Kaner *et al.* 2007; Nelson *et al.* 2007; O'Brien *et al.* 2009; Bunge *et al.* 2010; Elwyn *et al.* 2011; Myers *et al.* 2011).

References

Audrey, S., Abel, J., Blazeby, J.M., Falk, S. & Campbell, R. (2008) What oncologists tell patients about survival benefits of palliative chemotherapy and implications for informed consent: Qualitative study. *BMJ*, 337, a752.

Beach, M.C., Duggan, P.S. & Moore, R.D. (2007) Is patients' preferred involvement in health decisions related to outcomes for patients with HIV? *Journal of General Internal Medicine*, 22, 1119–1124.

Beaver, K., Luker, K.A., Owens, R.G., Leinster, S.J., Degner, L.F. & Sloan, J.A. (1996) Treatment decision making in women newly diagnosed with breast cancer. *Cancer Nursing*, 19, 8–19.

Bensing, J.M., Tromp, F., van Dulmen, S., van den Brink-Muinen, A., Verheul, W. & Schellevis, F.G. (2006) Shifts in doctor–patient communication between 1986 and 2002: A study of videotaped general practice consultations with hypertension patients. *BMC Family Practice*, 7, 62.

Brown, R.F., Butow, P.N., Dunn, S.M. & Tattersall, M.H. (2001) Promoting patient participation and shortening cancer consultations: A randomised trial. *British Journal of Cancer*, 85, 1273–1279.

Bunge, M., Muhlhauser, I. & Steckelberg, A. (2010) What constitutes evidence-based patient information? Overview of discussed criteria. *Patient Education and Counseling*, 78, 316–328.

Castro, C.M., Wilson, C., Wang, F. & Schillinger, D. (2007) Babel babble: Physicians' use of unclarified medical jargon with patients. *American Journal of Health Behavior*, 31 (Suppl. 1), S85–95.

Charles, C., Gafni, A. & Whelan, T. (1997) Shared decision making in the medical encounter: What does it mean? (Or it takes at least two to tango). *Social Science & Medicine*, 44, 681–692.

Chewning, B., Bylund, C.L., Shah, B., Arora, N.K., Gueguen, J.A. & Makoul, G. (2012) Patient preferences for shared decisions: A systematic review. *Patient Education and Counseling*, 86, 9–18.

Claramita, M., Utarini, A., Soebono, H., Van Dalen, J. & van der Vleuten, C. (2011) Doctor–patient communication in a Southeast Asian setting: The conflict between ideal and reality. *Advances in Health Sciences Education*, 16, 69–80.

Coulter, A. (1999) Paternalism or partnership? Patients have grown up – and there's no going back. *BMJ*, 319, 719–720.

Coulter, A. (2012) Patient engagement – what works? *Journal of Ambulatory Care Management*, 35, 80–89.

Degner, L.F., Kristjanson, L. J., Bowman, D., Sloan, J. A., Carriere, K. C., O'Neil, J., Bilodeau, B., Watson, P. & Mueller, B. (1997) Information needs and decisional preferences in women with breast cancer. *JAMA*, 277, 1485–1492.

Dimoska, A., Butow, P.N., Dent, E., Arnold, B., Brown, R.F. & Tattersall, M.H.N. (2008) An examination of the initial cancer consultation of medical and radiation oncologists using the Cancode interaction analysis system. *British Journal of Cancer*, 98, 1508–1514.

Dunn, S.M., Butow, P.N., Tattersall, M.H., Jones, Q.J., Sheldon, J.S., Taylor, J.J. & Sumich, M.D. (1993) General information tapes inhibit recall of the cancer consultation. *Journal of Clinical Oncology*, 11, 2279–2285.

Elwyn, G., Edwards, A., Gwyn, R. & Grol, R. (1999) Towards a feasible model for shared decision making: Focus group study with general practice registrars. *BMJ*, 319, 753–756.

Elwyn, G., Edwards, A., Mowle, S., Wensing, M., Wilkinson, C., Kinnersley, P. & Grol, R. (2001) Measuring the involvement of patients in shared decision making: A systematic review of instruments. *Patient Education and Counseling*, 43, 5–22.

Elwyn, G., Kreuwel, I., Durand, M A., Sivell, S., Joseph-Williams, N., Evans, R. & Edwards, A. (2011) How to develop web-based decision support interventions for patients: A process map. *Patient Education and Counseling*, 82, 260–265.

Fink, A.S., Prochazka, A.V., Henderson, W.G., Bartenfeld, D., Nyirenda, C., Webb, A., Berger, D.H., Itani, K., Whitehill, T., Edwards, J., Wilson, M., Karsonovich, C. & Parmelee, P. (2010) Enhancement of surgical informed consent by addition of repeat back: A multicenter, randomized controlled clinical trial. *Annals of Surgery*, 252, 27–36.

Gattellari, M., Butow, P.N. & Tattersall, M.H. (2001) Sharing decisions in cancer care. *Social Science & Medicine*, 52, 1865–1878.

Hagerty, R.G., Butow, P.N., Ellis, P.A., Lobb, E.A., Pendlebury, S., Leighl, N., Goldstein, D., Lo, S.K. & Tattersall, M.H.N. (2004) Cancer patient preferences for communication of prognosis in the metastatic setting. *Journal of Clinical Oncology*, 22, 1721–1730.

Holmes-Rovner, M., Valade, D., Orlowski, C., Draus, C., Nabozny-Valerio, B. & Keiser, S. (2000) Implementing shared decision making in routine practice: Barriers and opportunities. *Health Expectations*, 3, 182–191.

Hudak, P.L., Armstrong, K., Braddock, C., 3rd, Frankel, R.M. & Levinson, W. (2008) Older patients' unexpressed concerns about orthopaedic surgery. *Journal of Bone & Joint Surgery – American Volume*, 90, 1427–1435.

Jenkins, V., Fallowfield, L. & Saul, J. (2001) Information needs of patients with cancer: Results from a large study in UK cancer centres. *British Journal of Cancer*, 84, 48–51.

Jenkins, V., Solis-Trapala, I., Langridge, C., Catt, S., Talbot, D.C. & Fallowfield, L.J. (2011) What oncologists believe they said and what patients believe they heard: An analysis of phase I trial discussions. *Journal of Clinical Oncology*, 29, 61–68.

Kaner, E., Heaven, B., Rapley, T., Murtagh, M., Graham, R., Thomson, R. & May, C. (2007) Medical communication and technology: A video-based process study of the use of decision aids in primary care consultations. *BMC Medical Informatics & Decision Making*, 7, 2.

Kaplan, S.H., Greenfield, S., Gandek, B., Rogers, W.H. & Ware, J.E. (1996) Characteristics of physicians with participatory decision making styles. *Annals of Internal Medicine*, 124, 497–504.

Kemp, E.C., Floyd, M.R., McCord-Duncan, E. & Lang, F. (2008) Patients prefer the method of 'tell back – collaborative inquiry' to assess understanding of medical information. *Journal of the American Board of Family Medicine*, 21, 24–30.

Koch-Weser, S., Dejong, W. & Rudd, R.E. (2009) Medical word use in clinical encounters. *Health Expectations*, 12, 371–382.

Langseth, M.S., Shepherd, E., Thomson, R. & Lord, S. (2012) Quality of decision making is related to decision outcome for patients with cardiac arrhythmia. *Patient Education and Counseling*, 87, 49–53.

Mulley, A.G., Trimble, C. & Elwyn, G. (2012) Stop the silent misdiagnosis: Patients' preferences matter. *BMJ*, 345, e6572.

Murphy, S.M., Donnelly, M., Fitzgerald, T., Tanner, W.A., Keane, F.B.V. & Tierney, S. (2004) Patients' recall of clinical information following laparoscopy for acute abdominal pain. *British Journal of Surgery*, 91, 485–488.

Myers, R.E., Daskalakis, C., Kunkel, E.J., Cocroft, J.R., Riggio, J.M., Capkin, M. & Braddock, C.H. 3rd. (2011) Mediated decision support in prostate cancer screening: A randomized controlled trial of decision counseling. *Patient Education and Counseling*, 83, 240–246.

Nelson, W.L., Han, P.K., Fagerlin, A., Stefanek, M. & Ubel, P.A. (2007) Rethinking the objectives of decision aids: A call for conceptual clarity. *Medical Decision Making*, 27, 609–618.

O'Brien, M.A., Whelan, T.J., Villasis-Keever, M., Gafni, A., Charles, C., Roberts, R., Schiff, S. & Cai, W. (2009) Are cancer-related decision aids effective? A systematic review and meta-analysis. *Journal of Clinical Oncology*, 27, 974–985.

O'Connor, A.M., Rostom, A., Fiset, V., Tetroe, J., Entwistle, V., Llewellyn-Thomas, H., Holmes-Rovner, M., Barry, M. & Jones, J. (1999) Decision aids for patients facing health treatment or screening decisions: Systematic review. *BMJ*, 319, 731–734.

Quill, T.E. (1983) Partnerships in patient care: A contractual approach. *Annals of Internal Medicine*, 98, 228–234.

Richard, C. & Lussier, M.T. (2007) Measuring patient and physician participation in exchanges on medications: Dialogue ratio, preponderance of initiative, and dialogical roles. *Patient Education and Counseling*, 65, 329–341.

Richard, R. & Lussier, M.T. (2003) *Dialogic index: A description of physician and patient participation in discussions of medications. National Association of Primary Care Research Group Annual Conference*, Banff, Alberta.

Robinson, A. & Thomson, R. (2001) Variability in patient preferences for participating in medical decision making: Implication for the use of decision support tools. *Quality in Health Care*, 10 (Suppl. 1), i34–38.

Roter, D.L. & Hall, J.A. (1992) Doctors *Talking with Patients, Patients Talking with Doctors*. Auburn House, Westport, CT.

Sanson-Fisher, R.W., Redman, S., Walsh, R., Mitchell, K., Reid, A.L.A. & Perkins, J.J. (1991) Training medical practitioners in information transfer skills: The new challenge. *Medical Education*, 25, 322–333.

Schofield, T., Elwyn, G., Edwards, A. & Visser, A. (2003) Shared decision making. *Patient Education and Counseling*, 50, 229–230.

Sepucha, K.R. & Mulley, A.G. (2003) Extending decision support: Preparation and implementation. *Patient Education and Counseling*, 50, 269–271.

Shaw, A., Ibrahim, S., Reid, F., Ussher, M. & Rowlands, G. (2009) Patients' perspectives of the doctor–patient relationship and information giving across a range of literacy levels. *Patient Education and Counseling*, 75, 114–120.

Sibley, A., Latter, S., Richard, C., Lussier, M.T., Roberge, D., Skinner, T.C., Cradock, S. & Zinken, K.M. (2011) Medication discussion between nurse prescribers and people with diabetes: An analysis of content and participation using MEDICODE. *Journal of Advanced Nursing*, 67, 2323–2336.

Slade, D., Scheeres, H., Manidis, M., Iedema, R., Dunston, R., Stein-Parbury, J., Matthiessen, C., Herke, M. & McGregor, J. (2008) Emergency communication: The discursive challenges facing emergency clinicians and patients in hospital emergency departments. *Discourse & Communication*, 2, 271–298.

Stewart, M., Belle Brown, J., Donner, A., McWhinney, I.R., Oates, J. & Weston, W. (1997) *The Impact of Patient-Centred Care on Patient Outcomes in Family Practice*. Thames Valley Family Practice Research Unit, Ontario.

Tuckett, D., Boulton, M., Olson, C. & Williams, A. (1985) *Meetings between Experts: An Approach to Sharing Ideas in Medical Consultations*. Tavistock, London.

van der Meulen, N., Jansen, J., van Dulmen, S., Bensing, J. & Van Weert, J. (2008) Interventions to improve recall of medical information in cancer patients: A systematic review of the literature. *Psycho-Oncology*, 17, 857–868.

CHAPTER 13

Communicating about Risk and Uncertainty

Katherine Joekes

St George's University of London, London, UK

Historical context

The shift towards patient-centred care in modern medicine has generated a requirement for effective shared decision making between clinician and patient about prevention, treatment options or management. In order for a patient to be able to give informed consent, he or she will need to understand associated risks, benefits and uncertainty. A pragmatic definition of risk is 'the probability that a hazard will give rise to harm' (Mohanna & Chambers 2008), which is therefore accompanied by a level of uncertainty about future outcomes. Uncertainty can be defined as 'the subjective perception of ignorance' (Han *et al.* 2011) and pervades health care at all levels.

It has become evident that effective communication of risk and uncertainty is challenging, for both patients and healthcare professionals, with a variety of factors contributing to this. Clinicians need to make sense of (population) data, interpret these accurately, and use this within their own clinical, ethical and organisational context. Poor health 'numeracy' (i.e. the ability to understand numerical information) (Golbeck *et al.* 2005) can lead to problems for healthcare providers (Gigerenzer *et al.* 2007) and patients (Smith *et al.* 2010). Similarly, dealing with uncertainty can be difficult for all parties involved (Han *et al.* 2011). The way in which people process (health) information (Tversky & Kahneman 1974; Reyna & Bainerd 2008) can result in cognitive biases, where information is interpreted inaccurately. Finally, the influence of emotions (Slovic *et al.* 2005) further muddies the waters for patients when trying to make sense of information about risk and uncertainty.

It is possible to identify theoretical foundations to explain how risk is perceived and interpreted. Models from cognitive science can be applied to the understanding of health-related risk perception and information processing and have arisen within the field of psychology, where theories of cognition, affect and health behaviour intersect. In particular the 'social cognitive models' (reviewed by Edwards 2009) have informed the design of interventions aimed at helping patients understand risk. However, Edwards (2009) identifies a lack of consistency in the theoretical models used, the risks explored, or the research methods employed to evaluate such interventions. Other theoretical approaches to understanding risk arise from sociocultural perspectives (described by Berry 2004), which view risk as a notion that is constructed within a

Clinical Communication in Medicine, First Edition. Edited by Jo Brown, Lorraine M. Noble, Alexia Papageorgiou and Jane Kidd.

cultural and political perspective. Such perspectives, however, have received less attention within the context of health-related risk. Furthermore, neither theoretical approach appears to be applied to the complex processes involved in oral risk communication in medical consultations.

Current practice

Materials to support clinicians' practice are being developed (e.g. British Medical Association 2012). This includes a variety of decision aids, which aim to increase patients' knowledge and realistic perceptions of outcomes and may support doctor–patient communication (Trevena *et al.* 2006; Stacey *et al.* 2011). Little is known, however, about impact on long-term behaviours or health outcomes (Akl *et al.* 2011).

Evidence-based 'best practices' for representation of statistical information (Gigerenzer & Edwards 2003; Akl *et al.* 2011) and verbal risk communication within the context of a medical consultation are reviewed in the literature (e.g. Paling 2006; Lipkus 2007; Fagerlin *et al.* 2011; Ahmed *et al.* 2012); however, these and other (e.g. Visschers *et al.* 2009) authors identify that the research in this field contains gaps and some contradictions. Nonetheless, there is agreement on certain recommendations, providing helpful guidance for clinicians. These include: use of natural frequencies versus percentages; use of absolute risk versus relative risk; 'framing' information in a balanced manner; personalising the risk information where possible; and using appropriate graphical/pictorial material. These strategies address the problems of numeracy and cognitive biases to some extent. It is important to remember that 'best practice guidelines' do not automatically translate into practical competencies or easy-to-implement skills. Students and clinicians still face the challenge of making the transition from 'knowing that' to 'knowing how' (Miller 1990).

The issue of uncertainty arises when discussing prognosis, and the literature shows that patients/relatives wish for honest, accurate information (which will inevitably involve uncertainty) and hope (Clayton *et al.* 2008); a delicate balance to strike for clinicians. Guidelines for effective communication around prognosis have been developed (Glare *et al.* 2008); however, these 'common sense' competencies lack both theoretical underpinning and evaluation of efficacy.

At the postgraduate level, a brief training programme, which focused on developing skills to implement shared decision making and the use of risk communication aids, was shown to be effective (Elwyn *et al.* 2004). In recent years, UK medical schools have addressed the task of teaching and assessing risk communication to varying degrees, ranging from (brief) didactic lectures to workshops containing experiential learning through role-play. Some evidence is available on the efficacy of these efforts (Sedgwick & Hall 2003; Joekes *et al.* 2009; Han *et al.* 2014). Communication about uncertainty may be touched upon implicitly in any clinical communication skills teaching session and explicitly in sessions dealing with discussion about prognosis and bad news consultations.

Future directions

Development of teaching and assessment of communication about risk and uncertainty in medical education requires further attention (Han *et al.* 2014). Using the existing evidence on 'best practice guidelines' for clinical practice can form the basis for teaching materials and provide a helpful starting point for learners who need to transition from 'knowing' to 'implementing'. Integration of teaching around clinical communication, evidence-based medicine and clinical reasoning would validate and contextualise 'communicating about risk and uncertainty' for students and clinicians. Evaluation of teaching methods is recommended, whilst it is important to recognise that developing skills for effective communication about risk and uncertainty cannot be achieved in a single teaching episode.

Continued development of skills within the clinical context is required. Because much of the formal clinical communication skills teaching currently takes place in the preclinical years – in a context removed from clinical practice (Brown 2012) – students may struggle to recognise the relevance and challenges of effective risk communication. It can be argued that this topic might better be dealt with in the later years of medical school and into postgraduate education, where 'situated learning' takes place (Yardley *et al.* 2012). (More on situated and work-based learning will be found in chapter 29.)

An increase in the number of decision aids (e.g. OPTIONS grids) (Elwyn *et al.* 2013) is expected, and best practice in their use needs to be clarified. How decision aids or tools, which provide both patient and clinician with accurate and up-to-date information, could most effectively be used to assist risk communication within the consultation requires further exploration.

References

Ahmed, H., Naik, G., Willoughby, H. & Edwards, A.G. (2012) Communicating risk. *British Medical Journal*, 344 (no. 7862), 40–44.

Akl, E.A., Oxman, A.D., Herrin, J., Vist, G.E., Terrenato, I., Sperati, F., Costiniuk, C., Blank, D. & Schünemann, H. (2011) Using alternative statistical formats for presenting risks and risk reductions. Cochrane Database of Systematic Reviews, 3 (Art. No.: CD006776).

Berry, D. (2004) *Risk, Communication and Health Psychology*. Open University Press, Maidenhead, Berkshire.

British Medical Association. (2012) *Risk: What's Your Perspective? A Guide for Healthcare Professionals*. BMA Science & Education Department, London.

Brown, J. (2012) Perspective: Clinical communication education in the United Kingdom: Some fresh insights. *Academic Medicine*, 87 (no. 8), 1101–1104.

Clayton, J.M., Hancock, K., Parker, S., Butow, P.N., Walder, S., Carrick, S., Currow, D., Ghersi, D., Glare, P., Hagerty, R., Oliver, I.N. & Tattersall, M.H. (2008) Sustaining hope when communicating with terminally ill patients and their families: A systematic review. *Psycho-Oncology*, 17 (no. 7), 641–659.

Edwards, A. (2009) Risk communication – making evidence part of patient choices. In: A. Edwards & G. Elwyn, *Shared Decision-Making in Health Care: Achieving Evidence-Based Patient Choice*, 2nd edn, pp. 135–142. Oxford University Press, Oxford.

Elwyn, G., Edwards, A., Hood, K., Robling, M., Atwell, C., Russell, I., Wensing, M., Grol, R. & the Study Steering Group. (2004) Achieving involvement: Process outcomes from a cluster randomized trial of shared decision making skill development and use of risk communication aids in general practice. *Family Practice*, 21 (no. 4), 337–346.

Elwyn, G., Lloyd, A., Joseph-Williams, N., Cording, E., Thomson, R., Durand, M.A. & Edwards, A. (2013) Option grids: Shared decision making made easier. *Patient Education and Counseling*, 90 (no. 2), 207–212.

Fagerlin, A., Zikmund-Fisher, B.J. & Ubel, P.A. (2011) Helping patients decide: Ten steps to better risk communication. *Journal of the National Cancer Institute*, 103 (no. 19), 1436–1443.

Gigerenzer, G. & Edwards, A. (2003) Simple tools for understanding risks: From innumeracy to insight. *British Medical Journal*, 327 (no. 7417), 741.

Gigerenzer, G., Gaissmaier, W., Kurz-Milcke, E., Schwartz, L.M. & Woloshin, S. (2007) Helping doctors and patients make sense of health statistics. *Psychological Science in the Public Interest*, 8 (no. 2), 53–96.

Glare, P., Sinclair, C., Downing, M., Stone, P., Maltoni, M. & Vigano, A. (2008) Predicting survival in patients with advanced disease. *European Journal of Cancer*, 44 (no. 8), 1146–1156.

Golbeck, A.L., Ahlers-Schmidt, C.R., Paschal, A.M. & Dismuke, S.E. (2005) A definition and operational framework for health numeracy. *American Journal of Preventive Medicine*, 29 (no. 4), 375–376.

Han, P.K., Klein, W.M. & Arora, N.K. (2011) Varieties of uncertainty in health care: A conceptual taxonomy. *Medical Decision Making*, 31 (no. 6), 828–838.

Han, P.K., Joekes, K., Elwyn, G., Mazor, K.M., Thomson, R., Sedgwick, P., Ibison, J. & Wong, J.B. (2014) Development and evaluation of a risk communication curriculum for medical students. *Patient Education and Counseling*, 94 (no. 1), 43–49.

Joekes, K., Sedgwick, P. & Hall, A. (2009) Assessment of risk communication by objective structured clinical examination. *Medical Education*, 43 (no. 5), 484.

Lipkus, I.M. (2007) Numeric, verbal, and visual formats of conveying health risks: Suggested best practices and future recommendations. *Medical Decision Making*, 27 (no. 5), 696–713.

Miller, G.E. (1990) The assessment of clinical skills/competence/performance. *Academic Medicine*, 65 (no. 9), S63–S67.

Mohanna, K. & Chambers R (eds.) (2008) *Risk Matters in Healthcare: Communicating, Explaining and Managing Risk*, 2nd edn. Radcliffe Medical Press, Abingdon.

Paling, J. (2006) *Helping Patients Understand Risks*. Risk Communication Institute, Gainesville, FL.

Reyna, V.F. & Bainerd, C.J. (2008) Numeracy, ratio bias, and denominator neglect in judgements of risk and probability. *Learning and Individual Differences*, 18 (no. 1), 89–107.

Sedgwick, P. & Hall, A. (2003) Teaching medical students and doctors how to communicate risk: Combining the teaching of statistics with communication skills. *BMJ*, 327 (no. 7417), 694.

Slovic, P., Peters, E., Finucane, M.L. & MacGregor, D.G. (2005) Affect, risk, and decision making. *Health Psychology*, 24 (no. 4S), S35.

Smith, S.G., Wolf, M.S. & Wagner, C.V. (2010) Socioeconomic status, statistical confidence, and patient–provider communication: An analysis of the Health Information National Trends Survey (HINTS 2007). *Journal of Health Communication*, 15 (no. S3), 169–185.

Stacey, D., Bennett, C.L., Barry, M.J., Col, N.F., Eden, K.B., Holmes-Rovner, M. & Thomson, R. (2011) Decision aids for people facing health treatment or screening decisions. Cochrane Database of Systematic Reviews, 10 (Art. No.: CD001431).

Trevena, L.J., Barratt, A., Butow, P. & Caldwell, P. (2006) A systematic review on communicating with patients about evidence. *Journal of Evaluation in Clinical Practice*, 12 (no. 1), 13–23.

Tversky, A. & Kahneman, D. (1974) Judgement under uncertainty: Heuristics and biases. *Science*, 185 (no. 4157), 1124–1131.

Visschers, V.H., Meertens, R.M., Passchier, W.W. & De Vries, N.N. (2009) Probability information in risk communication: A review of the research literature. *Risk Analysis*, 29 (no. 2), 267–287.

Yardley, S., Teunissen, P.W. & Dornan, T. (2012) Experiential learning: AMEE guide No. 63. *Medical Teacher*, 34 (no. 2), e102–e115.

CHAPTER 14

Responding to Emotions

Theano V. Kalavana

University of Nicosia Medical School, Nicosia, Cyprus

Historical context

The topic of physicians responding to patient's emotions incorporates terms such as 'empathy' (Zinn 1993), 'sympathetic vibrations' (Stone 1993), 'affective connection' (Halpern 1993), 'connexion' (Matthews *et al*. 1993) and 'emotional resilience' (Coulehan 1995). There is strong evidence supporting the importance of physicians' responses to patients' emotions in the latter's positive health outcomes (Hojat *et al*. 2011). More specifically, evidence with outpatients showed that when doctors respond to patients' emotions and distress, this is positively associated with patients' decreased anxiety, improvement of medical outcomes and satisfaction (Roter *et al*. 1995; Epstein *et al*. 2007; Rakel *et al*. 2009; Hojat *et al*. 2011).

Empathy was introduced for the first time by Theodor Lipps (1935), an experimental psychologist who referred to empathy as a state in which an individual puts self into another person's experience (Hayward 2005). Michael Balint (1957) was the first to introduce empathy and the psychoanalytic concepts of transference and countertransference into medical practice. Based on his observations and experiences, he argued that almost all problems that a patient presents to the doctor are partially psychological in nature and must be explored. Furthermore, through his work with small groups of physicians who were presenting their cases anonymously, Balint (1957) outlined the importance of 'the doctor as the drug', meaning the effect that a doctor's responses, feelings and personality can have on a patient's recovery.

In medical terms, distinction is made between cognitive empathy, affective empathy and sympathy (or compassionate care). Cognitive empathy has been identified as the process in which the doctor shows genuine understanding to the patient's condition (physiological and nonphysiological) (Pedersen 2008), whereas affective empathy is defined as the doctors' ability to reflect back on a patient's experienced emotion (feeling with) (Cox *et al*. 2011). On the other hand, sympathy refers to the situation in which doctors experience intense feelings that are related to a patient's condition, such as pain – that is, suffering with the patient (feeling into) (Hojat *et al*. 2001; Khanuja *et al*. 2011).

The disagreement regarding the importance of responding to patients' emotions

Even though empathy is essential within doctor–patient communication, some scholars disagreed with the expression of affective clinical empathy, basically because it would prohibit, as they argued, objective diagnosis and treatment. More specifically,

Clinical Communication in Medicine, First Edition. Edited by Jo Brown, Lorraine M. Noble,
Alexia Papageorgiou and Jane Kidd.
© 2016 John Wiley & Sons, Ltd. Published 2016 by John Wiley & Sons, Ltd.

Blumgart (1964) supported the necessity of 'neutral empathy' in doctors' responses because empathizing with patients may remove objectivity and the scientific clinical perspective. 'Neutral empathy' is when the doctor proceeds with what needs to be done without experiencing any emotions (Blumgart 1964). Furthering Blumgart's argument, other researchers suggest that doctors should only present cognitive empathy, instead of affective empathy, as their acknowledgement of patients' emotions during consultation. Affective empathy is similar to sympathy and it involves emotions that in the end will work against an objective diagnosis and treatment (Landau 1993; Hojat *et al.* 2001). Also, a recent cross-sectional study with 294 general practitioners, in which the researchers investigated the general practitioners' empathic concerns in relation to burnout, found that sharing patients' emotions was related to physicians' personal distress, and that this was also associated with their decisions and performance (Lamothe *et al.* 2014). Furthermore, similar results were found in a third of 740 members of the Clinical Oncological Society of Australia who have reported high levels of emotional exhaustion due to their direct patient contact and the lack of appropriate communication skills training (Girgis *et al.* 2009).

On the other hand, Stone (1993) used the term "sympathetic vibrations" in order to explain that physicians must not only use cognitive empathy, but that they do need to sound as if they are sharing the patients' concerns. In addition, Irving and Dickson (2004) used three social psychological terms to explain empathy. They describe empathy as a process that involves the following dimensions: cognitive empathy (understanding – "know how"), affective empathy (feelings – know how it feels) and behaviour (as the result of the previous two dimensions – e.g. trying to imagine what the patient is going through). To date most models, such as Calgary-Cambridge Guide to Consultation Skills (Kurtz *et al.* 2003), the Three-Function Approach of the Medical Interview (Cole & Bird 2000), the BATHE Method (Stuart & Lieberman 1993), the PEARLS Method (Clark *et al.* 1996) advocate the importance of doctors' responses to patients' emotional needs.

Evidence on doctors' responses to patients' emotion

Positive outcomes from doctors' responses to patients' emotion

One of the very early studies looking into several aspects of the doctor–patient relationship showed that patient satisfaction results from a combination of medical care and significant support of patients' emotional and psychological needs (Caterinicchio 1979). Today there are many studies showing the benefits of physicians' responses to patients' emotions. Specifically, Bensing *et al.* (2011) and Mazzi *et al.* (2013) suggest patients perceive the consultation as more successful when doctors respond to their emotions. Furthermore, evidence shows that physicians' responses to patients' emotional problems can create a stronger therapeutic relation between the two parts, reduce symptoms of anxiety, increase patients' satisfaction and encourage better management of the disease (Butow *et al.* 2002; Zachariae *et al.* 2003; Shields *et al.* 2005; Uitterhoeve *et al.* 2009). Research on the consequences of physicians responding to patients' negative emotions indicated that when physicians invite further discussion of emotions, they establish a more positive doctor–patient relationship that contributes positively to treatment outcomes (Adams *et al.* 2012). Thus, physicians' effectiveness does not only rely on the medical/physical care they provide but also on the warm, comforting and friendly atmosphere they create (Di Blasi *et al.* 2001). Furthermore, Halpern (2001) noted three points about empathy that can be beneficial for both the patient and the physician. First, empathy encourages patients to talk more about their condition and symptoms and helps the physician to gather substantial information; second, it encourages patients' self-efficacy, which enables them to actively participate in their treatment; and third, it helps establish an efficient therapeutic interaction that has beneficial results on the patients' recovery process.

Additionally, even though the literature presents contradictory evidence in regards to doctors' empathic concerns and their effect on doctors' well-being (Lamothe *et al.* 2014), there is also evidence underlining the importance of empathy in doctors' well-being and job satisfaction. For instance, higher levels of cognitive empathy were associated with greater levels of well-being among therapists (Linley & Joseph 2007), and with personal growth and career satisfaction (Hojat 2007). On the other hand, lack of empathy or sympathy was related to burnout, compassion fatigue and medical errors (Shanafelt *et al.* 2005; Hojat 2007; West *et al.* 2009).

Why do physicians fail to respond to patients' emotion?

There has been an increased exploration of patients' emotions and psychological problems since the 1990s. However, the reality today is that a physician's work environment is not conducive to responding to patients' emotions. This is particularly due to heavy workloads and the dependence of doctors on technology for diagnosis instead of relying on information from patients (Butalid *et al.* 2014). Furthermore, evidence shows that medical students' empathy declines as students enter the final years of their studies (Chen *et al.* 2012).

More specifically, earlier studies have argued about several factors involved in physicians' missed empathic opportunities. These factors vary from focusing only on patients' medical symptoms and condition (Byrne & Long, 1976; Goldberg *et al.* 1982), to feeling uncomfortable dealing with patients' emotions, lack of confidence (Buckman 1984), and lack of time (Coulehan *et al.* 2001). Other possible factors that contribute to missed empathic opportunities are gender differences (female clinicians' responses are more emotionally focused) (Roter & Hall 2004); and how physicians address their questions regarding their patients' emotions (Detmar *et al.* 2000).

More recent studies show that doctors are perceived as not showing more empathy or asking more psychosocial questions. This suggests that doctors' responses to patients' emotions are limited to personal remarks and that there is a noticeable decline in empathy (Butalid *et al.* 2014). Furthermore, a more recent approach suggests that in order for physicians to be able to respond to patients' emotions, they must be able to detect them first. Not all patients express their emotions directly, and thus there is a need for physicians to read behind patients' words and body language. For this reason, terms such as 'cues' (verbal or nonverbal indications of an unpleasant emotion) and 'concerns' (clear verbalized statement of an emotion) have been introduced in the literature. Studies support the importance of a physician's ability to detect emotion; medical students who were sensitive to nonverbal cues were rated as more compassionate by simulated patients (Hall *et al.* 2009). When physicians address patients' emotional cues and concerns through empathic response, patients are more likely to adhere to treatment (Butow *et al.* 2002) and less likely to need to repeat their concerns. Additionally, shared decision making regarding patients' health goals is enhanced (Hulsman 2009; Pollak *et al.* 2007).

Thus, regarding physicians' responses to patients' emotional cues and concerns, there is evidence showing that accurate detection of patients' emotional cues (or even incorrect detection of emotional cues) is related to increased patient satisfaction compared to the nondetection of emotion cues. More specifically, Blanch-Hartigan (2013) investigated patient satisfaction with physician errors in detecting and identifying patient emotion cues. It was found that accurate identification of emotions, and inaccurate identification of emotions, did not significantly differ from each other. It was only the failure to detect patients' emotions that was related to patients' lower satisfaction. On the other hand, it has been noted by Mjaaland *et al.* (2011) that when patients express negative emotion cues, or even clear negative emotional concerns, physicians tended to avoid such communication and focus on the medical content instead of the affective issue. There are also other studies discussing the different ways that physicians respond to patients' emotions, such as the use of silence, encouragement of the discussion of emotions through exploration or verbally identifying the patients' specific emotion (Del Piccolo *et al.* 2011). Finally, some other factors that can influence the physicians' responses to patients' emotions involve the initiation of the concerns or cues (whether physicians or patients start a discussion on emotions), the emotional content of the concern and the time that the concern was expressed in the consultation (Zimmermann *et al.* 2007).

Addressing patients' emotions is an important process within a consultation, and it is related to patients' satisfaction, but still this is not enough! Evidence shows that apart from responding to patients' emotions during a consultation, it is important to encourage patients to manage their illness and be active; otherwise, they will not be able to cope efficiently with their health and risk factors (Kinmonth *et al.* 1998). In other words, doctors' responses to emotions are of great importance for patients' satisfaction; however, the physician's ability to encourage the patient to take action, and to jointly decide on appropriate therapy, will ultimately lead to adherence to the treatment (Smith *et al.* 2011).

Future directions

There is no doubt that doctors' responses to patients' emotions is one of the most important aspects of doctor–patient relations, of patients' increased adherence to treatment plans and of positive health outcomes. Even though medical students are often taught cognitively based empathic skills – such as understanding the patient's situation, perspective and feelings; communicating that understanding and checking its accuracy and acting on that understanding (Mercer & Reynolds 2002) – evidence shows that medical students' empathy declines as students enter the final years (Chen *et al.* 2012). Therefore, several researchers have insisted that further training must be provided in order for physicians to have successful consultation sessions with their patients.

For instance, Blanch-Hartigan (2012) argued that physicians and medical students must be taught the skills needed to detect emotion cues; she proposed the DIREC Model (Detection, Identification, Response to Emotion Cue) for this purpose as a useful tool. On the other hand, Satterfield and Hughes (2007) argued that identifying emotion cues is not enough and that students/physicians must also go through training on emotion processing. This means that they need first to be able to identify the emotional meaning of the cue, and second to be able to respond according to this emotional meaning. Finally, Stone *et al.* (2012) argued that physicians must all invest time to practice and receive feedback on their empathic skills through (self-) observation (videos etc). It was contended that to become a great physician one must have the ability to perceive the ambiguity within patients' emotion cues, to allow the patients to express their feelings and then be assured that these feelings were explicitly understood.

References

Adams, K. Cimino, J.E.W., Arnold, R.M. & Anderson, W.G. (2012) Why should I talk about emotion? Communication patterns associated with physician discussion of patient expressions of negative emotion in hospital admission encounters. *Patient Education and Counseling*, 89, 44–50.

Balint, M. (1957) *The Doctor, His Patient and the Illness*. International Universities Press, London.

Bensing, J.M., Deveugele, M., Moretti, F., Fletcher, I., Van Vliet, L., Van Bogaert, M. & Rimondini, M. (2011) How to make the medical consultation more successful from a patient's perspective? Tips for doctor and patients from lay people in the United Kingdom, Italy, Belgium and the Netherlands. *Patient Education and Counseling*, 84, 287–293.

Blanch-Hartigan, D. (2012) An effective training to increase accurate recognition of patient emotion cues. *Patient Education and Counseling*, 89, 274–280.

Blanch-Hartigan, D. (2013) Patient satisfaction with physician errors in detecting and identifying patient emotion cues. *Patient Education and Counseling*, 93, 56–62.

Blumgart, H. (1964) Caring for the patient. *New England Journal of Medicine*, 270, 449–456.

Buckman, R. (1984) Breaking bad news: Why is it still so difficult? *British Medical Journal*, 288, 1597–1599.

Butalid, L., Bensing, J.M. & Verhaak, P.F.M. (2014) Talking about psychosocial problems: An observational study on changes in doctor–patient communication in general practice between 1977 and 2008. *Patient Education and Counseling*, 94 (no. 3), 314–321. doi:10.1016/j.pec.2013.11.004.

Butow, P.N., Brown, R.F., Cogar, S., Tattersall, M.H.N. & Dunn, S.M. (2002) Oncologists' reaction to cancer patients' verbal cues. *Psycho-Oncology*, 11, 47–58.

Byrne, P. & Long, B. (1976) *Doctors Talking to Patients*. HMSO, London.

Caterinicchio, R.P. (1979) Testing plausible path models of interpersonal trust in patient-physician treatment relationships. *Social Science & Medicine*, 13(A), 81–99.

Chen, D.C.R., Kirshenbaum, D.S., Yan, J., Kirshenbaum, E. & Aseltine, R.H. (2012) Characterizing changes in student empathy throughout medical school. *Medical Teacher*, 34, 305–311.

Clark, W., Hewson, M. & Fry, M. (1996) *The Medical Interview. American Academy on Physician and Patient*, St Louis, MO.

Cole, S. & Bird, J. (2000) *The Medical Interview: The Three Function Approach*. Mosby, St Louis, MO.

Coulehan, J.L (1995) Tenderness and steadiness: Emotions in medical practice. *Literature and Medicine*, 14 (no. 2), 222–236.

Coulehan, J.L., Platt, F.W., Egener, B., Frankel, R., Lin, C.T., Lowen, B. & Salazar, W.H. (2001) 'Let me see if I have this right': Words that help build empathy. *Annual Internal Medicine*, 135, 221–227.

Cox, C.L., Uddin, L.Q., Di Martino, A., Castellanos F.X., Milham, M.P. & Kelly, C. (2011) The balance between feeling and knowing: Affective and cognitive empathy are reflected in the brain's intrinsic functional dynamics. *Social Cognitive and Affective Neuroscience*, 5, 1–11.

Del Piccolo, L., De Haes, H., Heaven, C., Jansen, J., Verheul, W., Bensing, J., Bergvik, S., Deveugele, M., Eide, H., Fletcher, I, Goss, C., Humpheris, G., Kim, Y.M., Langewitz, W., Mazzi, M., Mjaaland, T., Moretti, F., Nuebling, M., Rimondini, M., Salmon, P., Sibbern, T., Skre, I., van Dulmen, S., Wissow, L., Young, B. & Zandbelt, L. (2011) Development of the Verona coding definitions of emotional sequences to code health provider's responses (VR-CoDES-P) to patient cues and concerns. *Patient Education and Counseling*, 82, 149–155.

Detmar, S.B., Aaronson, N.K., Wever, L.D.V., Muller, M. & Schornagel, J.H. (2000) How are you feeling? Who wants to know? Patients' and oncologists' preferences for discussing health-related quality of life issues. *Journal of Clinical Oncology*, 18, 3295–3301.

Di Blasi, Z.D., Harkness, E., Ernst, E., Georgiou. A & Kleijnen, J. (2001) Influence of context effects on health outcomes: A systematic review. *Lancet*, 357, 757–762.

Epstein, R.M., Hadee, T., Carroll, J., Meldrum, S.C., Lardner, J. & Shields, C.G. (2007) 'Could this be something serious?' Reassurance, uncertainty, and empathy in response to patients' expression of worry. *Journal of General Internal Medicine*, 22, 1731–1739.

Girgis, A., Hansen, V. & Goldstein, D. (2009) Are Australian oncology health professionals burning out? A view from the trenches. *European Journal of Cancer*, 45, 393–399.

Goldberg, D., Steele, J.J., Johnson, A. & Smith, A.H.W. (1982) Ability of primary care physicians to make accurate ratings of psychiatric symptoms. *Archives of General Psychiatry*, 39, 829–833.

Hall, J.A., Roter, D.L., Blanch, D.C. & Frankel, R.M. (2009) Nonverbal sensitivity in medical students: Implications for clinical interactions. *Journal of General Internal Medicine*, 24 (no. 11), 1217–1222.

Halpern, J. (1993) Empathy: Using resonance emotions in the service of curiosity. In H.M. Spiro *et al.* (eds), *Empathy and the Practice of Medicine: Beyond Pills and the Scalpel*, pp.160–173. Yale University Press, New Haven, CT.

Halpern, J. (2001) *From Detached Concern to Empathy: Humanizing Medical Practice*. Oxford University Press, New York.

Hayward, R. (2005). Historical keywords: Empathy. *Lancet*, 366 (no. 9491), 1071.

Hojat, M. (2007) *Empathy in Patient Care: Antecedents, Development, Measurements, and Outcomes*. Springer, Berlin.

Hojat, M., Mangione, S., Gonnella, J.S., Nasca, T., Veloski, J.J. & Kane, G. (2001) Empathy in medical education and patient care. *Academic Medicine*, 76, 669.

Hojat, M., Louis, D.Z., Markham, F.W., Wende, R., Rabinowitch, C. & Gonnella, J.S. (2011) Physicians' empathy and clinical outcomes for diabetic patients. *Academic Medicine*, 86, 359–364.

Hulsman, R.L. (2009). Shifting goals in medical communication: Determinants of goal detection and response formation. *Patient Education and Counseling*, 74, 302–308.

Irving, P. & Dickson, D. (2004) Empathy: Towards a conceptual framework for health professionals. *International Journal of Health Care Quality Assurance*, 17 (no. 4), 212–220

Khanuja, S., Dongalikar, V., Arora, R. & Gupra, A. (2011) Empathy and sympathy in the medical profession: Should we stop the desertion? *Pravara Medical Review*, 3 (no. 3), 37–39.

Kinmonth, A.L., Woodcock, A., Griffin, S., Spiegal, N. & Campbell, M.J. (1998) Randomised controlled trial of patient centered care of diabetes in general practice: Impact on current wellbeing and future disease risk. *The diabetes care from diagnosis research team. BMJ*, 317, 1202–1208.

Kurtz, S., Silverman, J., Benson, J. & Draper, J. (2003) Marrying content and process in clinical method teaching: Enhancing the Calgary-Cambridge Guides. *Academic Medicine*, 78 (no. 8), 802–809.

Lamothe, M., Boujut, E., Zenasni, F. & Sultan, S. (2014) To be or not be empathic: The combined role of empathic concern and perspective taking in understanding burnout in general practice. *BMC Family Practice*, 15 (no. 15), 1–7.

Landau, R.L. (1993) And the least of these is empathy. In H.M. Spiro *et al.* (eds), *Empathy and the Practice of Medicine: Beyond Pills and the Scalpel*, pp.103–109. Yale University Press, New Haven, CT.

Linley, P.A. & Joseph, S. (2007) Therapy work and therapists' positive and negative well-being. *Journal of Social and Clinical Psychology*, 26, 385–403.

Lipps, T. (1935) Empathy, inner imitation, and sense-feelings. In: M. Rader (ed), *A Modern Book of Esthetics, 291–304*. Holt, Rinehart and Winston, New York.

Matthews, D., Suchman, A.L. & Branch, W.T. (1993) Making 'connexions': Enhancing the therapeutic potential of patient–clinician relationships. *Annals of internal Medicine*, 118 (no. 12), 973–977.

Mazzi, M.A., Bensing, J., Rimondini, M., Fletcher, I, Van Vliet, L., Zimmerman, C. & Deveugele, M. (2013) How do lay people assess the quality of physicians' communicative responses to patients' emotional cues and concerns? An international multicenter study based on video-taped medical consultations. *Patient Education and Counseling*, 90 (no. 3), 347–353.

Mercer, S.W. & Reynolds, W.J. (2002) Empathy and quality of care. *British Journal of General Practice*, 52, 9–13.

Mjaaland, T.A., Finset, A., Jensen, B.F. & Gulbrandsen, P. (2011) Physicians' responses to patients' expression of negative emotions in hospital consultations: A video-based observational study. *Patient Education and Counseling*, 84, 332–337.

Pedersen, R. (2008) Empathy: A wolf in sheep's clothing? *Medical Health Cara Philosophy*, 11, 325–335.

Pollak, L.I., Arnold, R.M., Jeffreys, A.S., Alexander, S.C., Olsen, M.K. & Abernethy, A.P. (2007) Oncologist communication about emotion during visits with patients with advanced cancer. *Journal of Clinical Oncology*, 25, 5748–5752.

Rakel, D.P., Hoeft, T.J., Barrett, B.P., Chewning, B.A., Craig, B.M. & Niu, M. (2009) Practitioner empathy and the duration of the common cold. *Family Medicine*, 41, 494–501.

Roter, D.L. & Hall, J.A. (2004) Physician gender and patient-centered communication: A critical review of empirical research. *Annual Review of Public Health*, 25, 497–519.

Roter, D.L., Hall, J.A., Kern, D.A., Barker, L.R., Cole, K.A. & Roca, R.P. (1995) Improving physicians' interviewing skills and reducing patients' emotional distress. A randomized clinical trial. *Archives of Internal Medicine*, 155, 1877–1884.

Satterfield, J.M. & Hughes, E. (2007) Emotion skills training for medical students: A systematic review. *Medical Education*, 41 (no. 10), 935–941.

Shanafelt, T.D., West, C., Zhao, X., Novotny, P., Kolars, J., Habermann, T. & Sloan, J. (2005) Relationship between increased personal well-being and enhanced empathy among internal medicine residents. *Journal of General Internal Medicine*, 20, 559–564.

Shields, C.G., Epstein, R.M., Franks, P., Fiscella, K., Duberstein, P., McDanniel, S.H. & Meldrum, S. (2005) Emotion language in primary care encounters: Reliability and validity of an emotion word count coding system. *Patient Education and Counseling*, 57, 232–238.

Smith, A., Juraskova, I., Butow, P., Miguel, C., Lopez, A.L., Chang, S., Brown, R. & Bernhard, J. (2011) Sharing vs caring – the relative impact of sharing decisions versus managing emotions on patient outcomes. *Patient Education and Counseling*, 82, 233–239.

Stone, A.L., Tai-Seale, M., Stults, C.D., Luiz, J.M. & Frankel, R.M. (2012) Three types of ambiguity in coding empathic interactions in primary care visits: Implications for research and practice. *Patient Education and Counseling*, 89, 63–68.

Stone, J. (1993) A deep dying. In H.M. Spiro *et al.* (eds), *Empathy and the Practice of Medicine: Beyond Pills and the Scalpel*, pp. 34–39. Yale University Press, New Haven, CT.

Stuart, M.R. & Lieberman, J.R. (1993) *The Fifteen Minute Hour: Applied Psychotherapy for the Primary Care Physician*. Praeger, New York.

Uitterhoeve, R., Bensing, J., Dilven, E., Donders, R., deMulder, P. & van Achterberg, T. (2009) Nurse–patient communication in cancer care: Does responding to patient's cues predict patient satisfaction with communication. *Psycho-Oncology*, 18, 1060–1068.

West, C.P., Tan, A.D., Habermann, T.M., Sloan, J.A. & Shanafelt, T.D. (2009) Association of resident fatigue and distress with perceived medical errors. *JAMA*, 302 (no. 12), 1294–1300.

Zachariae, R., Pedersen, C.G., Jensen, A.B., Ehrnrooth, E., Rossen, P.B. & von der Maase, H. (2003) Association of perceived physician communication style with patient satisfaction, distress, cancer-related self-efficacy, and perceived control over the disease. *British Journal of Cancer*, 88, 658–665.

Zimmermann, C., Del Piccolo, L. & Finset, A. (2007) Cues and concerns by patients in medical consultations: A literature review. *Psychological Bulletin*, 133, 438–463.

Zinn, W. (1993) The empathic physician. *Archives of Internal Medicine*, 153 (no. 3), 306–312.

CHAPTER 15

Breaking Bad News

Rob Lane

School of Medicine, University of Leeds, Leeds, UK

Historical context

Sharing adverse diagnoses with patients has always been a feature of medical practice. In the past it has been done badly and insensitively. As medicine focused on communication as a key component of professional practice, breaking bad news became an area of interest. Bad news was defined by Buckman (1984) as 'any information likely to alter drastically a patient's view of his or her future'.

The term 'breaking bad news' is paternalistic, implying it is something that a professional does to a patient, and in some of the literature it is now referred to as 'delivering difficult news'. This still does not go far enough to acknowledge that it is a two-way process, and the term should perhaps be 'sharing difficult news'.

Sharing difficult news is not different from any information sharing in a clinical context and should follow the same principles of establishing current understanding, listening to the patient to establish the level of language and the informational needs and delivering information in a logical way that is chunked, with checking of understanding and screening for new concerns. The big difference with sharing difficult news is the likelihood of strong emotional responses being experienced.

The aims of the sharing difficult news consultation are to help the patient retain important information and to reduce the psychological distress; the methodologies described are more aimed at managing the immediate emotional impact. Paul *et al.* (2009) in a review of the breaking bad news literature concluded that less than 2% were rigorous intervention studies, which addressed longer-term psychosocial outcomes, and that the evidence base was weak in this respect. Where long-term psychological outcomes were included there was little evidence to suggest a beneficial effect, although this is probably not surprising in light of the adversity and emotional distress faced by many receivers of bad news in the natural journey of their illness.

There is evidence that some clinicians have difficulty or lack the skills to share difficult news (Dosanib *et al.* 2001; Amiel *et al.* 2006), and that poor delivery of bad news has consequences for both patients (Lobb *et al.* 1999; Baile *et al.* 2000; Lamont and Christakis 2001) and doctors (Ramirez *et al.* 1995). For patients the outcomes include increased stress, poor adjustment and generally poorer health outcomes, whereas for doctors there is an increased risk of anxiety and burnout. A UK study of the helpfulness to patients of breaking bad news consultations (Barnett 2002) showed that just over 25% of patients were negative or very negative about the consultation, with doctors in surgical specialities most likely to be rated as unhelpful.

Clinical Communication in Medicine, First Edition. Edited by Jo Brown, Lorraine M. Noble, Alexia Papageorgiou and Jane Kidd.
© 2016 John Wiley & Sons, Ltd. Published 2016 by John Wiley & Sons, Ltd.

Overall the literature indicates that there are still problems in sharing difficult news despite a multitude of interventions over the past 3 decades, and this continues to have consequences for both patients and professionals.

Current practice

An important question is, what do patients want? A French study (Sastre *et al.* 2011) retrospectively surveying patients who had received bad news demonstrated that the acceptability of the interview was related to the quality of the information (understandability, personalisation and completeness) and the demonstration of emotional support, these two factors accounting for 95% of the variation. Wittmann *et al.* (2011) showed that 79% of patients with stomach or oesophageal cancer wanted as much information as possible; however, only 35% of doctors were willing to give this. It still left 21% of patients who did not want such complete information.

A number of studies support the requirement of patient-centredness and empathy in the process (Randall & Wearn 2005; Schmid *et al.* 2005; Martins & Carvalho 2013). Brown *et al.* (2011), in a survey of British cancer patients, showed that most dissatisfaction arose from doctors who were perceived as unsympathetic or pessimistic in manner. The survey also demonstrated that most patients wanted a collaborative role in decision making.

Doctors tend to focus on disease-related matters: Vail *et al.* (2011) showed that this was not related to age, sex, place of qualification or specialty. To overcome this a number of protocols have been devised to guide clinicians through the process of sharing difficult news; examples include SPIKES (Baile *et al.* 2000), ABCDE (VandeKieft 2001) and BREAKS (Narayanan *et al.* 2010). Details of these and other protocols can be found in the work of Buckman (1984), Maguire and Faulkner (1988), Kaye (1996), Rabow and McPhee (2000), Hagerty *et al.* (2005b) and Kaplan (2010).

Silverman *et al.* (2013) summarise the components of the common protocols. The majority include:

- establishing the patient's current knowledge and willingness to receive bad news;
- using a warning shot;
- making a direct and simple statement;
- addressing the patient's agenda in terms of feelings and concerns and
- the giving of professional information.

Whatever protocol is used there is evidence that doctors are more willing to communicate about a serious illness if the prognosis is good (Wittmann *et al.* 2011).

The need to uncover a patient's concerns to lessen anxiety and preoccupation when the professional is giving information is emphasised by Baile and Beale (2003). Sep *et al.* (2014), using healthy volunteers, demonstrated that physiological arousal declined more quickly when empathy was used and that this led to better retention of information, a finding that needs testing with real patients.

Whitney *et al.* (2008) make the case for hope and hopefulness in sharing bad news encounters, stating that maintaining hopefulness helps the patient adjust to the news. They discuss the changing role of hope and what can be hoped for as a disease progresses. The importance of realistic hope is also emphasised by VandeKieft (2001).

Work by Burgers *et al.* (2012) suggests that patients respond more favourably to positively framed statements; for example, 40% of patients will be alive after 5 years as opposed to 60% of patients will die from this illness within 5 years.

Shaw *et al.* (2012) used simulated consultations to show that doctors tended to use one of three styles when sharing difficult news that they described as blunt (information given within 30 seconds), forecasting (staged delivery within first 2 minutes) and stalling (news delayed more than 2 minutes). It was noted that in the stalling style the doctor rarely delivered the news directly but relied on the patient to come to a conclusion. Of the 31 doctors studied, just over a third used the blunt style, 45% the forecasting and 20% the stalling style. The blunt and forecasting styles gave clarity of information, with forecasting giving more descriptive information. Those using stalling used medical terminology and euphemisms more. Stalling increased consultation time, led to inconsistencies in the message and created more anxiety, confusion and distress in the simulated patients. Patient support and tailored information giving followed both the blunt and forecasting style; the blunt style led to fewer questions from patients. On balance it would appear that the forecasting style gives best results.

When discussing prognosis there is evidence that a majority of patients wish to be told but that a significant minority do not (Kapowitz *et al.* 2002; Hagerty *et al.* 2005a). Hagerty *et al.* (2005a) revealed that almost half of patients with cancer recurrence who wanted to know about prognosis wished the doctor to bring up the topic but that oncologists, in general, preferred the topic to be raised by the patient. There was also a difference in the type of information that patients wanted, the postal survey by Kapowitz *et al.* (2002) showed that 80% of patients wanted qualitative information (e.g. will I die from this disease?) but that only about half wanted quantitative information (e.g. how long will I survive?); 90% of those wanting qualitative information got it but only half of those who wanted quantitative information got it. However, over 60% of those not wanting quantitative information were given it. Failure of the patient to ask was a key contributor to not getting information (15% of those wanting qualitative and 33% of those wanting quantitative information). When quantitative information was given it tended to be an overestimate (Lamont & Christakis 2001). Step and Ray (2011) found changes in communication style when cancer recurred, with professionals becoming more business-like and less emotionally supportive than during prognosis discussions when cure was possible.

Much of the literature covers Western society and the question has to be asked – is it different elsewhere? There is evidence that attitudes are moving towards an open approach to sharing difficult information with patients, although resistance still exists. Adeleye and Fatiregun (2013) showed that there was a willingness in Nigerian neurosurgery patients (97%) to accept bad news, which is said to reflect a change in attitude. Similarly, in a Malaysian study Eng *et al.* (2012) showed that cancer patients in a tertiary centre were seeking honest, open and face-to-face disclosure of information. This contrasts with a Pakistani study (Ishaque *et al.* 2010) where only 40% of patients believed it was a patient's right to know bad news. Khalil (2013) reviewed the situation in Middle Eastern countries and found pressure from relatives to withhold truth, with physicians seeming confused and demonstrating mixed practice.

Sharing difficult news has an impact on professionals. Brown *et al.* (2009), using simulated bad news consultations, showed that less experienced doctors showed higher stress levels and those showing signs of burnout or fatigue performed less well. Shaw *et al.* (2013) conducted semistructured interviews with doctors and explored their experience of breaking bad news. Most described it as stressful and stated that they had physical and emotional symptoms (including sweating, palpitations, and feeling drained, distressed and anxious) that included anticipatory stress and that for some continued long after the event and impacted on their social life. Views were expressed that acknowledging this would lead to them being seen as weak by peers. A range of coping strategies was used, which included planning for the interview, structuring the work environment to minimise exposure, avoiding delivery altogether, focusing on nonemotional aspects of care, positive reframing, setting themselves realistic expectations of their role and accepting their limitations, distancing and social support. Senior doctors were more likely to use positive reframing than juniors; for example, looking at palliative treatment as something that would improve quality of life rather than at treatment that would not cure. Myers *et al.* (2007) similarly looked at the impact of delivering a positive HIV result on professionals. The majority reported a pronounced impact on themselves, describing the event as stressful or dramatic and attributing a negative change over time on their emotional state. Similar coping strategies were used but with comment also made on the use of alcohol, snack foods and black humour.

Future directions

From the literature it can be seen that patients want information that is understandable, personalized and complete; professional training needs to focus on these components of information giving and individuals given feedback to allow practice and improvement. Shaw *et al.* (2012) showed that a stalling style of delivery rarely gave clarity of information and this needs to be addressed in training. Patients are indicating a desire to hear news that is positively framed (Burgers *et al.* 2012).

Professional training needs to focus on the giving of emotional support as well as the delivery of information if patients' needs are to be met. In particular the skills of empathy and cue recognition and response need to be emphasised. Cue recognition and response ensures that the patient's agenda is made explicit and dealt with as the priority, reducing patient anxiety and increasing ability to hear professional information (Baile & Beale 2003).

Having shared difficult news there is a need for professionals to be more inclusive in involving patients in decision making at the level they desire. It may help for doctors to have models for sharing difficult information; the model used will depend on personal preference and comfort. It is just as important that doctors can be flexible in sharing information and that models are for guidance only and not always rigidly followed.

Patients' needs around prognostic information do not seem to be being met; this may in part be due to the difficulties of giving accurate quantitative information but also suggests that professionals do not proactively seek out the information needs of their patients in this area. Being aware that a significant minority of patients are not seeking prognostic information may inhibit professionals from exploring these issues.

Future training needs to focus on developing the skills to establish the informational needs of patients, particularly the need for qualitative and quantitative information and for doctors to feel skilled to initiate more of these conversations. It needs to be recognised that sharing difficult information has an emotional impact on the professional; just recognising this and making it explicit would be a helpful step forward. It is only by openly acknowledging the difficulties for professionals that barriers to communication can be addressed and more open communication established. The culture of healthcare needs to change and become more supportive to individuals.

References

Adeleye, A.O. & Fatiregun, A.A. (2013) Is breaking of bad news indeed unacceptable to native Africans? A cross-sectional survey of patients in a Nigerian neurosurgical service. *Acta Neurologica Scandinavica*, 127, 175–180.

Amiel, G. Ungar, L. & Alperin, M. (2006) Ability of primary care physicians to break bad news: A performance based assessment of an educational intervention. *Patient Education and Counseling*, 60, 10–15.

Baile, W.F. & Beale, E.A. (2003) Giving bad news to cancer patients: Matching process and content. *Journal of Clinical Oncology*, 21, 49s–51s.

Baile, W.F. Buckman, R., Lenzi, R., Glober, G., Beale, E.A. & Kudelka, A.P. (2000) SPIKES – a six-step protocol for delivering bad news: Application to the patient with cancer. *Oncologist*, 5, 302–311.

Barnett, M.M. (2002) Effect of breaking bad news on patients' perceptions of doctors. *Journal of the Royal Society of Medicine*, 95 (no. 7), 343–347.

Brown, R., Dunn, S., Byrnes, K., Morris, R., Heinrich, P. & Shaw, J. (2009) Doctors' stress responses and poor communication performance in simulated bad-news consultations. *Academic Medicine*, 84 (no. 11), 1595–1602.

Brown, V.A., Parker, P.A., Furber, L. & Thomas, A.L. (2011) Patient preferences for the delivery of bad news – the experience of a UK Cancer Centre. *European Journal of Cancer Care*, 20 (no. 1), 56–61.

Buckman, R. (1984) Breaking bad news: Why is it still so difficult? *BMJ*, 288, 1597–1599.

Burgers, C., Beukeboom, C.J. & Sparks, L. (2012) How the doc should (not) talk: When breaking bad news with negations influences patients' immediate responses and medical adherence intentions. *Patient Education and Counseling* 89 (no. 2), 267–273.

Dosanjh, S., Barnes, J. & Bhandari, M. (2001) Barriers to breaking bad news amongst medical and surgical residents. *Medical Education*, 35, 197–205.

Eng, T.C., Yaakup, H., Shah, S.A., Jaffar, A. & Omar, K. (2012) Preferences of Malaysian cancer patients in communication of bad news. *Asian Pacific Journal of Cancer Prevention*, 13 (no. 6), 2749–2752.

Hagerty, R.G., Butow, P.N., Ellis, P.M., Dimitry, S. & Tattersall, M.H.N. (2005a) Communicating prognosis in cancer care: A systematic review of the literature. *Annals of Oncology*, 16, 1005–1053.

Hagerty, R.G., Butow, P.N., Ellis, P.M., Lobb, E.A., Pendlebury, S., Leigh, N. & Tattersall, M.H. (2005b) Communicating with realism and hope: Incurable cancer patients' views on the disclosure of prognosis. *Journal of Clinical Oncology*, 23, 1278–1288.

Ishaque, S., Saleem, T., Khawaja, F.B. & Qidwai, W. (2010) Breaking bad news: Exploring patient's perspective and expectations. *Journal of Pakistan Medical Association*, 60 (no. 5), 407–411.

Kaplan, M. (2010) SPIKES: A framework for breaking bad news to patients with cancer. *Clinical Journal of Oncology Nursing*, 14 (no. 4), 514–516.

Kapowitz, S., Campo, S. & Chiu, W. (2002) Cancer patients' desires for communication of prognosis information. *Health Communication*, 14 (no. 2), 221–241.

Kaye, P. (1996) *Breaking Bad News: A 10 Step Approach*. EPL Publications, Northampton, UK.

Khalil, R.B. (2013) Attitudes, beliefs and perceptions regarding truth disclosure of cancer-related information in the Middle East: A review. *Palliative and Supportive Care*, 11 (no. 1), 69–78.

Lamont, E. & Christakis, N. (2001) Prognostic disclosure to patients with cancer near the end of life. *Annals of Internal Medicine*, 134, 1096–1105.

Lobb, E., Butow, P., Kenny, D. & Tattersall, M. (1999) Communicating prognosis in early breast cancer: Do women understand the language used? *Medical Journal of Australia*, 171, 290–294.

Maguire, P. & Faulkner, A. (1988) Communicate with cancer patients: 1. Handling bad news and difficult questions. *BMJ*, 297 (no. 6653), 907–909.

Martins, G.R. & Carvalho, I.P. (2013) Breaking bad news: Patients' preferences and health locus of control. *Patient Education and Counseling*, 92, 67–73.

Myers, T., Worthington, C., Aguinaldo, J.P., Haubrich, D.J., Ryder, K. & Rawson, B. (2007) Impact on HIV test providers of giving a positive test result. *AIDS Care*, 19 (no. 8), 1013–1019.

Narayanan, V., Bista, B. & Koshy, C. (2010) 'BREAKS' protocol for breaking bad news. *Indian Journal of Palliative Care*, 16 (no. 2), 61–65.

Paul, C.L., Clinton-McHarg, T., Sanson-Fisher, R.W., Douglas, H. & Webb, G. (2009) Are we there yet? The state of the evidence base for guidelines on breaking bad news to cancer patients. *European Journal of Cancer*, 45, 2960–2966.

Rabow, M. & McPhee, S. (2000) Beyond breaking bad news: Helping patients who suffer. *Student BMJ*, 8, 45–88.

Ramirez, A., Graham, J., Richards, M. & Gregory, W.M. (1995) Burnout and psychiatric disorder amongst cancer clinicians. *British Journal of Cancer*, 71, 1263–1269.

Randall, T. & Wearn, A. (2005) Receiving bad news: Patients with haematological cancer reflect upon their experience. *Palliative Medicine*, 19 (no. 8), 594–601.

Sastre, M.T.M., Sorum, P.C. & Mullet, E. (2011) Breaking bad news: The patient's viewpoint. *Health Communication*, 26, 649–655.

Schmid Mast, M., Kindlimann, A. & Langewitz, W. (2005) Recipients' perspective on breaking bad news: How you put it really makes a difference. *Patient Education and Counseling*, 58 (no. 3), 244–251.

Sep, M.S.C., van Osch, M., van Vliet, L.M., Smets, E.M.A. & Bensing J.M. (2014) The power of clinicians' affective communication: How reassurance about non-abandonment can reduce patients' physiological arousal and increase information recall in bad news consultations. An experimental study using analogue patients. *Patient Education and Counseling*, 95, 45–52.

Shaw, J.M., Brown, R.F. & Dunn, S.M. (2013) A qualitative study of stress and coping responses in doctors breaking bad news. *Patient Education and Counseling*, 91, 243–248.

Shaw, J.M., Dunn, S.M. & Heinrich, P. (2012) Managing the delivery of bad news: An in-depth analysis of doctors' delivery style. *Patient Education and Counseling*, 87 (no. 2), 186–192.

Silverman, J., Kurtz, S. & Draper, J. (2013) *Skills for Communicating with Patients*, third edn. Radcliffe Publishing, London.

Step, M.M. & Ray, E.B. (2011) Patient perceptions of oncologist–patient communication about prognosis: Changes from initial diagnosis to cancer recurrence. *Health Communication*, 26, 48–58.

Vail, L., Sandhu, H., Fisher, J., Cooke, H., Dale, J. & Barnett, M. (2011) Hospital consultants breaking bad news with simulated patients: An analysis of communication using the Roter Interaction Analysis System. *Patient Education and Counseling*, 83, 185–194.

VandeKieft, G.K. (2001) Breaking bad news. *American Family Physician*, 15, 64 (no. 12), 1975–1978.

Whitney, S.N., McCullough, L.B., Fruge, E., McGuire, A.L. & Volk, R.J. (2008) Beyond breaking bad news: The roles of hope and hopefulness. *Cancer*, 113 (no. 2), 442–445.

Wittmann, E., Beaton, C., Lewis, W.G., Hopper, A.N., Zamawi, F., Jackson, C., Dave, B., Bowen, R., Willacombe, A., Blackshaw, G. & Crosby, T.D. (2011) Comparison of patients' needs and doctors' perceptions of information requirements related to a diagnosis of oesophageal or gastric cancer. *European Journal of Cancer Care*, 20 (no. 2), 187–195.

CHAPTER 16

Facilitating Behaviour Change through Motivational Interviewing

Eva Doherty

Royal College of Surgeons in Ireland, Dublin, Ireland

Historical context

Motivational interviewing has its roots in the treatment of substance use disorders and was described in 1983 by William Miller (Miller 1983). It was recently defined to be a 'collaborative, person-centred form of guiding to elicit and strengthen motivation to change' (Miller & Rollnick 2009, p. 137). The method has been evaluated in hundreds of outcome studies, and meta-analyses of the effectiveness of the method have reported small to medium effects in indicators of change in health-related behaviours (Rubak *et al.* 2005; Lundahl *et al.* 2013). Motivational interviewing has been shown to be particularly effective for substance use disorders, smoking, weight loss, gambling and medical outcomes such as blood pressure, cholesterol, dental cavities, HIV viral load and improving risk of mortality following a stroke (Miller & Rollnick 2014). Motivational interviewing is a specific clinical method used to enhance personal motivation and at the time of its inception was not intended to be a conceptual theory of change. Thus the motivational interviewing method sits alongside and complements theories of behaviour change such as the transtheoretical model (TTM) of change (Prochaska & DiClemente 1984) but should not be confused with it (Miller & Rollnick 2009).

Current practice

The motivational interviewing method requires the doctor to engage in an empathic conversation with patients about their motivation and their confidence in the possibility of change. The skills are not easy and can feel counter-intuitive (Miller & Rollnick 2009). To use them effectively, one must inhibit a natural inclination to tell the individual the 'right thing to do for their own good', as the aim is to elicit the individual's own motivation to change and support the individual in setting and achieving realistic goals, thus enabling him or her to be in control of long-term change. Miller and Rollnick advise that users should ideally have proficiency in a person-centred counselling style and specifically in the therapeutic skills of accurate empathy (Miller & Rollnick 2009). Training in motivational interviewing is widely available and an organisation known as MINT (Motivational Interviewing Network of Trainers) provides resources and training (www.motivationalinterviewing.org). Clinicians who do not consider

Clinical Communication in Medicine, First Edition. Edited by Jo Brown, Lorraine M. Noble, Alexia Papageorgiou and Jane Kidd.

themselves to be skilled counsellors can still achieve clinically significant results using the principles of motivational interviewing (Rubak *et al.* 2005). Motivational interviewing is attractive for doctors who struggle with time constraints; however, it is important to be clear about what doctors can reasonably achieve and when it is appropriate to refer patients to other healthcare professionals for follow-up counselling (Campos-Outcalt & Calonge 2012).

The Institute of Medicine, a not-for-profit nongovernment organisation in the United States dedicated to the provision of national advice on issues relating to biomedical science, medicine and health, has reported that medical schools do not provide sufficient training in behavioural counselling methods despite the fact that patient health behaviours account for half of all deaths in the United States (Institute of Medicine 2004). A recent systematic review of behaviour change counselling curricula for medical trainees identified 109 studies (61: medical students; 47: postgraduate, 1: both) and concluded that 77 of these demonstrated improved learner performance and 12 showed actual benefit to patients or organisational practice (Hauer *et al.* 2012). There is also good evidence to show that motivational interviewing skills can be taught to doctors and that their behaviours change as a result of this training: a systematic review of the effectiveness of motivational interviewing training for health and mental health professionals concluded that significant practitioner behaviour change occurred in 17 of the 22 studies identified (Barwick *et al.* 2012).

The method of motivational interviewing involves the following four overlapping processes:
1 engaging is the process by which both parties establish a helpful connection and a working relationship;
2 focussing is the process by which the direction of behaviour change, if desired, is clarified;
3 evoking is the process by which the motivation for change is made explicit and
4 planning is the process that encompasses the development of the commitment to change and formulation of a specific plan of action.
The reader is referred to the third edition of Miller and Rollnick's book, *Motivational Interviewing* (Miller & Rollnick 2013), for detailed descriptions of these four processes.

A combination of didactic teaching accompanied with role-playing with actors or colleagues has been recommended as a useful technique in the delivery of motivational interviewing teaching courses (Hauer *et al.* 2012). Experiencing the difference between being told what to do about a problem versus the experience of being listened to in an empathic, nonconfrontational and nonjudgemental manner helps the learner to understand the difference between traditional methods and the motivational interviewing approach. One of the aims of motivational interviewing is to help the individual to explore the benefits of changing behaviour and the real differences these changes can make to one's life. The following five questions can be used to demonstrate to beginners the essence of a motivational conversation with someone about changing a behaviour (Miller & Rollnick 2013, p. 11):
1 'Why would you want to make this change?'
2 'How might you go about it in order to succeed?'
3 'What are the three best reasons for you to do it?'
4 'How important is it for you to make this change and why?'
…following a brief synopsis of the answers to the above four questions, the fifth and final question can be asked (if deemed appropriate):
5 'So what do you think you'll do?'

Group discussions with learners focus on how challenging it feels to resist giving advice and how rewarding it feels to be understood and not to be told what to do. The training can be enhanced with videos of patients discussing a problem, with demonstrations of the use of the motivational interviewing skills that helped them to achieve their behaviour change. Accurate empathy is a critical component of the motivational interviewing method, and role-playing exercises can be used to demonstrate this skill.

Using motivational interviewing skills may feel like a paradigm shift to the learners who may be more used to traditional methods of medical history taking, and so the trainer can watch out for resistance in the group and use this as an opportunity to demonstrate the principle of 'rolling with the resistance' (Miller & Rollnick 2013). Issues around confidence and belief in the possibility of achieving this change in their skill set may surface in the learners' minds, and these doubts need to be understood and empathy demonstrated. As with patients, 'change talk' may only progress if the learners indicate a motivation to change; that is, that they wish to learn these skills, and if this is not forthcoming, the training can adapt to this resistance. It may be important to make the existence of any resistance explicit to the learners and thereby model the technique in real time. Childers *et al.* (2012) have published a motivational interviewing curriculum for junior doctors in training that is 12 hours duration and can be taught over a total of three 4-hour sessions.

Motivational interviewing training can be assessed by the change in learners' skills following the course and also by the assessment of change in learners' knowledge and attitudes and their satisfaction with the training. Previous evidence indicates that the opportunity to practise the skills through the use of simulation and role-play are highly rated by learners (Childers *et al.* 2012; Hauer *et al.* 2012). In addition to the assessment tools described in cited literature, there are also a number of tools available on the MINT website (www.motivationalinterviewing.org) to assist with the evaluation of motivational interviewing skills.

Future directions

Supporting patients to care for themselves and empowering them to maintain healthy lifestyles is a significant challenge for effective healthcare delivery, and so the acquisition of a set of skills that have been proven to help patients to make lifestyle changes is invaluable for both doctors and patients. Future training programmes can include discussion of the limitations to what can be realistically achieved and training can focus on the enhancement of doctors' awareness of when to intervene and when to refer on for specialist counselling.

References

Barwick, M.A., Bennett, L.M., Johnson, S.N., McGowan, J. & Moore, J. (2012) Training health and mental health professionals in motivational interviewing: A systematic review. *Children and Youth Services Review*, 34, 1786–1795.

Campos-Outcalt, D. & Calonge, N. (2012) Adding realism and perspective to behavioural counselling curricula for medical students. *Academic Medicine*, 87, 840–841.

Childers, J.W., Bost, J.E., Kraemer, K.L., Cluss, P.A., Spagnoletti, C.L., Gonzaga, A.M.B. & Arnold, R.M. (2012) Giving residents tools to talk about behavior change: A motivational interviewing curriculum description and evaluation. *Patient Education and Counselling*, 89, 281–287.

Hauer, K.E., Carney, P.A., Chang, A. & Satterfield, J. (2012) Behavior change counseling curricula for medical trainees: A systematic review. *Academic Medicine*, 87, 956–968.

Institute of Medicine. (2004) *Improving Medical Education: Enhancing the Behavioural and Social Science Content of Medical School Curricula*. National Academies Press, Washington, DC.

Lundahl, B., Moleni, T., Burke, B.L., Butters, R., Tollefson, D., Butler, C. & Rollnick, S. (2013) Motivational interviewing in medical care settings: A systematic review and meta-analysis of randomized controlled trials. *Patient Education and Counselling*, 93, 157–168.

Miller, W.R. (1983) Motivational interviewing with problem drinkers. *Behavioural and Cognitive Psychotherapy*, 11, 147–172.

Miller, W.R. & Rollnick, S. (2009) Ten things that motivational interviewing is not. *Behavioural and Cognitive Psychotherapy*, 37, 129–140.

Miller, W.R. & Rollnick, S. (2013) *Motivational Interviewing: Helping People Change*, third edn. Guildford Press, New Yok.

Miller, W.R. & Rollnick S. (2014) The effectiveness and ineffectiveness of complex behavioral interventions: Impact of treatment fidelity. *Contemporary Clinical Trials*, 37, 234–241.

Prochaska, J.O. DiClemente, C.C. (1984) *The Transtheoretical Approach: Crossing Traditional Boundaries of Therapy*. Dow/Jones Irwin, Homewood, IL.

Rubak, S, Sandboek, A., Lauritzen, T. & Christensen, B. (2005) Motivational interviewing: A systematic review and meta-analysis. *British Journal of General Practice*, 55, 305–312.

CHAPTER 17

Responding to Medical Error and Complaints

Lucy Ambrose[1] and Lindsey Pope[2]

[1]*General practitioner, The Tutbury Practice, Tutbury, Staffordshire, UK*
[2]*Undergraduate Medical School, College of Medical, Veterinary and Life Sciences, University of Glasgow, Glasgow, UK*

Historical overview

The relationship between healthcare professionals and patients is not equal when it comes to error. Historically, healthcare professions have been seen to close ranks to defend their reputations when things go wrong. Patients and families in repeated events where people were harmed have been left fighting for information about errors and details of what has happened (Kennedy 2001; Francis 2013). Sadly this defensive culture is still present in healthcare.

Error

An error is defined as something incorrectly done through ignorance or inadvertence; a mistake, for example, in calculation, judgment, speech, writing, action and so forth (*Oxford English Dictionary* 2014). Therefore errors are closely linked to communication in all its various forms. Error in healthcare is a complex phenomenon and there are different taxonomies that try to explain why errors occur (Croskerry 2003; Reason 2008). A widely used framework, outlining error in practice, has been described by Reason (2008). It shows that errors occur as a result of:
- skill-based behaviours; for example, completing a physical examination;
- rule-based behaviours; for example, following a management guideline; and
- knowledge-based behaviours; for example, making a decision about prescribing.

Research over a 20-year period has demonstrated that medical error is a common problem (Leape 1994). Approximately 10–20% of patients will experience an adverse event as they pass through healthcare systems (Leape 1994; Kohn *et al.* 2000; Vincent *et al.* 2001). This evidence, alongside investigations into situations where patients have been harmed (Francis 2013), has highlighted the central role of communication in maintaining a safe environment for patients. Errors in communication, both with patients and colleagues, are a frequent cause of harm to patients. Conversely, good communication is key to resolving the consequences of medical error.

Clinical Communication in Medicine, First Edition. Edited by Jo Brown, Lorraine M. Noble, Alexia Papageorgiou and Jane Kidd.
© 2016 John Wiley & Sons, Ltd. Published 2016 by John Wiley & Sons, Ltd.

How does communication cause error?

Communication skills are most often seen as a core component in resolving error, but they are also a central cause of error. These can occur in a number of situations in health care and each is discussed below.

Errors in communication between health professionals and patients

The main errors that are identified in the literature relate to the following features of communication skills, specifically insufficient or inappropriate skills in:

1 information gathering, leading to errors in clinical reasoning; for example, making the wrong diagnosis because of premature closure of information gathering;
2 relationship building; for example, anger and frustration from the patient about unmet expectations or a lack of empathy within the consultation; and
3 information sharing, leading to errors in management; for example, consent for surgical procedures and information giving about drug interactions and the side effects of medications.

Reducing error in communication with patients

Good communication and a positive relationship between a patient and his or her healthcare professional results in less error and better outcomes (Rodriguez *et al.* 2008; Buetow *et al.* 2010; Longtin *et al.* 2010; Hojat *et al.* 2011).

There is evidence to suggest that relationship building is the most important aspect from the patient's perspective (Rodrigeuz *et al.* 2008; Hojat *et al.* 2011). If health professionals have high-quality interactions with patients and coordinate well with other health professionals, then patients are less likely to complain or to initiate litigation (Rodriguez *et al.* 2008). Empathy is specifically associated with better patient outcomes (Hojat *et al.* 2011).

Therefore, developing proficiency in communication skills is a key aspect of error reduction. Understanding how to structure information gathering, alongside developing knowledge about the different types of presentation of illness, allows healthcare professionals to gather appropriate and full information. When sharing information, using structured tools can help reduce error. The SPIKES framework was developed for breaking bad news (Buckman 2005) but is applicable to all instances of information sharing. It was designed as a gold standard for situations where poor communication and errors could be harmful to patients and their carers. All the evidence in this area suggests a thorough and empathetic health professional who listens is less likely to be involved in error (Rodriguez *et al.* 2008; Buetow *et al.* 2010; Longtin *et al.* 2010; Hojat *et al.* 2011).

Errors in communication between health professionals

The negative impact of poor communication is not only seen in health professional–patient communication but also in communication between health professionals. Poor coordination of care is a trigger for complaints and litigation (Rodriguez *et al.* 2008).

Handover is a common situation in which errors occur, and this has resulted in structured protocols and checklists being developed to improve communication between healthcare professionals. (Leonard *et al.* 2004; Haynes *et al.* 2009). The SBAR tool (Situation, Background, Assessment and Recommendation) is an example where using a structured tool can improve the content and structure of handover communication

Box 17.1 Example of Interprofessional Communication Using the SBAR Handover Checklist.

Situation	Identify yourself and the site/unit you are calling from. Identify the patient by name and the reason for your call. Describe your concern.	My name is Andrea Brown, I am a staff nurse on the children's ward 104. I am ringing about Jack Jones, who has abdominal pain and is now showing signs of sepsis.
Background	Give the patient's reason for admission. Explain significant medical history. Inform them of the patient's background: admitting diagnosis, date of admission, prior procedures, current medications, allergies, pertinent results and other relevant diagnostic results.	Jack Jones is a 12-year-old boy who was admitted 2 hours ago with abdominal pain starting in his right iliac fossa. Initial bloods were taken on admission and he has an elevated white cell count at 16.4 and C reactive protein of 48. He was started on intravenous fluids and we are awaiting radiology. He is normally fit and well and does not take any regular medication and has no known allergies.
Assessment	Vital signs. Relevant positive and negative findings. Clinical impressions, concerns.	Jack Jones's vital signs have deteriorated within the last 30 minutes. His temperature is 39.5°C, his pulse is 145, his respiratory rate is 28 and his blood pressure is 96/60. His oxygen saturations are 95%. I am concerned that he is now showing signs of sepsis.
Recommendations	Explain what you need (be specific and give a time frame). Clarify expectations.	I am very concerned about this child as I believe he is septic. I would like an immediate review by a senior doctor. How long will it be before you can get here? Is there anything you would like me to do before you get here?

(Leonard *et al.* 2004; NHS Institute for Innovation and Improvement 2008; Marshall *et al.* 2009; Institute for Healthcare Improvement 2015).

Box 17.1 gives an example of how this might be used. A staff nurse is concerned about a 12-year-old boy on surgical ward who has abdominal pain. His vital signs have deteriorated and she would like him to be reviewed urgently.

The WHO Surgical Safety checklist uses a team-based approach to structure communication of information within operating theatres. It improves communication across the theatre team, reducing error and improving patient outcomes (Haynes *et al.* 2009; de Vries *et al.* 2010; Einav *et al.* 2010). The checklist has three steps for every patient:

- sign in;
- time out and
- sign out.

Each checklist enables a comprehensive overview of critical safety issues for each patient, from elements such as patient identity and allergy status to surgical site infection prevention and recovery requirements. This level of detailed communication and coordination between health professionals is shown to reduce error and improve outcomes.

How can communication help to resolve the consequences of error?

Communication is central to all aspects of responding to error (O'Connor *et al.* 2010). Once an error has occurred, the way that communication is handled can have either a positive or negative impact on outcomes for patients and health professionals. The literature highlights that patients need an acknowledgement that an incident has occurred alongside information about how the incident happened, how a recurrence will be prevented and an apology (O'Connor *et al.* 2010). There is also evidence to suggest that there is a gulf between the information and attitudes patients and their families wish for (O'Connor *et al.* 2010) and what actually happens (Kaldjian *et al.* 2007; Kroll *et al.* 2008).

Openness about error

The lack of openness about error is thought to result from health professionals' fear of medico-legal action being initiated against them, and this distances them from patients, who desire transparency and openness (Crane 2001). Patients are likely to feel fewer distressing psychological after-effects if health professionals are open with them about what has happened (Vincent & Coulter 2002). Open disclosure is an example of a communication strategy that encourages health professionals to discuss errors with patients after an adverse event occurs (Australian Commission for Safety and Quality in Healthcare 2013). Box 17.2 provides a summary of steps in open disclosure where direct communication is important.

Example: being open about a medication error

Here is an example of a scenario and possible responses that a doctor might make that could be used as a basis for discussion in a training session.

You are a junior doctor and you are called to see an 81-year-old woman, Mrs Irene Smith, who has just been admitted with a kidney infection and is confused. She was admitted by your colleague, Dr John, who has prescribed a penicillin-based antibiotic to treat her. You are called by the ward staff, who tell you that her husband has just arrived and informed them that she has had an adverse reaction to penicillin previously. She has been given a single dose intravenously. He has asked to speak to a doctor and asks how this could have happened.

Scenario A. The adverse reaction experienced previously was diarrhoea and vomiting.
'I am very sorry that this has happened. It is clear that something unexpected has occurred but fortunately you were able to point this out to us quickly and I hope that Mrs Smith will not suffer harm from it. However, we will keep an eye on her for the next 24 hours and will ask you to let us know if you think she is getting any problems from the medication. We do not expect that Mrs Smith will need to stay here any longer than originally planned.'

Scenario B. The adverse reaction experienced previously was a severe rash that needed hospital admission for 72 hours.
'I am very sorry that this has happened. It is clear that something went wrong. It is fortunate that you were able to point this out to us quickly. We have given Mrs Smith treatment to help reduce any allergic reaction she might develop. She has not shown any signs of an allergic

Box 17.2 Direct Communication in Open Disclosure.

Steps in Open Disclosure	Communication Tips
Demonstrate honesty and candour.	The effectiveness of being open is linked to sincerity, including the health professional's tone of voice and his or her nonverbal communication, such as body language, gestures and facial expression.
A sincere and unprompted apology or expression of regret.	Using the words 'I am sorry' or 'we are sorry' is important for both patients and health professionals. The distinction between an apology or expression of regret and a factual explanation of the adverse event is important, as both can occur in the same conversation. An apology or expression of regret can be given once harm has been recognised, but a full explanation needs the facts to be established.
Tell the patient and family what has happened, including a clear explanation of the incident.	Gather accurate information before the discussion. You will need facts to be established before you can give a full explanation. If you do not have full facts it is important to be honest about what you do not know. Avoid speculating on the causes of the incident. Try not to attribute blame to any individual, group or system. Avoid preempting results of reviews and investigations.
Give the patient and his or her family or carers a chance to tell their story and to describe the personal effects of the adverse event.	Use active listening techniques. Ask open questions.
Explain what has happened to address the event and what will happen to prevent future events.	Give clear information about what has been done to help the patient and what will be done to prevent the incident happening again.
Provide a written document or record.	This should be available to both the patient and family and other health professionals.

reaction so far, but we will monitor her closely to identify if any problems arise. Please tell us if you think she is experiencing any side effects or a reaction to the antibiotic. We are also investigating the incident right now to find out how this happened. We will give you information as it comes to hand. It is very important for us to understand what you think happened. We can go through this now if you like, or we can wait until you are ready to talk about it.'

Responding to complaints

Responding to complaints involves the same principles as open disclosure. Frequently at this stage the two parties involved may be distant, and strong negative emotions are often present on both sides. What is key is acknowledging that something has gone wrong and apologising (O'Connor *et al.* 2010). Many regulatory bodies offer advice about how to respond to a complaint, and they include the elements of open disclosure with additional suggestions about professional behaviours linked to communication such as being patient focused, being open and accountable, acting fairly and proportionately and putting things right (Parliamentary and Health Service Ombudsman 2009).

Supporting colleagues after errors occur

A final component in medical error is communication between health professionals in coping with error and handling the anxiety that it brings. Communication skills are vital in supporting colleagues and enabling them to continue in caring for patients. In the literature, the health professional is sometimes referred to as a second victim (Wu 2000). The principles of supporting a colleague include encouraging the clinician involved to talk and reflect on the error (College of Emergency Medicine 2013). This involves the core communication skills of demonstration of empathy and active listening.

Future directions

It is inevitable with the complexity and uncertainty of medical practice that errors will occur. The defensive approach adopted historically by health professions when errors occur is changing in response to public expectations, guidance from professional bodies and health professionals themselves identifying the need for change. Good communication can minimise the occurrence of error and reduce the impact of errors when they occur. Therefore the widespread focus on the development and maintenance of communication skills across health professions is key both to minimising error in the future and to managing errors when they arise in a way that is acceptable for patients and their families.

References

Australian Commission for Safety and Quality in Healthcare. (2013) *Open disclosure framework* [WWW document]. URL http://www.safetyandquality.gov.au/our-work/open-disclosure/ [accessed on 10 April 2014].

Buckman, R. (2005) Breaking bad news: The S-P-I-K-E-S strategy. *Community Oncology*, 2 (no. 2), 138–142.

Buetow, S., Kiata, L., Liew, T., Kenealy, T., Dovey, S. & Elwyn, G. (2010) Approaches to reducing the most important patient errors in primary health-care: Patient and professional perspectives. *Health and Social Care in the Community*, 18 (no. 3), 296–303.

College of Emergency Medicine. (2013) *Supporting the second victim* [WWW document]. URL https://secure.collemergencymed.ac.uk/code/document.asp?ID=7172 [accessed on 1 October 2014]

Crane, M. (2001). What to say if you made a mistake. *Medical Economics*, 78, 26–28, 33–36.

Croskerry, P. (2003) The importance of cognitive errors in diagnosis and strategies to minimise them. *Academic Medicine*, 78 (no. 8), 775–780.

de Vries, E.N., Prins, H.A., Crolla, R.M., den Outer, A.J., van Andel, G., van Helden, S.H., *et al.* (2010) Effect of a comprehensive surgical safety system on patient outcomes. *New England Journal of Medicine*, 363, 1928–1937.

Einav, Y., Gopher, D., Kara, I., Ben-Yosef, O., Lawn, M., Laufer, N., Liebergall, M. & Donchin Y. (2010) Preoperative briefing in the operating room: Shared cognition, teamwork, and patient safety. *Chest*, 137, 443–449.

Francis, R. (2013) *The Mid Staffordshire NHS Foundation Trust public inquiry* [WWW document]. URL http://www.midstaffspublicinquiry.com/report [accessed on 28 January 2014].

Haynes, A., Weiser, T., Berry, W.R., Lipsitz, S., Breizat, A., Dellinger, P., *et al.* (2009) A surgical safety checklist to reduce morbidity and mortality in a global population. *New England Journal of Medicine*, 360, 491–499.

Hojat, M., Louis, D.Z., Markham, F.W., Wender, R., Rabinowitz, C. & Gonnella, J.S. (2011) Physicians, empathy and clinical outcome for diabetic patients. *Academic Medicine*, 86 (no. 3), 359–364.

Institute for Healthcare Improvement. (2015) *SBAR technique for communication: A situational briefing model* [WWW document]. URL http://www.ihi.org/resources/Pages/Tools/SBARTechnique forCommunicationAsituationalBriefingModel.aspx [accessed on 30 November 2014].

Kaldjian, L.C., Jones, E.W., Wu, B.J., Forman-Hoffman, V.L., Levi, B.H. & Rosenthal, G.E. (2007) Disclosing medical errors to patients: Attitudes and practices of physicians and trainees. *Journal of General Internal Medicine*, 22, 988–996.

Kennedy, I. (2001) *The report of the public inquiry into children's heart surgery at the Bristol Royal Infirmary 1984–1995: Learning from Bristol* [WWW document]. URL http://webarchive.nationalarchives.gov. uk/+/www.dh.gov.uk/en/Publicationsandstatistics/Publications/PublicationsPolicyAndGuidance/ DH_4005620 [accessed on 23 May 2014].

Kohn, L.T., Corrigan, J.M. & Donaldson, M.S. (eds). (2000) *To Err Is Human: Building a Safer Health System*. National Academies Press, Washington, DC.

Kroll, L., Singleton, A., Collier, J. & Rees Jones I. (2008) Learning not to take it seriously: Junior doctors' accounts of error. *Medical Education*, 42, 982–990.

Leape, L.L. (1994) Error in medicine. *JAMA*, 272 (no. 23), 1851–1857.

Leonard, M., Graham, S. & Bonacum, D. (2004) The human factor: The critical importance of effective teamwork and communication in providing safe care. *Quality and Safety in Health Care*, 13, 85–90.

Longtin, Y., Sax, H., Leape, L.L., Sheridan, S., Donaldson, L. & Pittet, D. (2010) Patient participation: Current knowledge and applicability to patient safety. *Mayo Clinic Proceedings*, 85 (no. 1), 53–62.

Marshall, S.D., Harrison, J. & Flanagan, B. (2009) The teaching of a structured tool improves the clarity and content of inter-professional clinical communication. *Quality and Safety in Health Care*, 18 (no. 2), 137–140.

NHS Institute for Innovation and Improvement. (2008) *SBAR* [WWW document]. URL http:// www.institute.nhs.uk/quality_and_service_improvement_tools/quality_and_service_ improvement_tools/sbar_-_situation_-_background_-_assessment_-_recommendation.html [accessed on 1 October 2014].

O'Connor, E., Coates, H., Yardley, I. & Wu, A. (2010) Disclosure of patient safety incidents: A comprehensive review. *International Journal for Quality in Health Care*, 22 (no. 5), 371–379.

Oxford English Dictionary (2014) *S.v. 'error'* [Online] URL http://www.oed.com/view/Entry/64126 ?rskey=JnW9o9&result=1#eid [accessed on 1 October 2014].

Parliamentary and Health Service Ombudsman. (2009) *Principles of good complaint handling* [WWW document]. URL http://www.ombudsman.org.uk/__data/assets/pdf_file/0005/1040/0188- Principles-of-Good-Complaint-Handling-bookletweb.pdf [accessed on 28 January 2014].

Reason, J. (2008) *The Human Contribution: Unsafe Acts*, Accidents and Heroic Recoveries. Ashgate Publishing, Farnham, Surrey, UK.

Rodriguez, H.P., Rodday, A.M., Marshall, R.E., Nelson, K.L., Rogers, W.H. & Safran, D.G. (2008) Relation of patients' experience with individual physicians to malpractice risk. *International journal of Quality in Health Care*, 20 (no. 1), 5–12.

Vincent, C.A. & Coulter, A. (2002) Patient safety: What about the patient? *Quality and Safety in Health Care*, 11, 76–80.

Vincent, C., Neale, G. & Woloshynowych, M. (2001) Adverse events in British Hospitals: Preliminary retrospective record review. *BMJ*, 322, 517–519.

Wu, A. (2000) Medical error: The second victim. *BMJ*, 320 (no. 7237), 726–727.

Diversity Issues in Clinical Communication and Cultural Diversity

CHAPTER 18

Overview of Diversity Issues in Clinical Communication

Costas S. Constantinou

University of Nicosia Medical School, Nicosia, Cyprus

Western modern medicine has been largely based on the biomedical model for understanding and treating ill health. Nettleton (2013) explained that the biomedical model understands ill bodies as reparable machines and the causes of diseases as purely natural. On this note, Western medicine has been criticised systematically since the 1970s for overlooking the importance of social forces and social background, such as education and socioeconomic status, in contributing to both the development of diseases and the volume of patients' adherence to treatment (Bury 1997; Nettleton 2013). It has also been criticised for downplaying patients' perspectives and the need for better communication with patients during therapies and consultation sessions (Vermeire *et al.* 2001; Morgan 2008).

An increasing recognition of social and cultural factors in health and illness has led to an acknowledgement of the need to incorporate more specialised training based on patients' background, such as age, family, ethnicity and so forth. It is these more specialised areas that this part of the book is addressing.

In this section, Margot Turner and Nisha Dogra discuss the meaning of 'diversity' and the specific communication challenges posed by loss of hearing or sight, learning disabilities or other differences such as cultural background and ethnicity (see chapter 19).

Communicating with families is discussed in chapter 20, where Xavier Coll asserts that families are dynamic groups and clinicians would benefit from learning about the functions of a family, social roles, gender issues and sensitive matters. In the following chapter. Coll explains that children should be approached differently from adults. For example, information and treatment stages need to be explained simply, while clinicians should establish a good rapport with children in order to improve children's understanding and adherence to treatment.

Consultations with older patients pose different challenges. As Andrew Tarbuck explains in chapter 22, there is a power and dependency relationship with healthcare professionals, and studies show that professionals may not pay as much attention as necessary to patients' specific health problems or concerns. Clinicians need to be aware of such challenges and overcome their own biases in order to communicate effectively with older patients.

Clinical Communication in Medicine, First Edition. Edited by Jo Brown, Lorraine M. Noble, Alexia Papageorgiou and Jane Kidd.
© 2016 John Wiley & Sons, Ltd. Published 2016 by John Wiley & Sons, Ltd.

Two issues that are often difficult for clinicians to discuss with patients – end of life issues and mental health matters – are discussed in chapters 23 and 24. Vinnie Nambisan and Jennifer Balls consider the core skills and attitudes that underpin effective communication in end of life care (chapter 23). Jonathan Wilson highlights the complex needs of the mental health consultation and the importance of the clinician having a sophisticated repertoire of advanced communication skills (chapter 24).

Reality is often more complicated than what is discussed in the separate chapters here, and integrating more diversity in medical curricula would better prepare medical students for their clinical practice. For example, a clinician may be faced with a case that combines multiple components of diversity, such as treating a child born in the UK to a migrant family from Ethiopia who do not embrace modern medicine and believe in the act of the 'evil eye'. The clinician must be able to understand the child's needs and way of thinking, communicate with the whole family, respond to family dynamics, and be cognisant of the family's cultural and religious background. Essentially, to be proficient, the doctor needs to be able to respond seamlessly to multiple challenges. Medical training needs to provide sufficient opportunities to practise in order for doctors to attain this proficiency.

References

Bury, M. (1997) *Health and Illness in a Changing Society*. Routledge, New York.

Morgan, M. (2008) The doctor–patient relationship. In: G. Scrambler, *Sociology as Applied to Medicine*, sixth edn, pp.55–70. Saunders Elsevier, London.

Nettleton, S. (2013) *The Sociology of Health and Illness*, third edn, Polity Press, Cambridge.

Vermeire E., Hearnshaw, H., Van Royen, P. & Denekens, J. (2001) Patient adherence to treatment: Three decades of research. *A comprehensive review. Journal of Clinical Pharmacy and Therapeutics*, 26, 331–342.

CHAPTER 19

Diversity Issues in Clinical Communication

Margot Turner[1] and Nisha Dogra[2]

[1] *St George's University of London, London, UK*
[2] *University of Leicester, Leicester, UK*

Historical context

In this section we outline the introduction of cultural competence and diversity into the medical curricula. We also consider the increasing diversity of medical students and how these factors set the context for current practice.

Recognising the importance of diversity issues in clinical communication and medical education is still a work in progress. The Declaration from the Conference on Primary Care in Alma Ata in 1978 emphasised that health was a state of well-being and a human right, and social factors that led to health inequalities needed to be tackled, with more emphasis given to primary care worldwide. This informed the principles that were incorporated into *Tomorrow's Doctors* (General Medical Council 1993), in which students are asked to respect patients and colleagues without prejudice to diversity of background. *Tomorrow's Doctors* concentrated more on diversity issues and communication skills and probably gave the most specific directions on how diversity issues could be incorporated into the communication curriculum; for example, encouraging sessions on British sign language, communication with patients with hearing or visual impairment, and use of interpreters with patients who could not speak English. It was less clear from *Tomorrow's Doctors* how students were going to be taught to *'communicate effectively with individuals regardless of their social cultural or ethnic background'* (General Medical Council 2003).

It is also relevant to consider the literature on diversity in medical education during the early 21st century. Diversity teaching was mainly referred to in literature in terms of 'cultural competence', which had various interpretations. In the USA, Betancourt (2003) referred to it as *'training and corporate development on how to better manage diversity in the work place'*. Kai *et al.* (1999) identified that cultural competence had grown out of multicultural training in nursing education. This training in nursing education was based on the model of learning knowledge about different cultures that critics suggested could lead to stereotyping or 'othering'. The concept of 'othering' is described effectively by Taylor (2003), who suggested that medical professionals often only perceive culture to be a descriptor of patients' experiences and ignore the fact that medical knowledge has a culture as well, one that may impact on behaviour and care. Tervalon and

Murray-Garcia (1998) suggested that 'cultural humility' was the way forward and that students should be taught to understand the power imbalance between patient and doctor and develop self-evaluation skills to help redress this power imbalance. Betancourt (2003) hypothesised that there is no 'manual' on how to care for patients from racial, ethnic or cultural groups. He suggested that attention needed to be given to knowledge, attitudes and skills, with each of these components being crucial to achieving cultural competence. The Association of American Medical Colleges (AAMC) (2005) published guidance on definition of cultural competence with a 'Tool for Assessing Cultural Competence Training'. There were five domains and under each domain, knowledge, skills and attitudes were identified. The skills outlined in the section 'Understanding the impact of stereotyping and cross-cultural clinical skills' are probably most relevant to clinical communication teaching, such as:
• demonstrate an ability to reflect on your own cultural beliefs and practices;
• demonstrate strategies for addressing stereotyping and
• recognise and manage the impact of bias, class and power on the clinical encounter.

The AAMC (2005) also identified models for 'Cross-Cultural Communication and Negotiation'. These could be seen as reductionist, as students may not address their own biases if they simply apply a formula.

Karnik and Dogra (2010) proposed cultural sensibility as an openness to emotional impressions, susceptibility and sensitiveness that allows one to reflect and change because of his or her interactions with people from different cultural backgrounds. The cultural sensibility framework focuses on students' understanding that culture is a complex compilation of numerous influences and emphasises developing students' understanding of how culture, in turn, influences interactions and knowledge. This approach considers whether students are able to use their understanding of culture to develop constructive and positive relationships or skills, including communicating with diverse communities and individuals.

Although there has been an increasing expectation that diversity education is included in the curriculum, Dogra *et al.* (2005) reported that whilst 75% of medical schools in the UK stated that they did so, the teaching was fragmented and there was uncertainty about the content. Hobgood *et al.* (2006) reported similar findings in the USA.

Another strand that needs to be considered is the changing profile and increasing diversity of medical students during the 20th and early 21st centuries. Lempp & Seale (2006), for example, identified that since 1996 over 50% of medical school intakes in the UK, USA and Canada have been women; this was a major change from previous decades. Esmail (2001) suggested there was a considerable increase in South Asian students in the 1960s as a result of Asian doctors being invited to come and work in the National Health Service. Some medical schools now have 40% of students from Asian backgrounds; however, students from black British backgrounds remain under represented (Esmail 2011).

The changing diversity of the student body and the implications of this for clinical communication, the whole curriculum and assessment have been explored in the literature. Several linguistic issues that might impact negatively on students from ethnic backgrounds have been identified (Roberts *et al.* 2000; Wass *et al.* 2003; Dewhurst *et al.* 2007).

There have also been a number of sociolinguistic studies in the USA that showed that black African Americans believed that white Americans spoke proper or correct English and black Americans spoke "slang English" (Fought 2006). Additionally there is the issue of the globalisation of medical education that has led to the massive increase in Western medical school outposts being set up all over the world. The question arises as to which context these students are being prepared to work in and who defines good medical practice. There have been concerns that such outposts reinforce colonialism and may lead to imitating the 'white doctor' and a lack of awareness of local contexts (Stegers-Jeger & Themmen 2013). However, there is a need to ensure that there is a balanced debate and there is no polarisation implying that all "Western" is bad and the rest is good or vice versa.

Current practice

Medical schools over the last 25 years have been trying different methods to increase teaching on cultural diversity in undergraduate education in order to address these three main objectives identified in Dogra *et al.* (2010):

1 enhancing cross-cultural patient doctor encounters;
2 eliminating health inequalities and
3 improving health outcomes of the marginalised.

Before exploring current practice regarding diversity and clinical communication, it is important to consider how to define the term 'culture', which underpins all of the teaching. Although there are many definitions, we use the following definition developed by a group of medical educators in the UK:

> Culture is a socially transmitted pattern of shared meanings by which people communicate, perpetuate and develop knowledge and attitudes about life. An individual's cultural identity may be based on heritage as well as individual circumstances and personal choice and is a dynamic entity.
>
> *(Diversity in Medicine and Healthcare 2014)*

This model moves away from the ever-lengthening and exhaustive lists of people's characteristics that can make both students and academics feel that this subject is insurmountable and often external to them and somewhat trivial (Dogra 2004). It encourages a more holistic approach to the curriculum, moving away from a tokenistic approach often described as 'political correctness'.

There is limited literature about how medical education addresses diversity issues in clinical communication. The majority of the literature is descriptive and not a critical evaluation of curricula. In part that reflects how diversity teaching has evolved in curricula in an ad hoc way with a lack of ownership by whole institutions (Murray-Garcia & Garcia 2008).

The UK Council's consensus statement (von Fragstein *et al.* 2008) on content of the communication curricula has been influential, and while it emphasises that diversity issues need to be addressed, they are identified as special issues rather than integrated into the core curriculum. Hargie *et al.* (2010), in their survey of current trends in clinical communication training in UK medical schools, commented that diversity issues were most effectively covered in relation to dealing with patients from culturally diverse backgrounds and those with disabilities. Later in the article they refer to a varied core clinical communications curricula that includes 'dealing with diversity', and yet examples appeared to be limited to ethnicity and disability.

McEvoy *et al.* (2009) describe a very comprehensive programme with sessions over 3 years, developing clinical communication with diverse communities with limited English proficiency and also including developing an ability to explore the patient's perspective and health beliefs.

The General Medical Council (2011b), in their supplement on public involvement, acknowledged the importance of recognising diversity and different perspectives with the caveat that it is important that members of the public can only really represent themselves and cannot necessarily speak for others. They gave seven examples of effective practice of working with diverse communities in the UK. One of those refers to medical schools such as Bristol who facilitate sessions raising awareness on disability, diversity and disadvantage, and many of these are run by people from different communities. However, while these are useful there is a danger that people may assume that simply by 'meeting' people different from themselves they will understand the complexities of diversity issues in healthcare. There is evidence that many medical students struggle with uncertainty, and if given some facts about specific groups will latch on to those rather than reflect on how to explore patient perspectives instead of relying on their assumptions (Dogra *et al.* 2007). Such activities need to be contextualised and integral to learning objectives on diversity that could challenge attitudes and stereotypes (Turner *et al.* 2014). The literature largely lacks any in-depth analysis or critique of how diversity issues are addressed in communication skills teaching. However, an article by Nazar *et al.* (2014) used qualitative research to evaluate the different cultural diversity models used in the curriculum and the impact it had on the students through individual student interviews. Their conclusions were that cultural competence led to the students perceiving certain patients as problematic and that cultural humility/sensibility was the optimum model, especially if educators were trained and encouraged to share their own cultural narratives and dilemmas with students throughout their training.

Medical educators are still struggling to assess diversity issues in the curriculum. Lurie (2012) suggested there may be 'staff resistance' to developing assessment in this area because there is a belief that questions or scenarios could be difficult to formulate and too reductionist, discouraging 'critical thinking'. Hamilton (2009) suggested that scenarios could equally be too complex and unrealistic and would require a level of rapport that would be too difficult to achieve in a short simulated consultation. He also felt that academics should look at where assessment on diversity happens in the curriculum, suggesting that if students are assessed too early they may be 'demotivated by the experience'. Many academics have recommended that diversity issues are best assessed either in stand-alone practical examinations in cultural competency or cultural diversity stations embedded into end-of-year clinical examinations (Altshuler & Kachur 2001; Rosen *et al.* 2004; Betancourt 2003). However, Dogra and Wass (2006) suggested that while standardised consultations in clinical examinations are an important part of cultural diversity assessment, they should not be the only approach. Miller and Green (2007) and Hamilton (2009) both emphasise the importance of ensuring that standardised patients are trained effectively, alongside examiner training and faculty development.

More recently, assessment guidance by the General Medical Council (2011a) highlighted the need for the inclusion of specific diversity training as part of any examiner training programme. There has been some research into student attitudes in order to inform diversity teaching and assessment but little or no work into faculty attitudes to diversity issues. The European Union has recently funded a project to consider how medical teachers across the curriculum can be trained to ensure that they integrate diversity issues across the curriculum (Academisch Medisch Centrum 2014).

It is important to complete this section with a brief overview of the key themes in diversity and medical education now. Bleakley *et al.* (2008) first suggested that given the globalisation of Western medical education, it is essential to explore medical education within a postcolonial paradigm, and without this there is a danger that imposing Western educational frameworks without questioning could appear imperialist. This suggestion is reinforced by research by Roberts *et al.* (2014), who identified in their sociolinguistic study of the UK membership of the Royal College of General Practitioners clinical examination that international medical graduates may be failing due to an unconscious weighting on a Western concept of empathy. More research is needed to ensure that certain members of our diverse student bodies are not being disadvantaged by certain communication assessments implying that there is only one way to communicate.

Stegers-Jeger & Themmen (2013) suggest that there is a wide cultural variation in clinical communication in Europe alone, and medical educators need to consider whether some communication skills that are described as 'poor' are in fact merely different. They thought more educators should consider whether international students in particular are being forced to fit in to the culture of the medical school, which may be different from the contexts they might ultimately practice in. Frambach *et al.* (2013) questioned whether Western frameworks of medical education were applicable to all contexts. Although they were not specifically considering communication skills, the argument is relevant and challenges the stance taken by von Fragstein *et al.* (2008), who suggested that their recommendations for the communication curricula were applicable throughout the world. This leaves an unresolved dilemma about how best to teach ever-increasing numbers of international medical students in diverse contexts.

The latest framework that has grown out of both the postcolonial and feminist discourses is the intersectional framework. Sears (2012) emphasises the importance of understanding that here are different 'social locations' that will have led to disparities in healthcare and discrimination. She suggests that it is important for clinicians to not only understand the complexity of these and the impact of multiple social statuses but also that they should be encouraged to reflect on their own intersectional identities, which may be similar or different to patients. Recognising the complexities and common identities might challenge the reductionist approach that can lead to 'othering'. Sears suggests that it is important to explore issues of intersectionality in a patient-centred interviewing model with the caveat that models can lead to premature assumptions. Educators need to be particularly aware that scenarios or clinical examination stations do not address one aspect of discrimination while dismissing and devaluing another aspect of prejudice (Verdonk & Abma 2013).

Future directions

This section offers suggestions to take the area of diversity and communication skills further. It will discuss the importance of the whole curriculum commitment, acknowledgement of student diversity, staff training and effective evaluation and assessment.

It may be useful to consider the similarities between diversity and clinical communication and then consider each in order to help integration:
- no one discipline or profession owns it;
- requires reflection that is ongoing and integral to practice;
- requires an awareness of own limitations;
- aided by openness and practice;
- requires congruence between 'what is said' and 'how it is said';
- those that most need the teaching often don't recognise the need;

- impact on outcomes is hard to measure and
- a tendency to teach both in abstract and reduce to checklist.

First, communication teachers need to consider that their own views on diversity are likely to be communicated to students through their teaching. For example, if the majority of case studies do not integrate diversity aspects but there are one or two cases that focus on diversity, the students may pick up that diversity only appears when there is obvious visible difference or a language barrier. If cases with communication difficulties usually have non-Western-sounding names, students may come to associate diversity issues with 'foreigners'.

Many authors (Wear 2003; Katchur & Alshuler 2004; Dogra *et al.* 2009; Seeleman *et al.* 2009) have argued for integration of cultural diversity across the whole curriculum, emphasising the importance of communication skills in a diversity curriculum. Diversity in Medicine and Healthcare recommends a minimum of 15 hours contact time across a medical undergraduate course with an additional 15 hours independent learning. The 15 hours of contact time should include dedicated small group work in which students can explore their views and how to manage the challenges they may face when working with perspectives very different from their own.

Dogra & Wass (2006) emphasised that diversity issues need to be assessed if students are going to give this aspect the same weight as other aspects of the curriculum. Accrediting bodies around the world have opportunities to take the lead on embedding diversity in the curriculum by working with teachers and academics in the area, helping with definitions of learning outcomes and being transparent about how this area is being evaluated. If accrediting bodies do not take a lead fully embedding diversity into the medical curriculum, it will remain a hobby often led by very committed individuals but without much institutional support. There is a need for medical schools to demonstrate their commitment by allowing adequate resources to develop an effective curriculum and assessment that in this era of globalisation does address patient needs and does not disadvantage any student group.

A challenge for clinical communication has been that while students can be taught the mechanisms of good practice, they cannot be given exact answers about how to integrate these mechanisms in a way that is congruent with them as individuals. This is important so that patients receive a genuine experience when communicating, as opposed to a technically correct performance devoid of congruity, warmth or humanity. In integrating diversity within clinical communication teaching, students could be enabled to reflect on aspects of communication they find difficult and specifically address these.

There is clearly a place for integration of many aspects of diversity and communication skills, and it is perhaps surprising that there are few teachers with responsibility for both. The way forward is to develop a solid evidence base for both areas, and by bringing teachers, patients and carers together, progress can be made in the development of outcomes. Lie *et al.* (2012) argued that framing diversity as a health literacy issue may be a useful way of advancing both areas.

References

Academisch Medisch Centrum. (2014) *Cultural competence in medical education* [WWW document]. URL http://www.amc.nl/web/Research/Major-projects-and-collaborations/Overview/Culturally-Competent-in-Medical-Education/Culturally-Competent-in-Medical-Education/Project-C2ME.htm [accessed 16 January 2014].

Altshuler, L. & Kachur E. (2001) A culture OSCE: Teaching residents to bridge different worlds. *Academic Medicine*, 76, 514.

Association of American Medical Colleges. (2005) *Cultural Competence Education*. Association of American Medical College, Washington, DC.

Betancourt, J. (2003) Cross-cultural medical education: Conceptual approaches and frameworks for evaluation. *Academic Medicine*, 78, 560–569.

Bleakley, A., Brice, J. & Bligh, J. (2008) Thinking post-colonial in medical education. *Medical Education* 42, 266–270.

Dewhurst, N., McManus, C., Mollon, J., Dacre, J. & Vale, A. (2007) Performance in MRCP (UK) examinations 2003–2004: Analysis of pass rates of UK graduates in relation to self declared ethnicity and gender. *BMC Medicine*, 5, 1186–1195.

Diversity in Medicine and Healthcare. (2014) URL www.dimah.co.uk.

Dogra, N. (2004) The learning and teaching of cultural diversity in undergraduate medical education in the UK. PhD Thesis, University of Leicester.

Dogra, N. & Wass, V. (2006) Can we assess students' awareness of 'cultural diversity'? A qualitative study of stakeholders' views. *Medical Education*, 40, 682–690.

Dogra, N., Conning, S., Gill, P.S., Spencer, J. & Turner, M. (2005) Teaching of cultural diversity in medical schools in the United Kingdom and Eire: Cross sectional questionnaire survey. *BMJ*, 360, 403–404.

Dogra, N., Giordano, J. & France, N. (2007) Cultural diversity teaching and issues of uncertainty: Findings of a qualitative study. *BMC Medical Education*, 7 (no. 8), 1472–1478.

Dogra, N., Reitmanova, S. & Carter-Pokras, O. (2009) Twelve tips for teaching diversity and embedding it in the medical curriculum current status. *Medical Teacher*, 31, 990–993.

Dogra, N., Reitmanova, S. & Carter-Pokras, O. (2010) Teaching cultural diversity: Current status in U.K., U.S., and Canadian medical schools. *Journal of General Internal Medicine*, 25, 164–168.

Esmail, A. (2001) Racial discrimination in medical schools. In: N. Coker (ed), *Racism and Medicine: An Agenda for Change*. King's Fund Publishing, London.

Esmail, A. (2011) Ethnicity and academic performance in the UK. *BMJ;* 342, 10.

Fought, C. (2006) *Language and Ethnicity: Key Topics in Socio Linguistics*. Cambridge Press, New York.

Frambach, J.M., Driessen, E.W., Chan, L.C. & van der Vleuten, C.P. (2013) Rethinking the globalistion of problem based learning: How culture challenges self directed learning. *Medical Education*, 46, 738–747.

General Medical Council. (1993) *Tomorrow's Doctors*. General Medical Council, London.

General Medical Council. (2003) *Tomorrow's Doctors*. General Medical Council, London.

General Medical Council. (2011a) *Assessment in Undergraduate Medical Education: Advice Supplementary to 'Tomorrow's Doctors' (2009)*. General Medical Council, London.

General Medical Council. (2011b) *Patient and Public Involvement in Undergraduate Medical Education: Advice Supplementary to 'Tomorrow's Doctors' (2009)*. General Medical Council, London.

Hamilton, J. (2009) Intercultural competence in medical education – essential to acquire difficult to assess. *Medical Teacher*, 31, 862–865.

Hargie, O., Boohan, M., McCoy, M. & Murphy, P. (2010). Current trends in communication skills training in UK schools of medicine. *Medical Teacher*, 32, 385–391.

Hobgood, C., Sawning, S., Bowen, J. & Savage, K. (2006) Teaching culturally appropriate care: A review of educational models and methods. *Academic Emergency Medicine*, 13, 1288–1295.

Kai, J., Spencer, J., Wilkes, M. & Gil, P. (1999) Learning to value ethnic diversity –what, why and how? *Medical Education*, 33, 616–623.

Karnik, N. & Dogra, N. (2010) The cultural sensibility model for children and adolescents: A process oriented approach. *Child and Adolescent Psychiatric Clinics of North America*, 19, 719–738.

Katchur, E. & Alshuler, L. (2004) Cultural competence is everyone's responsibility! *Medical Teacher*, 26, 101–105.

Lie, D., Carter-Pokras, O., Braun, B. & Coleman, C. (2012) What do health literacy and cultural competence have in common? Calling for a collaborative health professional pedagogy. *Journal of Health Communication*, 17, 13–22.

Lempp, H. & Seale, C. (2006) Medical student perceptions in relation to ethnicity and gender: Qualitative study. *BMC Medical Education*, 6, 1472–1483.

Lurie, S. (2012) History and practice of competency based assessment. *Medical Education*, 46, 49–57.

McEvoy, M., Santos, M., Marzan, M., Green, E.H. & Milan, F.B. (2009) Teaching medical students how to use interpreters: A three-year experience. *Medical Education Online*, 14, 12.

Miller, E. & Green A.R. (2007) Student reflections on learning cross cultural skills through a cultural competence OSCE. *Medical Teacher*, 29, 76–84.

Murray-Garcia, J.L. & Garcia, J.A. (2008) The institutional context of multicultural education: What is your institutional curriculum? *Academic Medicine*, 83, 646–652.

Nazar, M., Kendal, K., Day, L. & Nazar, H. (2014) Decolonising medical curricula through diversity education: Lessons from students. *Medical Teacher*, 37 (no. 4), 1–9.

Roberts, C., Atkins, S. & Hawthorne, K. (2014) *Performance Features in Clinical Skills*. Centre of Language Discourse and Communication Kings College London with University of Nottingham.

Roberts, J.H., Sarangai, S., Southgate, L., Wakeford, R. & Wass, V. (2000) Oral examinations – equal opportunities, ethnicity, fairness, in the MRCGP. *BMJ*, 320 (no. 7231), 320–337.

Rosen, J., Spatz, E., Gaserud, A., Abramovitch, H., Weinreb, B., Wenger, N.S. & Margolis, C.Z. (2004) A new approach to developing cross-cultural communication skills. *Medical Teacher*, 26, 126–132.

Sears, K.P. (2012) Improving cultural competence education: The utility of an intersectional framework. *Medical Education*, 46, 545–551.

Seeleman, C., Suurmond, J. & Stronks, K. (2009) Cultural competence: A conceptual framework for teaching and learning. *Medical Education*, 43, 229–237.

Stegers-Jeger, K. & Themmen, A. (2013) Dealing with diversity. *Medical Education*, 47, 752–759.

Taylor, J. (2003) Confronting 'culture' in medicine's 'culture of no culture'. *Academic Medicine*, 78, 555–559.

Tervalon, M. & Murray-Garcia, J. (1998) Cultural humility versus cultural competence: A critical distinction in defining physician training outcomes in medical education. *Journal of Health Care for the Poor and Underserved*, 9, 117–125.

Turner, M.A., Kelly, M., Leftwick, P. & Dogra, N. (2014) *Tomorrow's Doctors* and diversity issues in medical education. *Medical Teacher*, 36, 743–745.

Verdonk, P. & Abma, T. (2013) Intersectionality and reflexivity in medical education research. *Medical Education*, 47, 754–756.

von Fragstein, M., Silverman, J., Cushing, A., Quilligan, S., Salisbury, H. & Wiskin, C. (2008) UK consensus statement on content of communication curricula in undergraduate medical education. *Medical Education*, 42, 1100–1107.

Wass, V., Roberts, C., Hoogenboom, R., Jones, R. & van der Vleuten, C. (2003) Effect of ethnicity on performance in objective structured clinical examination: Qualitative and quantitative study. *BMJ*, 326 (no. 7393), 800–803.

Wear, D. (2003) Insurgent multiculturalism: Rethinking how and why we teach culture in medical education. *Academic Medicine*, 78, 549–554.

CHAPTER 20

The Family Consultation

Xavier Coll

Norwich Medical School, University of East Anglia; Children, Families, and Young People Service, Norwich, Norfolk, UK

Historical context

Consultations with families have been present throughout history, sometimes including the extended family as well as non-kin members of the community. As a distinct professional practice within Western cultures, the origins of family consultations could be traced back to the work of clinicians such as John Bowlby (1953; 1988) and Nathan Ackerman (1959), amongst others, who began seeing family members together for consultations, reporting it and articulating various theories about the nature and functioning of the family.

Family consultations received an important boost in the mid-1950s through the work of anthropologist Gregory Bateson (1980) and some of his colleagues, such as Jay Haley (1967) and John Weakland (Weakland & Ray 1995), who introduced ideas from cybernetics (Wiener 1948) and general systems theory (von Bertalanffy 1968). As a result, a number of distinct approaches to family consultation emerged by the late 1960s. Of special relevance to doctor–family communications have been the Palo Alto Mental Research Institute of Brief Therapy (Weakland & Ray 1995), Strategic Therapy (Nichols & Tafuri 2013), Salvador Minuchin's (1974) Structural Family Therapy, and the Milan's Systemic Model (Bateson 1971).

The late 1960s and early 1970s saw the development of Network Therapy (which bears some resemblance to traditional practices such as Ho'oponopono, an ancient Hawaiian practice of reconciliation and forgiveness) and the emergence of behavioural couple and family therapy, as models in their own right (Sholevar 2003).

Since the 1980s there has been a progressive move towards integration of the ideas of the different models and eclecticism (Franck & Callery 2004).

Current practice

Key features of communication in doctor–family consultations include the awareness of observing the patient in context, the task of understanding who the patient regards as family (taking care not to make assumptions), the identification of the family's influence on care and treatment, and the role of family beliefs in treatment adherence (Lloyd & Bor 2004; Coll & Maxwell 2012).

Clinical Communication in Medicine, First Edition. Edited by Jo Brown, Lorraine M. Noble, Alexia Papageorgiou and Jane Kidd.

It is not the number of people present that transform an individual interview into a family consultation. The difference is how the clinician thinks about the nature of the problem, how it evolved, how its presence is maintained and the implications for change in the wider social context (Kinston & Loader 1988; Coll & Maxwell 2012).

Brown and Rutter (1966) showed that, with the use of interviewing techniques, sensitive, reliable and valid measures of subtle aspects of family life and relationships can be obtained from a single interview with one parent.

Nevertheless, the emotional tone, the alliances between family members and the family's influence on how to manage the difficulties (Kinston *et al.* 1979; Kinston & Loader 1988) are more effectively assessed by observation during family interviews. Aspects such as the consultation's venue and the presence or absence of family members will affect both the process and content of the consultation.

In addition to the verbal aspects of a family consultation, the genogram (or family tree) is one of the most useful techniques at our disposal, as it allows the clinician to gain a clear overview of the family as well as help engaging all family members. Clinical experience informs us that it is not uncommon that new information emerges when drawing a family tree, and 'forgotten events', patterns over generations (which may be important in terms of inherited physical vulnerabilities) or perhaps how individuals have left the family in the past reveal themselves. This view is also supported by research, in that patients reported that they felt the genogram helped their physicians understand them better and thus provide better healthcare (Rogers & Durkin 1984; Puskar & Nerone 1996).

Increasingly, clinicians use the techniques that fit with the needs of the family, over and above the school of family consultation they originated from. In doing so, a generic family consultation that seeks to incorporate the best of the accumulated knowledge in the field, and which can be adapted to many different contexts (Franck & Callery 2004), has been developed.

Ill health can destabilise relationships within the family or create a closer bond (Levetown 2008). Factors such as the nature of the health problem, the recognition (or not) that the problem exists, previous personal and family experience of coping with difficulties, the expectations of different family members and the vulnerabilities or resilience of each member of the group will determine the different dynamics that could arise (Lloyd & Bor 2004).

Finally, there has been a growing interest in assessing the training in using the skills needed (Coll & Maxwell 2012) in family consultations. Examples of this would be in working with cancer patients and their families (Moore *et al.* 2009; Zwaanswijk *et al.* 2011), in our daily practice with children when breaking bad news (Harrison & Walling 2010), in using genograms (Shore *et al.* 1994), or in primary care family consultations (Sanders *et al.* 2003).

Future directions

In a rapidly changing world, aspects such as culture and ethnicity (Coll 1998), variations in family composition (with adoption, fostering, separation, divorce and remarriage) becoming commonplace, appearance of massive socio-economic differences between people, ever-increasing geographical mobility, and neighbourhood violence, as well as the influence of the electronic media and social networks, should all be taken into consideration and will be key to family consultations over the coming decades.

We are all likely to be baffled by technological advances. Clinicians will need common sense when assessing problems associated with electronic media, gaming, social networking and their effects on families, so that the energies are focused appropriately.

In order to care for these challenges, practitioners will need to shift from a linear cause-and-effect model to one that reflects on clinical practice. Doctors can also promote positive change by informing families about ways of using new technology effectively (Greenberg *et al.* 2006; Rodríguez-Idígoras *et al.* 2009; Akpose 2011), including advocating access to quality resources in the media.

The advantages of working, whenever possible, with the whole family will continue to include the opportunity to deal with dynamics and with more than one problem at the same time. Skills specific to family consultations will be needed when there are unspoken 'secrets' between family members, since those can and probably will jeopardise the clinician's effectiveness (Coll & Maxwell 2012).

Often, difficulties experienced by different family members are related (Aarthun & Akejurdet 2014). Therefore, this approach will become more and more important in a cost-efficient-driven health service.

References

Aarthun, A. & Akerjurdet, K. (2014) Parent participation in decision-making in health-care services for children: An integrative view. *Journal of Nursing Management*, 22, 177–191.

Ackerman, N.W. (1959) *The Dynamics of Family Treatment*. Basic, New York.

Akpose, W. (2011) *10 things you may not know about social networking and social networking sites* [WWW document]. URL http://www.todaysengineer.org/2011/Jan/social-networking.asp [accessed on 11 January 2011].

Bateson, G. (1971) A systems approach. *International Journal of Psychiatry*, 9, 242–244.

Bateson, G. (1980) *Mind and Nature*. Fontana, Glasgow.

Bowlby, J. (1953) *Child Care and the Growth of Love*. Penguin Books, London.

Bowlby, J. (1988) *A Secure Base: Clinical Applications of Attachment Theory*. Routledge, London.

Brown, G. W. & Rutter, M. (1966) The measurement of family activities and relationships: A methodological study. *Human Relations*, 19, 241–263.

Coll, X. (1998) Importance of acknowledging racial and cultural differences: Please don't let me be misunderstood. *Psychiatric Bulletin*, 22, 370–372.

Coll, X. & Maxwell, S. (2012) Working with families and young people. In: X. Coll, A. Papageorgiou, A. Stanley & A. Tarbuck (eds), *Communication Skills in Mental Health Care*, pp. 69–82. Radcliffe, London.

Franck, L.S. & Callery, P. (2004) Re-thinking family-centred care across the continuum of children's healthcare. *Child: Care, Health & Development*, 30 (no. 3), 265–277.

Greenberg, N., Boydell, K.M. & Volpe, T. (2006) Pediatric telepsychiatry in Ontario: Caregiver and service provider perspectives. *Journal of Behavioural Health Sciences & Research*, 33 (no. 1), 105–111.

Haley, J. (1967) Toward a theory of pathological systems. In: G. Zuk & I. Boszormneyi-Nagy (eds), *Family Theory and Disturbed Families*, pp. 1–27. Science and Behaviour Books, Palo Alto, CA.

Harrison, M.E. & Walling, A. (2010) What do we know about giving bad news? A review. *Clinical Pediatrics*, 49 (no. 7), 619–626.

Kinston, W. & Loader, P. (1988) The family task interview: A tool for the clinical research in family interaction. *Journal of Marital and Family Therapy*, 14, 67–87.

Kinston, W., Loader, P. & Stratford, J. (1979) Clinical assessment of family interactions: A reliability study. *Journal of Family Therapy*, 1, 291–312.

Levetown, M. (2008) Communicating with children and families: From everyday interactions to skill in conveying distressing information. *Pediatrics*, 121, 1441–1460.

Lloyd, M. & Bor, R. (2004) Communication with a patient's family. In: M. Lloyd & R. Bor, (eds), *Communication Skills for Medicine*, second edn, pp. 120–132. Churchill Livingstone, London.

Minuchin, S. (1974) Families and Family Therapy. Harvard University Press, Cambridge, MA.

Moore, P.M., Wilkinson, S.S.M. & Rivera Mercado, S. (2009) *Communication Skills Training for Healthcare Professionals Working with Cancer Patients, Their Families, and/or Carers: A Cochrane Collaboration Review.* John Wiley & Sons, Oxford.

Nichols, M. & Tafuri, S. (2013) Techniques of structural family assessment: A qualitative analysis of how experts promote a systemic perspective. *Family Process*, 52 (no. 2), 207–215.

Puskar, K. & Nerone, M. (1996) Genogram: A useful tool for nurse practitioners. *Journal of Psychiatric & Mental Health Nursing*, 3 (no. 1), 55–60.

Rodríguez-Idígoras, M.I., Sepúlveda-Muñoz, J., Sánchez-Garrido, E.R., Martínez-González, J.L., Escolar-Castelló, J.L., Paniagua-Gómez, I.M., Bernal-López, R., Fuentes-Simón, M.V. & Garófeno-Serrano, D. (2009) Telemedicine influence on the follow-up of type 2 diabetes patients. *Diabetes Technology & Therapeutics*, 11 (no. 7), 431–437.

Rogers, J. & Durkin, M. (1984) The semi-structured genogram interview. I: Protocol. II: Evaluation. *Family Systems Medicine*, 2 (no. 2), 187.

Sanders, M.R., Murphy-Brennan, M. & McAuliffe, C. (2003) The development, evaluation and dissemination of a training programme for general practitioners in evidence-based parent consultation skills. *International Journal of Mental Health Promotion*, 5 (no. 4), 13–20.

Sholevar, G.P. (2003). Family theory and therapy. In: G.P. Sholevar & L.D. Schwoeri, *Textbook of Family and Couples Therapy: Clinical Applications.* American Psychiatric Publishing, Washington, DC.

Shore, W.B., Wilkie, H.A. & Croughan-Minihare, M. (1994) Family of origin genograms: Evaluation of a teaching programme for medical students. *Family Medicine*, 26 (no. 4), 238–243.

von Bertalanffy, L. (1968) *General Systems Theory*. Penguin, Harmondsworth.

Weakland, J. & Ray, W. (1995) *Propagations: Thirty Years of Influence from the Mental Research Institute.* Haworth, New York.

Wiener, N. (1948) Cybernetics. *Scientific American*, 179, 14–18.

Zwaanswijk, M., Tates, K., van Dulmen, S., Hoogerbrugge, P.M., Kamps, W.A., Beishuizen, A. & Bensing, J.M. (2011) Communicating with child patients in pediatric oncology consultations: A vignette study on child patients', parents' and survivors' communication preferences. *Psycho-Oncology*, 20 (no. 3), 269–277.

CHAPTER 21

Consulting with Children and Young People

Xavier Coll

Norwich Medical School, University of East Anglia; Children, Families, and Young People Service, Norwich, Norfolk, UK

Historical context

There have been many models underpinning effective communication with children and young people (Table 21.1), but, clearly, the past two decades have witnessed a growing recognition that children and young people have a right to participate in matters that affect their lives. There is now widespread acceptance that every child has a right to self-determination, dignity, respect and the right to make informed decisions (United Nations 1989; International Association for Youth Mental Health 2013). Hospital policies accept that services should be child-centred, with children being encouraged to become active partners in decisions about their health and care, and where possible, being able to exercise choice (UNICEF 2003; Hemingway & Redsell 2011).

However, despite the importance of consulting with children, literature reviews suggest that often children are not active participants in their own consultations (Coyne 2008) and that their views are rarely sought or acknowledged within the heathcare setting (Cavet & Sloper 2004; Savage & Callery 2007), although this problem might be less pervasive in tertiary mental health services (Day 2008).

With regards to the reasons for their exclusion, studies suggest that divergent opinions exist among health professionals on whether children and young people should be encouraged to have a say in matters that affect them (Coyne 2008), and that generally they have been given a marginal role in the information-exchange process. Reviews (Coyne 2008; Moore & Kirk 2010) indicate that children and doctors reported different reasons for the children's limited involvement (Table 21.2).

Current practice

Most literature reviews (Tates & Meeuwesen 2001; Epstein *et al.* 2005; Cahill & Papageorgiou 2007; Coyne 2008; Coyne *et al.* 2013) outline that current practices direct healthcare services to give children and young people greater choice and participation in decisions about their healthcare.

All models described in Table 21.1 have contributed to more patient-centred paediatric consultations, helping, for example, to manage behaviour change

Clinical Communication in Medicine, First Edition. Edited by Jo Brown, Lorraine M. Noble, Alexia Papageorgiou and Jane Kidd.
© 2016 John Wiley & Sons, Ltd. Published 2016 by John Wiley & Sons, Ltd.

Table 21.1 Models underpinning effective communication with children and young people.

Models	Names attached	Main ideas
Developmental	Freud, Piaget, Erikson, Bowlby	Emphasis on the child moving from one stage (by completing a set of tasks) to the next
Systemic	Von Bertalanffy 1968	Understands the child as part of a bigger reality or 'system'
Triadic consultations	Cahill & Papageorgiou 2007	Three-way consultations involving children and parents, opening the room to narrative-based medicine, where different parties bring their own individual context
Biopsychosocial	Engel 1978	Holistic integration to increase understanding of difficulties
Calgary-Cambridge model in children and young people	Coll & Maxwell 2012	Guide to communicate with children and young people
Transactional analysis	Berne 1964	Understanding and identifying the parent, adult, and child 'ego-states' to improve communication
Consultations as learning	Pendleton *et al.* 1984	Describes a sequence of tasks for any consultation with ideas, concerns and expectations
Transtheoretical, cycle of change, or motivational interviewing	Prochaska & DiClemente, 1984	Model describing several stages of intentional change (precontemplation, contemplation, preparation, action and maintenance)

Table 21.2 Key reasons for the children's limited involvement, as reported by children and doctors (adapted from Coyne 2008 and Moore & Kirk 2010).

Children's reasons	Doctor's reasons
Not wanting to hear bad news	Lack of time
Fear of 'being in trouble' by asking questions	A threat of loss of power and control
Time pressure in the interaction with health professionals	Having their views and approaches questioned
Difficulty understanding medical terminology	Not agreeing with the children's wishes
The actions from their parents	Lack of communication skills with children

(e.g. transtheorethical model in diabetes; Huang & Tang 2007). Likewise, the Calgary-Cambridge model provides a guideline to communicate with children and their parents, and more medical schools are incorporating either this or similar models into their curricula, so that the new graduates will carry these skills with them (Coll & Maxwell 2012).

With regards to consent to treatment in children and young people, the general principle is that children should be involved as much as possible in decisions about their care, even if they are not able to make decisions on their own (General Medical Council 2013). When obtaining consent, the doctor must establish whether the child is legally competent (in legal terms 'has capacity' to give consent).

Some clinicians have argued that children over 5 years should be considered competent to be involved in healthcare decisions concerning them (Coyne 2008; Moore & Kirk 2010), in partnership with their adult carer and health professionals.

In the UK, according to the Family Law Reform Act 1969 children over 16 are presumed to have capacity to consent to treatment unless there is evidence to the contrary (National Archives 1969). However, just because someone is aged over 16, this does not, as with adults (aged 18 or over), necessarily mean that the person is competent. In England, 'Gillick competence' defines the threshold at which children are able to independently consent to treatment, based on understanding and maturity, which could be much younger than 14 years of age (Gillick v West Norfolk and Wisbech Health Authority and the Department of Health and Social Security 1985).

Nevertheless, the UK Department of Health recommends that it is good practice to encourage children and young people to involve their families in decisions about their care, unless it would not be in their best interests to do so. If, however, a competent child under the age of 16 is insistent that his or her family should not be involved, the child's right to confidentiality must be respected, unless such an approach would put him or her at serious risk of harm. This legal framework applies to England, Wales and Northern Ireland. In Scotland, there is no statutory legislation, but there is clear case law to guide practitioners. A child aged 16 and 17 cannot refuse treatment if it has been agreed by a person with parental responsibility or the court, and it is in his or her best interests (General Medical Council 2013). Therefore, children do not have the same status as adults. Special situations, such as the clinician disagreeing with the parents, would require an application to the court.

In essence, the doctor's role is to integrate the views of the carers and the young person. The challenge here is to maintain an effective clinical relationship while the health responsibilities transfer from the adults to the young person. Our awareness that in triadic consultations the needs of the parent could inadvertently take priority (despite the guidance from good medical practice stating that doctors need to have the best interests of their patient, the child, as their first concern), and our ability to deal sensitively with the needs of the parent while assessing and treating the child, will be essential skills to maintain a good therapeutic alliance.

Doctors also need to know about adolescent development (both physical and psychosocial, including the development of abstract thinking) to assess key issues that influence clinical communication, such as:

- the young person's adherence to the medical advice;
- adolescent risk-taking behaviours;
- worries about confidentiality, the relationships between the young person and his or her family and
- the young person's difficulties in understanding the impact of his or her behaviour on others.

To facilitate the assessment, doctors must be aware that knowledge "handed down" by adults perceived to be in authority is likely to be given very little value. Here, involving the young person in formulating a plan might help to overcome this block (Coll & Maxwell 2012).

Future directions

Parents and health professionals play a key role in the consultation process and have the power to facilitate children's participation. The devolution of responsibility to the child and young person, empowering them to make decisions about care, raises a need to train doctors and educate young people to achieve this participation, and then design studies to measure its effectiveness, because patient-centred consultations with children and young people are key in any successful health service redesign (International Association for Youth Mental Health 2013).

Clinicians working with children and young people will also need to adapt and respond to new clinical environments, financial constraints and technological advances. In 1971, the first email was delivered. More than 40 years on, social media has taken the world by storm. Social networking sites, such as Facebook, MySpace, Bebo and Twitter, are now used by 1 in 4 people worldwide (1 in 2 for people under the age of 25). Such activity may seem harmless, but some researchers suggest that social media may affect our mental health and well-being (Kross 2013).

But, what is social media? Social media is an array of Internet sites that enable people from all over the world to interact through discussion, photos, video and audio. It is a means of communicating that has become pervasive for young people all over the world. Therefore, it would be a good exercise to look at the evidence for its pros and cons:

Positives
- Social networking can help develop new social connections and friendships and keeps young people connected to friends and family (Solis 2011).
- Can be used to discuss educational topics, offering teachers a platform for collaboration with other teachers and communication with students outside the classroom (National School Boards Association 2007; Stansbury 2011).
- Social networking sites can facilitate face-to-face interaction (Morgan 2012).
- Can maximise support groups and networks for young people, also making easier to organise events.
- Source of employment (e.g. LinkedIn).
- Assist police to catch criminals who declare their offences online (LexisNexis Risk Solutions 2012).
- Contribute to health services boosting their image as leaders in the field.
- Improve communication with young people. We have a Facebook account in our youth service and we also use the site to make important announcements on the services we offer, the therapeutric groups we run, the teaching we do and so forth.
- Use of virtual worlds as role-play simulations as a communication, therapeutic and teaching tool (Vallance *et al.* 2014).

Negatives
- Spending too much time has been linked with lower academic grades (Daly 2012), wasting time (Rideout *et al.* 2010).
- Rauch *et al.* (2014) concluded that the main reasons that young people use social media are for self-distraction and boredom relief because it delivers a reinforcement when they log on, in the form of supportive comments and 'likes'. This behaviour could lead to addiction.
- It has also become a way of gaining attention, since social media tends to create excessive drama.
- Many people on social media sites present an idealised version of their lives, leading others to make upward social comparisons, which can lead to negative emotions (Rauch *et al.* 2014).
- Perceived need to be electronically connected and available at all times. This could be related to becoming even more sleep deprived (texting and gaming until early hours).
- Cyberbullying (Mishna *et al.* 2010).

- Social networking sites enable 'sexting', which can lead to criminal charges and the unexpected proliferation of personal images (Wolak *et al.* 2012).
- Misinformation (Marino 2012).
- Desensitisation to aggressive behaviour after exposure to aggression (Krahé *et al.* 2011).
- Takes time out of face-to-face communication, both at home (families who reported spending less time with one another rose from a level of 8% in 2000 to 32% in 2011; USC 2012) and with peers. This could lead to young people losing out on the ability to learn about and read social cues of nonverbal communication and interact mindfully in the moment.
- Relatively easy to make a fake account.
- Increased vulnerability to security attacks such as hacking, identity theft (Topping 2012) and viruses (Waugh 2012).

Social media can lead to both positive and negative communication experiences with children and young people, but it is essential that as doctors we understand new technologies and the promise they offer to revolutionise education and communication.

Away from the virtual world, the development of youth services, covering the ages of 14 to 25, alongside under-14s services, should help to consolidate developmentally appropriate consultations. This is a radical change in organising health services, aiming at brindging gaps and smoothing transitions. Norwich in the UK and Melbourne in Australia are two prime examples of this approach (McGorry *et al.* 2013), which has communicating effectively at its core.

References

Berne, E. (1964) *Games People Play: The Basic Handbook of Transactional Analysis*. Ballantine Books, New York.

Cahill, P. & Papageorgiou, A. (2007) Triadic communication in the primary care paediatric consultation: A review of the literature. *British Journal of General Practice*, 57, 904–911.

Cavet, J. & Sloper, P. (2004) The participation of children and young people in decisions about UK service development. *Child: Care, Health & Development*, 30 (no. 6), 613–621.

Coll, X. & Maxwell, S. (2012) Working with families and young people. In: X. Coll, A. Papageorgiou, A. Stanley & A. Tarbuck (eds), *Communication Skills in Mental Health Care*, pp. 69–82. Radcliffe, London.

Coyne, I. (2008) Children's participation in consultations and decision-making at health service level: A review of the literature. *International Journal of Nursing Studies*, 45, 1682–1689.

Coyne, I., Mathúna, D.P.O., Gibson, F., Shields, L. & Sheaf, G. (2013) *Interventions for Promoting Participation in Shared Decision-Making for Children with Cancer: A Review*. Cochrane Collaboration, 6. doi:10.1002/14651858.CD008970.pub2.

Daly, J. (2012) *How Is Facebook Affecting College Students' Grades* [Infographic]. URL www.edtechmagazine.com [accessed on 2 July 2012].

Day, C. (2008) Children's and young people's involvement and participation in mental health care. *Child and Adolescent Mental Health*, 13 (no. 1), 2–8.

Engel, G.L. (1978) The biopsychosocial model and the education of health professionals. *Annals of the New York Academy of Sciences*, 310, 169–187.

Epstein, R.M., Fiscella, K., Shields, C.G., Meldrum, S.C., Kravitz R.L. & Duberstein, P.R. (2005) Measuring patient-centered communication in patient–physician consultations: Theoretical and practical issues. *Social Science & Medicine*, 61 (no. 7), 1516–1528

General Medical Council. (2013) *0–18 Years Guidance: Other Sources of Information and Guidance*. GMC Publications, London.

Gillick v West Norfolk and Wisbech Area Health Authority and the Department of Health and Social Security. (1985) URL http://www.bailii.org/uk/cases/UKHL/1985/7.html.

Hemingway, P. & Redsell, S. (2011) Children and young people's participation in healthcare consultations in the emergency department. *International Emergency Nursing*, 19 (no. 4), 192–198.

Huang, C. & Tang, S. (2007) An experience using the transtheorethical model of health behaviour change to promote exercise in a type 2 diabetes patient. *Journal of Nursing*, 54 (no. 5), 99–103.

International Association for Youth Mental Health. (2013) *International Declaration on Youth Mental Health*. International Association for Youth Mental Health, Victoria, Australia.

Krahé, B., Möller, I., Huesmann, L.R, Kirwil, L., Felber, J. & Berger, A. (2011) Desensitization to media violence: Links with habitual media violence exposure, aggressive cognitions, and aggressive behavior. *Journal of Personality and Social Psychology*, 100 (no. 4), 630–646.

Kross, E. (2013) *Social Media in the Public Interest*. University of Michigan's Institute for Social Research [WWW document]. URL http://home.isr.umich.edu/isrinnews/ethan-kross-2.

LexisNexis Risk Solutions. (2012) *Role of Social Media in Law Enforcement Significant and Growing* [WWW document]. URL www.lexisnexis.com [accessed on 18 July 2012].

Marino, K. (2012) *Social Media: The New News Source* [WWW document]. URLwww.schools.com [accessed on 16 April 2012].

McGorry, P., Bates, T. & Birchwood, M. (2013) Designing youth mental health services for the 21st century: Examples from Australia, Ireland and the UK. *British Journal of Psychiatry*, 202, s54–s40.

Mishna, F., Cook, C., Gadalla, T., Daciuk, J. & Solomon, S. (2010) Cyber bullying behaviors among middle and high school students. *American Journal of Orthopsychiatry*, 80 (no. 3), 362–374.

Moore, L. & Kirk, S. (2010) A literature review of children's and young people's participation in decisions relating to health care. *Journal of Clinical Nursing*, 19, 2215–2225.

Morgan, J. (2012) *5 Ways Social Media Can Facilitate Offline Networking* [WWW document]. URL www.sociableboost.com [accessed on 8 May 2012].

National Archives. (1969) *Family Law Reform Act 1969* [WWW document]. URL http://www.legislation.gov.uk.

National School Boards Association. (2007) *Creating and Connecting: Research and Guidelines on Online Social – and Educational – Networking* [WWW document]. URL www.nsba.org.

Pendleton, D., Schofield, T., Tate, P. & Havelock, P (1984) *The Consultation: An Approach to Learning and Teaching*. Oxford University Press, Oxford, UK

Prochaska, J.O. & DiClemente, C.C. (1984) *The Transtheoretical Approach: Towards a Systematic Eclectic Framework*. Dow Jones Irwin, Homewood, IL.

Rauch, S.M., Strobel, C., Bella, M., Odachowski, Z. & Bloom, C. (2014) Face to face versus Facebook: Does exposure to social networking websites augment or attenuate physiological arousal among the socially anxious? *Cyberpsychology, Behavior, and Social Networking*, 17 (no. 3), 187–190. doi:10.1089/cyber.2012.0498.

Rideout, V.J., Foehr, U.G. & Roberts, D.F. (2010) *Generation M2L Media in the Lives of 8- to 18-Year-Olds* [WWW document]. URL www.kff.org [accessed on 24 January 2010].

Savage, E. & Callery, P. (2007) Clinic consultations with children and parents on the dietary management of cystic fibrosis. *Social Science & Medicine*, 64, 363–374.

Solis, B. (2011) *People Use Social Networks to Connect with Friends and Family, Sometimes Brands* [WWW document]. URLwww.briansolis.com [accessed on 13 September 2011].

Stansbury, M. (2011) *Ten Ways Schools Are Using Social Media Effectively* [WWW document]. URL www.eschoolnews.com [accessed on 21 October 2011].

Tates, K. & Meeuwesen, L. (2001) Doctor–patient–child communication. A (re)view of the literature. *Social Science & Medicine*, 52, 839–851.

Topping, A. (2012) *Social Networking Sites Fuelling Stalking, Report Warns* [WWW document]. URL www.guardian.co.uk [accessed on 1 February 2012].

UNICEF. (2003) *The State of the World's Children*. UNICEF, New York.

United Nations. (1989) *Convention on the Rights of the Child*. United Nations, Geneva.

USC Annenberg School Center for the Digital Future. (2012) *Special Report: America at the Digital Turning Point* [WWW document]. URL www.annenberg.usc.edu [accessed on 27 January 2012].

Vallance, A.K., Hemani, A., Fernandez, V., McCusker, K. & Toro-Troconis, M. (2014) Using virtual worlds for role play simulation in child and adolescent psychiatry: An evaluation study. *Psychiatric Bulletin*, 38, 204–210.

von Bertalanffy, L. (1968) *General Systems Theory*. Penguin, Harmondsworth, UK.

Waugh, R. (2012) *Beware the New Computer Virus Spreading via Chat Messaging Window on Facebook* [WWW document]. URL www.dailymail.co.uk [accessed on 21 May 2012].

Wolak, J., Finkelhor, D. & Mitchell, K.J. (2012) How often are teens arrested for sexting? Data from a national sample of police cases. *Pediatrics*, 129, 4–12.

CHAPTER 22

The Older Patient

Andrew Tarbuck

Norfolk and Suffolk NHS Foundation Trust; University of East Anglia; Dementias & Neurodegenerative Diseases Local Research Network in East Anglia, Norfolk, UK

Historical context

As a result of increasing longevity and changes in population structure, health services are providing care to increasing numbers of older people. In the UK, 66% of hospital inpatients are over 70 years of age and approximately half of them will have cognitive impairment due to delirium or dementia (Goldberg *et al.* 2012).

Older people often have multiple and complex health issues (e.g. combinations of physical and mental health conditions, side effects from polypharmacy and speech and language problems resulting from stroke or Parkinson's disease), which may be further complicated by social problems such as loneliness and poverty. Communication and joint decision making with older patients is more difficult due to poor 'health literacy' resulting from limited education and access to information (Kriplani & Weiss 2006) and high rates of cognitive and sensory impairments (Williams *et al.* 2007).

Unfortunately, doctors and medical students often demonstrate poor communication skills when dealing with older people; for example, failing to compensate for cognitive and sensory changes, taking the interview too rapidly, providing insufficient information, using jargon and failing to allow or encourage the patient to ask questions (Intrieri *et al.* 1993; Shue *et al.* 2005; Belcher *et al.* 2006). Communication with people who have dementia is often poor (e.g. 'talking over the patient' to relatives or carers and adopting a paternalistic, dismissive or intimidating manner) and this can result in significant harm, including the hastening of cognitive decline, by reinforcing perceived deficits whilst failing to support and encourage preserved abilities (Tullo & Allan 2011; Young *et al.* 2011). Surveys of medical students and junior doctors have demonstrated perceived training gaps in communication with patients who have dementia and with their families (Drickamer *et al.* 2006; Manu *et al.* 2012; Griffiths *et al.* 2013).

Doctors and medical students have also been demonstrated to hold negative attitudes about working with elderly patients; holding stereotyped, ageist beliefs; underestimating patients' cognitive abilities and willingness to engage; having a lack of knowledge regarding ageing and demonstrating little desire to work with or treat older people (Higashi *et al.* 2012).

Current practice

In the UK, the General Medical Council (GMC) sets out the outcomes and standards for undergraduate medical education in *Tomorrow's Doctors* (General Medical Council 2009). This document contains a number of general statements, such as requiring the ability to 'communicate sensitively and effectively with individuals...regardless of age', but it does not specifically cover communication skills with older people. The GMC is clear that it is up to each medical school to design its own curriculum and it is therefore very difficult to know exactly what is being taught across the country, particularly in specialist areas such as dementia (Tullo & Gordon 2013).

The 'UK Consensus Statement on the Content of Communication Curricula in Undergraduate Medical Education' (von Fragstein *et al.* 2008) and a proposed 'European Undergraduate Curriculum in Geriatric Medicine' (Masud *et al.* 2014) make very general statements about the need to cover communication with elderly patients and people with cognitive impairment and with sensory deficits, although the latter document also refers to the importance of being able to assess cognition and capacity.

The competencies and skills required by qualified doctors vary with their level of training and medical specialty. In the UK, doctors in Foundation Year 1 and 2 posts are expected to have adequate communication skills to assess capacity and consent, manage three-way consultations (i.e. interviews involving doctor, patient and carer) and compensate for sensory deficits (UK Foundation Programme Curriculum 2012). Senior trainees (Specialist Trainees in years 4–6) in geriatric medicine and old age psychiatry are required to be competent in a range of more complex tasks relating to the care of older people, including modifying their interview to compensate in patients with communication difficulties, assessing cognitive function and mental capacity and discussing end-of-life issues (Joint Royal Colleges of Physicians Training Board 2010; Royal College of Psychiatrists 2013). In these documents the communication skills aspects are often not stated explicitly but are dealt with as joint requirements in knowledge, skills and attitudes.

In the USA until recently only 70% of residency training programmes in internal medicine included any recognised training in geriatric medicine (Institute of Medicine 2008). It was generally assumed that trainees would encounter sufficient numbers of older patients during their rotation through various medical specialties. However, this has been demonstrated to be much less effective than spending a period within a service specialising in the treatment of older patients (Diachun *et al.* 2010). Such training is now being substantially expanded (Eleazer & Brummel-Smith 2009) and a recommended set of essential geriatric competencies have now been developed for medical students (Leipzig *et al.* 2009) and for internal medicine and family medicine residents (Williams *et al.* 2010). These include communication skills with patients who have cognitive or sensory impairment, limited health literacy and chronic/life-limiting illness and cover the areas of cognitive and capacity assessment and advance care planning.

Although communication with patients who have sensory impairment is mentioned frequently in these documents, there appears to be relatively little research on communication skills in age-related sensory loss. Most work is focussed on patients with early onset deafness who use sign language or on specialist situations such as patients who have received cochlear implants. There is some guidance on what should be covered in teaching communication skills with deaf and hard-of-hearing patients (Erber & Scherer 1999; Barnett 2002), and communication skills workshops and training for medical students have been described (Smith & Hasnip 1991; Lock 2003).

Other specialist areas developing training curricula (that include communication skills elements) of relevance to the care of older patients include oncology (Kissane *et al.* 2012), palliative care (Just *et al.* 2010) and old age psychiatry (Robinson *et al.* 2010; Beer *et al.* 2011; Young *et al.* 2011).

Initially the vast majority of educational and training interventions were based upon 'expert opinion' and experience. More recently there has been a trend to undertake an initial assessment of training needs and then to design an evidence-based intervention based upon educational principles to fill these gaps (Robinson *et al.* 2010; Clayton *et al.* 2012; Kissane *et al.* 2012; Schulz *et al.* 2013).

The majority of interventional studies regarding communication skills with older patients have included this work as part of an 'educational package' with a broader remit. Such programmes also include elements designed to foster more positive attitudes towards older people, improve knowledge and understanding of conditions such as dementia and develop practical skills such as cognitive assessment. A wide variety of different educational approaches have been used to address these issues and to teach communication skills to medical students/doctors. Some studies aimed at nurses and other nonmedical staff have demonstrated even greater ingenuity of approach. The areas covered and techniques that have been used are summarised in Box 22.1.

There is also great variation in the length of courses. For medical students this ranges from a single 4-hour session (Adelman *et al.* 2007) to 31 sessions, each of 45 minutes, delivered over two semesters (Schulz *et al.* 2013) and for doctors from three sessions of 1 hour (Clayton *et al.* 2012) to 'an intensive 2-day retreat' (Kelley *et al.* 2012). Other variables include the number of participants involved, the breadth and scope of the intervention, whether or not the sessions are embedded within day-to-day practice and the use of 'homework' between sessions. Because of these differences it is extremely difficult to compare across studies. Replication of the intervention could also be problematic as the exact content of the sessions is often not provided in sufficient detail – although more recent studies have provided comprehensive descriptions either in the paper itself (Shield *et al.* 2011; Kelley *et al.* 2012) or in a separate file accessible via the Internet (Schulz *et al.* 2013).

Evaluation of the effectiveness of the communication skills training has largely depended on self-assessment by the participants themselves, often at the end of the course. This is clearly unsatisfactory as it is very open to bias and does not clearly demonstrate that the intervention has actually produced any meaningful change in behaviour. Slightly better is a comparison of self-assessment scores pre- and posttraining (Kelley *et al.* 2012; Schulz *et al.* 2013), which can at least demonstrate that, in the opinion of the trainee, the intervention has produced a change. Some studies have used more robust outcome measures, principally scoring of an observed or recorded interview with a simulated patient (Intrieri *et al.* 1993; McFarland *et al.* 2006) or using the simulated patient to score the trainee's performance (Schlaudecker *et al.* 2013). The best studies have compared blinded ratings of videotaped interviews with simulated patients obtained before and after training (Clayton *et al.* 2012) or have included control groups (Intrieri *et al.* 1993; Schulz *et al.* 2013).

Studies looking at communication skills training in nurses and care workers in dementia care settings have used patient/carer reported outcome measures, looking for effects of the intervention on quality of life, prevalence of problem behaviours or patient and carer satisfaction (see reviews by Caris-Verhallen *et al.* 1997; Vasse *et al.* 2010; Eggenberger *et al.* 2013). Because of the high turnover of patients and the nature

Box 22.1 Components of educational and communication skills training programmes related to older people.

(1) Areas covered

Knowledge

Assessment & provision of information
- Changes associated with ageing (sensory, cognitive & socio-demographic)
- Specific conditions (e.g. dementia, delirium, physical health conditions)
- Cognitive assessment (including rating scales)
- Medico-legal aspects (capacity, consent, etc.)
- Psychology of ageing
- Ethical issues
- Understanding behaviour as a means of communication in advanced dementia

Treatment/management of age-related conditions

Attitudes

Increasing empathy
- Exploring the patient experience
- Understanding the challenges associated with ageing

Increasing enthusiasm
- Exposure to fit & active older people
- Developing positive attitudes to ageing
- Challenging negative stereotypes

Encouraging reflective practice

Skills

Increasing confidence in talking with older people/ people with dementia/sensory loss, etc.

Maximising opportunities for communication & conversation during healthcare interventions

Structuring the environment
- Appropriate arrangement of seating
- Minimisation of distractions/noise
- Adequate lighting

Technical aspects of how to compensate for sensory problems
- Insertion & use of hearing aids
- Ensuring patients have spectacles
- Use of amplifier systems, induction loop systems, etc.
- Using correct volume & pitch of voice, clear pronunciation, use of visual cues

Structuring the consultation
- Checking prior levels of knowledge & understanding
- Negotiating of the agenda
- Clear signposting, summarising, chunking & checking

Eliciting & providing information
- Using simple language, avoiding jargon & matching vocabulary to educational level of patient
- Dealing with one point at a time
- Pacing the interview appropriately
- How & when to clarify
- Using open versus closed questions
- Use of nonverbal cues
- Assessing cognitive function sensitively & providing appropriate feedback

Empathy
- Using appropriate verbal & nonverbal techniques
- Validating the patient's perspective

Triadic consultations
- Structuring & controlling the interview
- Dealing with different agendas, expectations & concerns
- Managing difficult dynamics

Skills in people with advanced dementia
- Using nonverbal techniques
- Using 'yes' and 'no' questions and prompts appropriately

Avoiding unnecessary correction or confrontation & using distraction

(2) Techniques employed

Knowledge
Didactic teaching
- Lectures
- Seminars
- Written information (booklets, handouts, etc.)
- Reading lists
- E-learning modules
Discussion groups & workshops

Attitudes
Group discussion
- Examination of real-life cases or incidents
- Review of prerecorded DVD material, case vignettes, examples of good & bad practice
Experiental theatre
Literature
Meeting older volunteers
Encouragement of reflective practice
- Mentorship, workshops
- Reflective diaries, essays
Role play
Simulated sensory loss

Skills
Didactic teaching
- Lectures
- Seminars
- Written information (booklets, handouts, etc.)
Group discussion
- Real-life events
- Case vignettes
- Examples of good & bad practice
Role play
- Using actors/simulated patients (sometimes with video or audio recording)
- Feedback (one to one or group discussion)
Rehearsal of skills
- With actors/simulated patients
- With real patients/elderly volunteers
- Using equipment (e.g. amplifiers, correct insertion of hearing aids, etc.)
Reflective practice & analysis
- Review of video recordings of clinics/consultations with real patients
Modelling – observation of experienced clinicians using:
- DVD recordings
- Interviews with simulated patients/volunteers
- 'Sitting in' on clinics/consultations

of doctor–patient interactions in acute hospital settings, such approaches would probably be difficult to apply in evaluating communication training interventions for medical students and doctors.

Future directions

Doctors working with older people need to have specialist knowledge and technical skills to deal with complex issues such as the assessment of cognitive function and mental capacity. Whilst these aspects of training are very important, communication skills training for doctors and medical students should also include more general skills (e.g. increasing confidence in talking with older people and how to maximise the opportunities for conversation), which have traditionally been 'assumed' in medical education but explicitly taught in nursing. Curricula need to state exactly what skills and competencies are required at each level of training, and it would be helpful if these communication skills elements could be identified explicitly. Older patients and carers should be included in reference groups involved in the design of curricula, communication skills training packages and research studies to ensure that areas of particular importance and relevance to them are covered in a meaningful way.

There is a need for further high-quality research to investigate which are the most effective and acceptable methods for teaching communication skills related to the care of older people to medical students and doctors. The evidence from nursing and other nonmedical staff suggests that such training programmes are most effective when they are longer (i.e. taking place over several sessions rather than being 'one-off' events), require the active participation of trainees, are embedded within usual day-to-day activities, include an element of individual feedback, are recognised within an individual's personal development programme (e.g. training is timetabled, attendance is mandatory and/or formally recognised) and are followed by periodic refresher sessions (Vasse *et al.* 2010). There is limited evidence from medical education that similar findings apply (van Weel-Baumgarten *et al.* 2013), although this was not focused on communication skills with older people.

Training programmes are expensive and time consuming and *there is a clear need to include measurements of cost and cost efficiency in future studies*. Teachers and trainers will be under increasing pressure to demonstrate that their interventions provide good value for money. There is also a need to use better outcome measures in studies; objective measures such as observed interviews with simulated patients, pre- and postintervention assessments and the use of control groups will provide much more robust evidence about the efficacy of training. If possible, measures that demonstrate meaningful outcomes for patients that persist over time should also be used.

Doctors and medical students are currently being trained to involve all patients in decisions about their healthcare as a matter of routine. However, the situation with older people is complex, and a "one size fits all" approach may not actually reflect the needs and wants of this group. Indeed, insisting that all clinicians adopt this way of working could itself be considered paternalistic (McNutt 2004)!

The available evidence suggests that, whilst older people wish to be listened to and informed about their illness and treatment so that they can understand what is happening, the majority of them do not want to be involved in making the medical decisions themselves (Ekdhal *et al.* 2010). This pattern appears to increase with advancing age (Levinson *et al.* 2005).

In teaching communication skills with older people there is a need to differentiate between involving the patient and actually expecting him or her to make decisions about treatment. In addition to taking factors such as the patient's cognitive state into account, we should also be teaching clinicians to make an assessment of an individual patient's preferred communication style and then adjust their approach accordingly.

Further work is required to investigate whether older patients are more willing to be involved in decision making in some areas rather than others (e.g. medical versus psychosocial aspects of care) and also whether the degree of involvement wanted may vary depending on the severity and length of the illness.

References

Adelman, R.D., Capello, C.F., LoFaso, V., Greene, M.G., Konopasek, L. & Marzuk, P.P. (2007) Introduction to the older patient: A 'first exposure' to geriatrics for medical students. *Journal of the American Geriatrics Society*, 55, 1445–1450.

Barnett, S. (2002) Communication with deaf and hard-of-hearing people: A guide for medical education. *Academic Medicine*, 77, 694–700.

Beer, C., Lowry, R., Horner, B., Almeida, O.P., Scherer, S., Lautenschlager, N.T., Bretland, N., Flett, P., Schaper, F. & Flicker, L. (2011) Development and evaluation of an educational intervention for general practitioners and staff caring for people with dementia living in residential facilities. *International Psychogeriatrics*, 23, 221–229.

Belcher, V.N., Fried, T.R., Agostini, J.V. & Tinetti, M.E. (2006) Views of older adults on patient participation in medication-related decision making. *Journal of General Internal Medicine*, 21, 298–303.

Caris-Verhallen, W.M.C.M., Kerkstra, A. & Bensing, J.M. (1997) The role of communication in nursing care for elderly people: A review of the literature. *Journal of Advanced Nursing*, 25, 915–933.

Clayton, J.M., Butow, P.N., Waters, A., Laidsaar-Powell, R.C., O'Brien, A., Boyle, F., Back, A.L., Tulskey, J.A. & Tattersall, M.H.N. (2012) Evaluation of a novel individualised communication-skills training intervention to improve doctors' confidence & skills in end-of-life communication. *Palliative Medicine*, 27, 236–243.

Diachun, L., van Bussel, L., Hansen, K.T., Charise, A. & Rieder, M.J. (2010) 'But I see old people everywhere': Dispelling the myth that eldercare is learned in non-geriatric clerkships. *Geriatric Medicine*, 85, 1221–1228.

Drickamer, M.A., Levy, B., Irwin, K.S. & Rohrbaugh, R.M. (2006) Perceived needs for geriatric education by medical students, internal medicine residents and faculty. *Journal of General Internal Medicine*, 21, 1230–1234.

Eggenberger, E., Heimerl, K. & Bennett, M.I. (2013) Communication skills training in dementia care: A systematic review of effectiveness, training content and didactic methods in different care settings. *International Psychogeriatrics*, 25, 345–358.

Ekdahl, A.W., Andersson, L. & Friedrichsen, M. (2010) 'They do what they think is best for me'. Frail elderly patients' preferences for participation in their care during hospitalisation. *Patient Education and Counseling*, 80, 233–240.

Eleazer, G.P. & Brummel-Smith, K. (2009) Commentary: Ageing America: Meeting the needs of older Americans and the crisis in geriatrics. *Academic Medicine*, 84, 542–544.

Erber, N.P. & Scherer, S.C. (1999) Sensory loss and communication difficulties in the elderly. *Australasian Journal on Ageing*, 18, 4–9.

General Medical Council. (2009) *Tomorrow's Doctors: Outcomes and Standards for Undergraduate Medical Education* [WWW document]. URL http://www.gmc-uk.org/static/documents/content/Tomorrow_s_Doctors_0414.pdf [accessed on 8 May 2014].

Goldberg, S.E., Whittamore, K.H., Harwood, R.H., Bradshaw, L.E., Gladman, J.R. & Jones, R.G. (2012) The prevalence of mental health problems among older adults admitted as an emergency to a general hospital. *Age & Ageing*, 41, 80–86.

Griffiths, A., Knight, A., Harwood, R. & Gladman, J.R.F. (2013) *Preparation to Care for Confused Older Patients in General Hospitals: A Study of UK Health Professionals* [WWW document]. URL http://ageing.oxfordjournals.org/content/early/2013/10/27/ageing.aft171.full.pdf+html?sid=5512e7f0-fb43-4aaa-9e5c-f04bd0891f7d [accessed on 8 May 2014].

Higashi, R.T., Tillack, A.A., Steinman, M., Harper, M. & Bree-Johnson, C. (2012) Elder care as 'Frustrating' and 'boring': Understanding the persistence of negative attitudes toward older patients among physicians-in-training. *Journal of Ageing Studies*, 26, 476–483.

Institute of Medicine. (2008) *Retooling for an Aging America: Building the Healthcare Workforce*. National Academies Press, Washington DC.

Intrieri, R.C., Kelly, J.A., Brown, M.M. & Castilla, C. (1993) Improving medical students' attitudes toward and skills with the elderly. *Gerontologist*, 33, 373–378.

Joint Royal Colleges of Physicians Training Board. (2010) *Specialty Training Curriculum for Geriatric Medicine Curriculum: August 2010 (Amendments August 2013)* [WWW document]. URL http://www.jrcptb.org.uk/trainingandcert/ST3-SpR/Documents/2010%20Geriatric%20Medicine%20Curriculum%20(AMENDMENTS%202013).pdf [accessed on 8 May 2014].

Just, J.M., Schulz, C., Bongartz, M. & Schnell, M.W. (2010) Palliative care for the elderly – developing a curriculum for nursing and medical students. *BMC Geriatrics*, 10, 66.

Kelley, A.S., Back, A.L., Arnold, R.M., Goldberg, G.R., Lim, B.B., Litrivis, E., Smith, C.B. & O'Neill, L.B. (2012) Geritalk: Communication skills training for geriatrics and palliative care fellows. *Journal of the American Geriatrics Society*, 60, 332–337.

Kissane, D.W., Bylund, C.L., Banerjee, S.C., Bialer, P.A., Levin, T.T., Maloney, E.K. & D'Agostino, T.A. (2012) Communication skills training for oncology professionals. *Journal of Clinical Oncology*, 30, 1242–1247.

Kriplani, S. & Weiss, B.D. (2006) Teaching about health literacy and clear communication. *Journal of General Internal Medicine*, 21, 888–890.

Leipzig, R.M., Granville, L., Simpson, D., Andreson, M.B., Sauvigne, K. & Soriano, R.P. (2009) Keeping granny safe on 1st July: A consensus on minimum geriatrics competencies for graduating medical students. *Academic Medicine*, 84, 604–610.

Levinson, W., Kao, A., Kuby, A. & Thisted, R.A. (2005) Not all patients want to participate in decision-making. *Journal of General Internal Medicine*, 20, 531–535.

Lock, E. (2003) A workshop for medical students on deafness and hearing impairments. *Academic Medicine*, 78, 1229–1234.

Manu, E., Marks, A., Berkman, C.S., Mullan, P., Montagnini, M. & Vitale, C.A. (2012) Self-perceived competence among medical residents in skills needed to care for patients with advanced dementia versus metastatic cancer. *Journal of Cancer Education*, 27, 515–520.

Masud, T., Blundell, A., Gordon, A.L., Mulpeter, K., Roller, R., Singler, K., Goeldlin, A. & Stuck, A. (2014) *European Undergraduate Curriculum in Geriatric Medicine Developed Using an International Modified Delphi Technique* [WWW document]. URL http://ageing.oxfordjournals.org/content/early/2014/03/05/ageing.afu019.full.pdf+html?sid=cdaf8685-9962-4a23-94ae-68b0371c7354 [accessed on 8 May 2014].

McFarland, K., Rhoades, D., Roberts, E. & Eleazer, P. (2006) Teaching communication and listening skills to medical students using life review with older adults. *Gerontology & Geriatrics Education*, 27, 81–94.

McNutt, R.A. (2004) Shared medical decision-making: Problems, process, progress. *JAMA*, 292, 2516–2518.

Robinson, L., Bamford, C., Briel, R., Spencer, J. & Whitty, P. (2010) Improving patient-centered care for people with dementia in medical encounters: An educational intervention for old age psychiatrists. *International Psychogeriatrics*, 22, 129–138.

Royal College of Psychiatrists. (2013) *A Competency Based Curriculum for Specialist Training in Psychiatry: Specialists in Old Age Psychiatry* (February 2010; Updated March 2014 [WWW document]. URL http://www.rcpsych.ac.uk/pdf/Old%20Age%20Psychiatry%20submission%20October%202010%20(2014%20Update).pdf [accessed 8 May 2014].

Schlaudecker, J.D., Lewis, T.J., Moore, I., Pallerla, H., Stecher, A.M., Wiebracht, N.D. & Warshaw, G.A. (2013) Teaching resident physicians chronic disease management: Simulating a 10-year longitudinal clinical experience with a standardised dementia patient and caregiver. *Journal of Graduate Medical Education*, 5, 468–475.

Schulz, C., Moller, M.F., Seidler, D. & Schnell, M.W. (2013) Evaluating an evidence-based curriculum in undergraduate palliative care education: Piloting a phase II exploratory trial for a complex intervention. *BMC Medical Education*, 13, 1.

Shield, R.R., Tong, I., Tomas, M. & Besdine, R.W. (2011) Teaching communication and compassionate care skills: An innovative curriculum for pre-clerkship medical students. *Medical Teacher*, 33, e408–e416.

Shue, C.K., McNeley, K. & Arnold, L. (2005) Changing medical students' attitudes about older adults & future older patients. *Academic Medicine*, 80 (10 Supp.), S6–S9.

Smith, M.C.A. & Hasnip, J.H. (1991) The lessons of deafness: Deafness awareness and communication skills training with medical students. *Medical Education*, 25, 319–321.

Tullo, E. & Allan, L. (2011) What should we be teaching medical students about dementia? *International Psychogeriatrics*, 23, 1044–1050.

Tullo, E. & Gordon, A.L. (2013) Teaching and learning about dementia in UK medical schools: A national survey. *BMC Geriatrics*, 13, 29.

UK Foundation Programme Curriculum. (2012) [WWW document]. URL http://www.foundationprogramme.nhs.uk/download.asp?file=Fp_Curriculum_2012_updated_for_2014_WEB_FINAL.pdf [accessed on 8 May 2014].

van Weel-Baumgarten, E., Bolhuis, S., Rosenbaum, M. & Silverman, J. (2013) Bridging the gap: How is integrating communication skills with medical content throughout the curriculum valued by students? *Patient Education and Counseling*, 90, 177–183.

Vasse, E., Vernooij-Dassen, M., Spijker, A., Rikkert, M.A. & Koopmans, R. (2010) A systematic review of communication strategies for people with dementia in residential and nursing homes. *International Psychogeriatrics*, 22, 189–200.

von Fragstein, M., Silverman, J., Cushing, A., Quilligan, S., Salisbury, H. & Wiskin, C. (2008) UK Consensus Statement on the Content of Communication Curricula in Undergraduate Medical Education. *Medical Education*, 42, 1100–1107.

Williams, B.C., Warshaw, G., Fabiny, A.R., Lundebjerg, N., Medina-Walpole, A., Sauvigne, K., Schwartzberg, J.G. & Leipzig, R.M. (2010) Medicine in the 21st century: Recommended essential geriatrics competencies for internal medicine and family medicine residents. *Journal of Graduate Medical Education*, 2, 373–383.

Williams, S.L., Haskard, K.B. & DiMatteo, M.R. (2007) The therapeutic effects of the physician–older patient relationship: Effective communication with vulnerable older patients. *Clinical Interventions in Aging*, 2, 453–467.

Young, T.J., Manthorp, C., Howells, D. & Tullo, E. (2011) Optimising communication between medical professionals and people living with dsementia. *International Psychogeriatrics*, 23, 1078–1085.

CHAPTER 23

End of Life Issues

Vinnie Nambisan[1,2] and Jennifer Balls[1]
[1]Saint Francis Hospice, Romford, Essex, UK
[2]University College London Medical School, London, UK

Historical overview

What is 'end of life care'?

End of life care refers to the treatment and care of children and adults who are likely to die within the next 12 months, due to an advanced progressive incurable condition, including both cancer and noncancer diagnoses, general frailty with coexisting conditions or life-threatening acute conditions. It aims to support the person to live as well as possible until they die and to die with dignity (General Medical Council 2010). It includes symptom control, psychological, social and spiritual support, care in the last few days of life and support and bereavement care for the person's family and carers.

End of life care has a relatively short history as a defined part of healthcare. The pioneering work of Dame Cicely Saunders in the 1960s, in the UK and USA, inspired by a recognition of deficiencies in hospital care of the dying at that time, was instrumental in the development of modern end of life healthcare. Her work built upon a history of care tailored to the needs of the dying that included the establishment of hospices in Europe and the USA in the mid-19th century. This, in turn, built upon a long tradition of care of the dying in some form, stretching back at least as far as the Aesculapian school of ancient Greece (Royal College of Physicians 2007).

More recently, in England, the *End of Life Care Strategy*, published in 2008, identified a need for high-quality end of life care for the approximately half a million people who die each year. It emphasised the importance of early identification of people approaching the end of life, treatment with dignity and respect and communication that is sensitive and responsive, with the aim of enabling preparation and planning for death (UK Department of Health 2008). Recent publications have again highlighted the importance of effective communication in end of life care (National Institute for Clinical Excellence 2013; UK Department of Health 2013).

Common examples of communication challenges in end of life care are shown in Box 23.1.

Clinical Communication in Medicine, First Edition. Edited by Jo Brown, Lorraine M. Noble, Alexia Papageorgiou and Jane Kidd.
© 2016 John Wiley & Sons, Ltd. Published 2016 by John Wiley & Sons, Ltd.

Box 23.1 Common Examples of Communication Challenges in End of Life Care.

Prognostication/diagnosing dying: 'How long have I got?' 'Am I dying now?'
Denial: 'I know I'm going to get better from this.'
Collusion: 'You won't tell them it's serious, will you?'
Addressing misconceptions about end of life care, including responding to requests for, or concerns about, euthanasia.
Advance care planning (e.g. discussing decisions about treatment escalation, whether or not to attempt cardiopulmonary resuscitation and preferred place of death).
Communicating about *best interests decisions* for patients who lack capacity *Ethically challenging situations*, such as withdrawal of life-sustaining treatment.*What to say when someone dies*.
Bereavement care.

Current practice

It is increasingly recognised that good end of life care should be available to all who need it, wherever it is needed, with emphasis on people being able to receive that care in their usual place of residence. It should be delivered by a wide multiprofessional team, including doctors, nurses and allied health professionals from primary and secondary care, and specialist palliative care including hospices, working together with social care professionals.

End of life care will involve the core tasks in clinical communication already discussed in this chapter, with perhaps additional challenges. Relationship building is crucial and may have to occur within a short time frame; information gathering and sharing may be more challenging at times of emotional or physical stress. End of life care will inevitably involve sharing bad news, communicating risk and uncertainty and responding to highly emotionally charged situations. The issues of diversity previously discussed are also commonly encountered in end of life care, which has a strong ethos of tailoring care to the needs of the individual.

Why might healthcare professionals find end of life care challenging?

Most healthcare professionals will be involved in the care of people near to the end of life at some stage of their careers (UK Department of Health 2008). End of life care is accepted as a core part of healthcare, albeit one that is different in aim from the more usual life-saving and life-prolonging ethos of healthcare. This difference, along with the still widely held view of death as a failure of healthcare rather than as an inevitable part of life, is one of many reasons that explain why end of life care is often viewed as disproportionately challenging and is closely linked to the societal, religious and cultural context of both healthcare and death and dying.

Healthcare professionals can feel daunted when faced with end of life issues. A lack of confidence may be related to uncertainty about one's own communication skills, knowledge of relevant law, professional guidance or ethics, or simply about which drug to use for pain control. Even with sound knowledge, healthcare professionals may worry that their lawful actions (for example, appropriate sedation of an agitated, dying patient) will be perceived as unlawful or unethical. Although training in end of life care must often compete for resources with training in other areas of healthcare, it is widely accepted as an essential to the provision of the best end of life care (UK Department of Health 2008; Royal College of Physicians 2012).

The impact of healthcare professionals' own attitudes towards, and experience of, death and dying often goes unnoticed but will influence their engagement with end of life issues. These might lead to avoidance behaviours that reflect a mistaken belief that they lack the necessary time or expertise to deal with such issues, or the conscious or unconscious setting of protective boundaries behind which one might hide from the emotional impact of caring for a dying person. These boundaries may also protect from feelings of anxiety about possible negative impacts of significant communications with people close to death and their loved ones, the fear of dealing with strong emotions, or blame (Whitehead 2012) and worries that giving bad news to a patient might take away his or her hope (Reinke *et al.* 2010). Professional support, whether formal or informal, is essential in supporting healthcare professionals' reflection and learning (Royal College of Physicians 2012).

Decisions not to attempt cardiopulmonary resuscitation (DNACPR) are commonly encountered in end of life care and serve to illustrate some of these points. A good outcome will depend on several factors, including:

- a healthcare professional's knowledge about the legal and professional framework in which such decisions must be made (e.g. whether or not a patient can ensure that cardiopulmonary resuscitation is attempted);
- the healthcare professional's confidence in talking to patients about sensitive issues relating to death (on which may impact, for example, worries about dealing with conflict, or about the effectiveness of the professional's own communication skills) or
- the attitudes and beliefs of all involved towards withholding life-sustaining treatment (which may reflect the professional's own, or the patient's, religious or cultural beliefs).

Anxiety about any of these factors may adversely affect the outcome.

In the face of such challenges, however, it is important to recognise the hugely positive impact that providing good end of life care can have (Whippen & Canellos 1991).

Conclusions and the way forward

Managing issues relating to end of life care can be amongst the most challenging, and the most rewarding, aspects of a healthcare professional's role. Good communication skills will enable professionals to successfully negotiate many challenging end of life issues (such as decisions about attempted resuscitation), in combination with training, confidence and reflection on one's own beliefs and attitudes. End of life issues need not be approached using communication skills that are specific to end of life care but instead through applying the core communication skills previously covered in this book and through reflection on and learning from experience. Good formal and informal professional support is a vitally important aspect of this process.

References

General Medical Council. (2010) *Treatment and Care towards the End of Life: Good Practice in Decision Making* [WWW document]. URL http://www.gmc-uk.org/guidance/ethical_guidance/end_of_life_care.asp. [accessed on 1 October 2014].

National Institute for Clinical Excellence. (2013) *Guidance, Quality Standards QS13 – End of Life Care for Adults*, November 2011 [WWW document]. URL http://publications.nice.org.uk/quality-standard-for-end-of-life-care-for-adults-qs13. [accessed on 1 October 2014].

Reinke, L.F., Shannon, S.E., Engelberg, R.A., Young, J.P. & Curtis, J.R. (2010) Supporting hope and prognostic information: Nurses' perspectives on their role when patients have life-limiting prognoses. *Journal of Pain and Symptom Management*, 39 (no. 6), 982–992.

Royal College of Physicians. (2007) *Palliative Care Services: Meeting the Needs of Patients* [WWW document]. URL http://www.rcplondon.ac.uk/sites/default/files/consultant_physicians_revised_5th_ed_full_text_final.pdf [accessed on 1 October 2014].

Royal College of Physicians, National End of Life Care Programme, Association for Palliative Medicine of Great Britain and Ireland. (2012) *Improving End-of-Life Care: Professional Development for Physicians. Report of a Working Party* [WWW documen]. URL http://www.rcplondon.ac.uk/resources/improving-end-life-care-professional-development-physicians [accessed on 1 October 2014].

United Kingdom Department of Health. (2008) *End of Life Care Strategy: Promoting High Quality Care for All Adults at the End of Life* [WWW document]. URL http://webarchive.nationalarchives.gov.uk/20130107105354/http://www.dh.gov.uk/en/Publicationsandstatistics/Publications/PublicationsPolicyAndGuidance/DH_086277 [accessed on 1 October 2014].

United Kingdom Department of Health. (2013) *More Care, Less Pathway: A Review of the Liverpool Care Pathway* [WWW document]. URL https://www.gov.uk/government/uploads/system/uploads/attachment_data/file/212450/Liverpool_Care_Pathway.pdf [accessed on 1 October 2014].

Whippen, D.A. & Canellos, G.P. (1991) Burnout syndrome in the practice of oncology: Results of a random survey of 1,000 oncologists. *Journal of Clinical Oncology*, 9 (no. 10), 1916–1920.

Whitehead, P.R. (2012) The lived experience of physicians dealing with patient death. *BMJ Supportive and Palliative Care*, 4, 271–276.

CHAPTER 24

Mental Health Matters

Jonathan Wilson

University of East Anglia, Norfolk, UK; St George's University, New York, USA; Child Family and Young Person Service, Norfolk, UK

Historical context

Contained within modern psychology and psychiatry, there are many hundreds of models that attempt to explain how the mind operates or at least understand the connections between thoughts and the resultant behaviour. Mental illness is unique in that it tends to be perceived not as a particular physical part of the body that needs to be treated but rather as an innate, almost existential aspect of oneself, often deemed in some way to be an inner, personal fault. To varying degrees, specific tests for mental illness remain hypothetical, and it is still the case that there are few, if any, reliable biological tests for successful diagnosis. Indeed, many of the conceptual stalwarts that underpin modern psychiatric practice, including the validity of concepts such as schizophrenia, personality disorder and the usefulness of modern medications, continue to be questioned by the public and increasingly by professionals alike (Van Os 2009; Allan 2011; Morrison *et al.* 2012).

This is no great surprise. Without reliable biological measures, many theories can abound. Modern psychiatry is forced to draw upon complex theoretical constructs and navigate through a maze of often competing ideas as to the causes of psychological distress and thereby a multitude of possible treatments in accordance with what might be considered the primary causal factor.

Modern psychiatry places the discovery of the primary causal factor, or formulation of the causal factors, at the centre of its philosophy. These can be biological, psychological or social in origin or a mixture of all three. In order to elicit and understand the relative impact of each factor, the relationship and interaction between the medical practitioner and patient is pivotal if a successful outcome is to be achieved. The concept of 'talking therapies' and the proposal that such practices lead to positive outcomes dates back to the earliest days of psychiatry. At its origins in the mid-19th century, interest was growing in the power of the mind, and following the early work of Franz Mesmer and others, hypnosis began to take Paris by storm in the 19th century (Ellenberger 1970). Subsequently, a young neurologist called Sigmund Freud was intrigued by what he encountered, and his work led to the start of a revolution in the exploration of the interface between the brain, mind and body (Ellenberger 1970), of which, in many ways, this book is a distant echo or legacy.

Clinical Communication in Medicine, First Edition. Edited by Jo Brown, Lorraine M. Noble, Alexia Papageorgiou and Jane Kidd.
© 2016 John Wiley & Sons, Ltd. Published 2016 by John Wiley & Sons, Ltd.

Early talking and physical therapies were led as much by desperation as by a sense of exploration, but many of the concepts that underpinned them still linger today, though in modified form. These ideas permeate not just medicine but also society in general, as can be evidenced not only by modern literature but also mass entertainment such as chat shows, films, medical dramas and lifestyle magazines. It is, of course, from such sources that the general public acquires most of its preconceptions about mental health and medicine in general. It follows, therefore, that any preconception that modern society holds will necessarily shape an individual's viewpoint and need to be at the heart of any ensuing treatment. Thus a more holistic approach to understanding a patient's life experience, perceptions and resultant condition has to take prominence in order to generate an effective, collaborative intervention or treatment plan.

Current practice

Modern medical practice now tends to use a biopsychosocial model (Engel 1980) in an attempt to explain the interrelationship between social (e.g. poverty, unhealthy life choices), psychological (e.g. stress) and biological (e.g. genetic expression) elements. In this respect psychiatry is no different. However, what is variable is the starting point of the treating clinician, dependent upon his or her training or background, with respect to the relative weight of importance that is placed upon the different elements within an assessment of a patient's life and condition.

To undertake a comprehensive psychiatric history, advanced consultation skills are undoubtedly needed (Coll *et al.* 2012). These skills may come from a variety of clinical communication models, for example, the Calgary-Cambridge model (Coll, *et al.* 2012; Silverman *et al.* 2013); the Three-Function Model (Bird & Cohen-Cole 1990); and arguably a variety of psychotherapeutic approaches such as cognitive behaviour therapy (Hawton *et al.* 1989), psychodynamic psychotherapy (Hughes 1999) and so on. The consultation style depends somewhat on the therapeutic model being used, but a successful outcome will result from an enhancement of the therapeutic relationship (Martin *et al.* 2000; Del Re *et al.* 2012) by providing skills to strengthen the relationship in a number of ways:
• by setting a clear agenda or goals;
• by ensuring a clear joint understanding is reached and
• by taking into account the myriad of preconceptions that mental health generates (Coll *et al.* 2012; Silverman *et al.* 2013).

These preconceptions influence the clinician–practitioner relationship in a number of ways. For example, a cognitive behavioural therapy trained practitioner might focus upon the interaction between how a person's past experience or 'core beliefs' about him- or herself and the world impact upon the assumptions and actions that he or she makes (Hawton *et al.* 1989). Take, for example, a patient who has been raised by what is perceived as an overly critical parent. One outcome *may* be that an individual begins to develop defensive strategies to prevent him- or herself from feeling uneasy because of real or imagined criticism. Such attitudes or procedures will occur in all aspects of that individual's life. However, the heightened anxiety felt by the patient due to the context of an 'authoritarian' medical consultation will more than likely result in such attitudes being brought to, and probably exaggerated by, the consultation environment. But one should not forget that the clinician will also bring his or her own

preconceptions and assumptions to the interaction. Such is the nature of being human. Expert consultation and rapport-building skills are therefore needed to ensure that a clear joint understanding is reached. For example:
- that an effective and agreed agenda is set (agenda setting);
- that preconceptions can be adeptly made explicit (clarifying);
- that all topics are covered (ideas, concerns and expectations – ICE) and
- that specific techniques are used to ensure that the interview achieves its goals (e.g. rapport building, empathising) (Coll *et al.* 2012; Silverman *et al.* 2013).

By contrast, a psychoanalytically or psychodynamically trained professional (broadly similar in their ethos) will be inherently more attuned to how a patient interacts with the clinician and from there will make hypotheses about why this might be so (Bateman 2010). Such a therapist will also notice how he or she is made to feel by a patient and attempt to interpret, contain or manage these feelings (Casement 1988; Wilson 2001; Bateman 2010). These therapists' ideas may or may not be made explicit and discussed logically depending upon the situation and whether the patient is able to bear acknowledging them. Therefore skills aimed at increasing empathy and rapport need to be learnt and utilised and are crucial to the attainment of a positive interview and treatment plan. In addition, and outside of the interview setting, clinicians should use supervision to help see the patterns set up by each interaction with patients and ensure that the interviews remain purposeful and useful (Casement 1988).

In reality, all such psychotherapeutic concepts are arguably somewhat flawed, but they still have their place throughout medicine, not just in psychiatry. All patients come with health beliefs but also complex and at times (particularly during moments of stress) exaggerated attitudes towards and assumptions about the world around them. The clinician's role is to understand these assumptions and use them to create a sense of meaning for the patient. The clinician holds the knowledge and experience, but throughout medical practice rarely does this translate into an effective treatment plan unless the clinician recognises the patient's understanding of how his or her particular biopsychosocial model of illness fits together in a way that is meaningful for the patient. This can be evidenced by the low levels of compliance with treatment plans in all branches of medicine (Zolnierek & Dimatteo 2009) if there is a mismatch between the patient and clinician, and the high placebo responses if there is good collaborative working relationship (Kirsch 2009). Both potential outcomes imply that the process by which an interview is conducted, and the techniques used to foster a good working alliance, are crucial if there is to be a positive outcome for both the patient and clinician. Where mental illness forms any part of the presentation, such sophisticated consultation skills are a necessary requirement if a successful outcome is to be found through the creation of a sound therapeutic alliance (Martin *et al.* 2000; Kirsch 2009; Del Re *et al.* 2012). Merely diagnosing a problem may or may not be of assistance, and depression is a classic example. It forms a part of many medical presentations but its presence is rarely explored despite clear evidence to suggest better health outcomes if it is addressed; for example, following myocardial infarction (Meijer *et al.* 2011).

Clearly, any diagnosis should lead to an optimal treatment. However, just as there remains debate about the role of diagnosis in modern psychiatry (Van Os 2009; Allan 2011), there are of course differing viewpoints as to what denotes 'optimal'. On the one hand, the prescription of medication too readily can overemphasise the 'bio' elements and not encourage a patient to address the causal or maintaining underlying psychosocial aspects. Alternatively, not recognising crushing biological symptoms that are causing an individual's underlying personality traits to be exaggerated and skewed can lead to unreasonable expectations for the patient to change his or her attitude or behaviour. As mentioned, clarifying ideas, concerns and expectations explicitly and actively working to a shared agenda (Coll *et al.* 2012; Silverman *et al.* 2013) should lead to a more realistic intervention, better compliance and better overall outcomes and satisfaction for clinician and patient alike.

Future implications

Understanding the underlying genesis or formulation of why 'this person is presenting at this time with these particular problems' is the key to a meaningful psychiatric consultation. For the clinician, it requires a full exploration or assessment of the person who is sitting in front of him or her, at least the best assessment possible. Specific techniques such as clarification seem to be one of the cornerstones to achieving a comprehensive understanding (McCabe *et al.* 2013), as it encourages the patient to feel able to participate in the formation of a shared understanding of the nature of the problem and the reasons why this problem is present and to develop a sensible and meaningful solution. To do this requires information from a person's past and present but also information about how he or she operates within and perceives the world and how he or she interacts and why and to make predictions about the person's future actions. Only once this shared understanding has been reached can a true treatment plan be devised, certainly one that will lead to optimal improvement for the patient. Enhancing the therapeutic relationship is known to improve outcomes (Martin *et al.* 2000; Del Re *et al.* 2012), and specific techniques such as collaborative agenda setting and the exploration and clarification of ideas, concerns and expectations are tools and skills specifically designed to assist with this (Coll *et al.* 2012; Silverman *et al.* 2013).

It follows, therefore, that because of the personalised nature of mental distress, when assessing and treating symptoms of mental illness, increased emphasis and attention needs to be paid to the subjective elements of the presentation. In order to achieve this, higher levels of consultation skills are required. Poor-quality interviews lead to poor-quality treatments, as ineffective communication skills within psychiatry can lead to alienation and disengagement from services, deterioration in mental health and the possibility of compulsory admission, and risk to self and others (Priebe *et al.* 2005).

It may be that in the future, biological tests will abound to help and guide clinicians towards accurate diagnoses within psychiatry. However, ideal treatment will only be achieved, in medical practice but particularly within psychiatry, if the human element is acknowledged as being a major factor leading to optimal treatment outcomes. For that reason, possibly above all other reasons, advanced consultation skills will always be an essential and indispensable part of medical practice.

References

Allan, C. (2011) British Psychological Society. 2011. *Response to the American Psychiatric Association: DSM-5 development* [WWW document]. URL apps.bps.org.uk/_publicationfiles/consultation-responses/DSM-5%202011%20-%20BPS%20response.pdf [accessed on 11 December 2014].
Bateman, A. (2010) *Introduction to Psychotherapy: An Outline of Psychodynamic Principles and Practice*, fourth edn. Routledge, London.
Bird, J. & Cohen-Cole, S.A. (1990) The three-function model of the medical interview: An educational device. *Advances of Psychosomatic Medicine*, 20, 65–88.

Casement, P. (1988) *On Learning from the Patient.* Routledge, London.

Coll, X., Papageorgiou, A., Stanley, A. & Tarbuck, A. (eds) (2012) *Communication Skills in Mental Health.* Radcliffe, London.

Del Re, A.C., Flückiger. C., Horvath, A.O., Symonds, D. & Wampold, B.E. (2012) Therapists' effects in the therapeutic alliance-outcome relationship: A restricted-maximum likelihood meta-analytic review. *Clinical Psychology Review,* 32 (no. 7), 642–649.

Ellenberger, H. (1970) *The Discovery of the Unconscious: The History and Evolution of Dynamic Psychiatry.* Basic Books, New York.

Engel, G.L. (1980) The clinical application of the biopsychosocial model. *American Journal of Psychiatry,* 137, 535–544.

Hawton, K., Salkovskis, P.M., Kirk, J. & Clark, D.M. (1989) *Cognitive Behavior Therapy for Psychiatric Problems: A Practical Guide.* Oxford University Press, New York.

Hughes, P. (1999) *Dynamic Psychotherapy Explained.* Radcliffe, London.

Kirsch, I. (2009) *The Emperor's New Drugs.* Bodley Head, London.

Martin, D.J., Garske, J.P. & Davis, M.K. (2000) Relation of the therapeutic alliance with outcome and other variables: A meta-analytic review. *Journal of Consulting and Clinical Psychology,* 68 (no. 3), 438–450.

McCabe, R., Healey, P.G., Priebe, S., Lavelle, M., Dodwell, D., Laughame, R., Snell, A. & Bremner, S. (2013) Shared understanding in psychiatrist–patient communication: Association with treatment adherence in schizophrenia. *Patient Education and Counseling,* 93 (no. 1), 73–79.

Meijer, A., Conradi, H.J., Bos, E.H., Thombs, B.D., van Melle, J.P. & de Jonge, P. (2011) Prognostic association of depression following myocardial infarction with morality and cardiovascular events: A meta analysis of 25 years of research. *General Hospital Psychiatry,* 33 (no. 3), 203–216.

Morrison, A.P., Hutton, P., Shiers, D. & Turkington, D. (2012) Antipsychotics: Is it time to introduce patient choice? *British Journal of Psychiatry,* 201, 83–84.

Priebe, S., Watts, J., Chase, M., and Matanov, A. (2005) Processes of disengagement and engagement in assertive outreach patients: a qualitative study. *British Journal of Psychiatry,* 187, 438–443.

Silverman, J., Kurtz, S. & Draper, J. (2013) *Skills for Communicating with Patients,* third edn. Radcliffe, London.

Van Os, J. (2009) A salience dysregulation syndrome. *British Journal of Psychiatry,* 194, 101–103.

Wilson, J. (2001) Starting out in psychodynamic psychotherapy. *Psychiatric Bulletin,* 25, 72–74.

Zolnierek, K.B. & Dimatteo, M.R. (2009) Physician communication and patient adherence to treatment: A meta-analysis. *Medical Care,* 47 (no. 8), 826–834.

PART 2C

Interprofessional Communication

CHAPTER 25

Interprofessional Communication and Its Challenges

Susanne Lindqvist

Norwich Medical School, University of East Anglia, Norfolk, UK

Overview

Historically, when things go wrong (or nearly go wrong) in the care setting, breakdown in communication between professionals is high on the list of factors contributing to the failure of the service (Kennedy *et al.* 2001; Laming 2003; Haringey Council Local Safeguarding Children Board 2009; Francis 2013). Statements made by the UK Department of Health (e.g. Department of Health 2001; 2008; 2011) and professional bodies such as the General Medical Council and Nursing and Midwifery Council (General Medical Council 2009; 2013; Nursing and Midwifery Council 2008) therefore highlight the need for and importance of effective communication and collaboration between professionals and agencies involved in care delivery. To date, there are no clear guidelines as to what education and training should be delivered to ensure development of key skills that enable interprofessional communication and underpin effective collaboration.

Most health and social care students will receive opportunities to learn and practise communication skills within their respective courses. According to Silverman and colleagues (2005), a doctor needs to adopt a person-centred, engaged and empathic approach whilst building rapport during a consultation. In parallel, a doctor also needs to follow a structured process to ensure all relevant information is collected and understood by both parties. In order to prepare future doctors, many medical schools have adopted the Calgary-Cambridge model (Kurtz *et al.* 1998; Silverman *et al.* 2005) as a framework for their communication skills teaching, whereas nonmedical courses often use less structured teaching sessions (Bachman *et al.* 2013). The focus of consultation skills teaching is on the students learning to communicate with the person seeking care, rather than with the colleagues they will work with.

In the practice setting, different professionals are expected to work together effectively, but rarely if at all will they have opportunities to learn how to do this in the most effective way (Watkin *et al.* 2009). In response to a call for professionals to be equipped with the necessary skills required for interprofessional communication and working, not only in the UK (Francis 2013) but also globally (Frenk *et al.* 2010; World Health Organization 2010), many universities now offer opportunities for students to learn and work together with peers from different health and social care courses.

Clinical Communication in Medicine, First Edition. Edited by Jo Brown, Lorraine M. Noble, Alexia Papageorgiou and Jane Kidd.

The Centre for the Advancement of Interprofessional Education recently published a guide to support those who wish to introduce interprofessional learning into their curricula (Barr & Low 2013). Despite growing evidence related to the effectiveness of interprofessional learning, there is still room for more research, evaluation and discussion amongst stakeholders to tease out what the challenges are for professionals as they communicate with each other and how educators can support the future workforce by providing high-quality education and training.

This chapter aims to look at some of the known challenges from the past, present examples of how they are currently addressed and provide suggestions of how future educators can support the development of effective interprofessional collaboration.

Challenges associated with interprofessional communication

As with any relationship, a key ingredient in the recipe for success is effective communication. In the health and social care arena, such communication can be particularly difficult to carry out and possibly even harder to maintain. Known challenges associated with communication between professionals are often linked to a lack of

- awareness of own role in communication;
- understanding of, and ability to deal with, rank dynamics between professions;
- understanding of different professions' roles and responsibilities;
- courage and being proactive;
- skills in dealing with conflict and emotional stress;
- common language and consistency in the interpretation of confidentiality;
- respect towards, and trust in, the abilities of other professions and time.

Awareness of own role in communication

The emphasis of self-awareness within the team and the importance of effective communication is more developed in other sectors such as the aviation (Gordon *et al.* 2012) and retail industries (Fill 2009). Within these areas, the main drivers for making sure professionals are sufficiently trained in communication skills are safety and customer satisfaction. For pilots and sales managers there is no doubt that it is not enough to have the skills in flying a plane or marketing a product. Rather, these professionals need to possess the skills that enable them to interact and communicate effectively with their team members and customers in order to successfully fulfil their professional role. Staff in these fields receives the necessary training to develop the required skills, which are monitored thereafter on an ongoing basis (Fill 2009; Gordon *et al.* 2012).

For each health and social care professional group there are a set of standards (Nursing and Midwifery Council 2008; General Medical Council 2013; Health and Care Professions Council 2014) that individuals need to meet in order to continue their current practice, but the literature is currently lacking evidence on how to develop their awareness of own role in communication.

In order to improve communication with others, Brent and Dent (2010) argue that the starting point is with the 'self'. Learners can complete inventories to gain an awareness of their personality style (e.g. Champagne & Hogan 1979) and preferred team role (e.g. Belbin 2013), which will help identify personal strengths and weaknesses and how they are perceived by others. Knowledge of self is hypothesised to enhance an individual's emotional intelligence (Goleman 1995) and thus optimise his or her ability to interact effectively with others, regardless of real or perceived rank between professions.

Understanding of, and ability to deal with, rank dynamics between professions

Issues around power between and within professions are frequent causes of communication breakdown (Collins & Lindqvist 2013). Rank dynamics are complex and well rooted in our society, also historically between health (Paley 2002) and social (McLaughlin 2012) care professions, creating a barrier to communication. The literature offers a wealth of insight into power struggles between care professions (McLaughlin 2012), many of which can be linked to the skills and behaviour of the team leader (Collins & Lindqvist 2013; Reeves *et al.* 2010b). It is therefore essential for team leaders to recognise the power of rank dynamics and the emotional labour (Humphrey *et al.* 2008) associated with dysfunctional teams where members do not feel free, or able, to challenge decisions, actions and interactions – yet are still expected to deliver compassionate care (Reeves *et al.* 2010a). They must also have the ability to create a safe and open environment that allows for this to happen. However, all team members need to actively engage in the process of working together and receive appropriate support to be able to communicate across ranks (Goleman 1995; Gordon *et al.* 2012).

Despite health and social care professionals being absolutely clear that their common goal is to deliver person-centred care, they do not always agree how this should be accomplished or have the ability to overcome the challenges linked to interacting with members of professions with perceived higher, or lower, rank (Collins & Lindqvist 2013). Tensions related to rank within the health and social work professions often derive from a lack of understanding of the roles and responsibilities of those contributing different aspects of care and how they depend on each other in order to provide a holistic service (Mizrahi & Abrahamson 2000; McLaughlin 2012).

Understanding of different professions' roles and responsibilities

Knowledge of different professional roles and responsibilities enables a team to provide a person with the care he or she needs by referring the person to the appropriate professional(s) with the most appropriate skills at the right time. This is a core aim of interprofessional education *when two or more professions learn with, from and about each other to improve collaboration and the quality of care* (Centre for the Advancement of Interprofessional Education 2002). Although the evidence is not conclusive as to when interprofessional learning should be introduced in order to gain most benefit (Barr & Low 2013), there is increasing support for early introduction (Hammick *et al.* 2007; Reeves *et al.* 2010a) so that positive attitudes (Lindqvist *et al.* 2005) and behaviours can develop that facilitate interprofessional collaboration.

According to Gordon (2009), the adult learner needs to take incremental steps to become a capable interprofessional worker. As roles and responsibilities evolve in response to changing demands on healthcare, tensions can arise unless everyone is aware of who does what, when, why and how. This is discussed by Hawkes *et al.* (2013), who also highlight the challenge in managing such change without diluting professional identities.

The National Health Service (NHS) Leadership Framework (NHS Leadership Academy 2011) emphasises the importance for future leaders in health and social care to be aware of their own and other's role and responsibilities within the team. However, in line with reports following past and recent incidents (Kennedy *et al.* 2001; Laming 2003; Haringey Council Local Safeguarding Children Board 2009; Francis 2013;

Berwick 2013), more attention needs to be placed on the responsibility of all team members being proactive and courageous with any concerns they may have about their own or other's ability to provide safe and effective care.

Courage and being proactive

Whistleblowing has been discussed at length in the literature since the report published by Kennedy and his team in 2001 and has recently been encouraged for the safety of care delivery (Francis 2013). However, many professionals find it difficult to address concerns related to a colleague, especially if this colleague is of a higher rank (Collins & Lindqvist 2013). The sad and unexpected death of Elaine Bromiley in 2005 highlighted this issue as well as the impact of human factors and how people sometimes behave in stressful situations (Harmer 2005). Taking lessons from the aviation industry, guides and checklists are now available to ensure care is delivered as safely as possible, such as the surgical safety checklist (World Health Organization 2009), which has proven to effectively save lives (de Vries *et al.* 2010). According to Gordon and colleagues (2012), we need to look beyond the checklists to ensure situational awareness and safety of patients, as well as the other members of the team.

The significance of keeping the team spirit high, avoiding a blame culture, and promoting open and transparent communication channels has been emphasised to support the workforce (Berwick 2013). On successful completion of the 2-year Foundation Programme (UK Foundation Programme 2012/2014), doctors are expected to encourage open communication in a blame-free environment where they understand the importance of learning from mistakes. Further to this, they are expected to be able to describe ways of identifying poor performance in self and in colleagues and use appropriate lines of communication when dealing with such situations – some of which can no doubt lead to conflict.

Skills to deal with conflict and emotional stress

Dealing with any kind of conflict is challenging (Goleman 1995; Patient Safety First Campaign 2009). Currently, students may be able to practise communication with patients who are angry or want to complain, but there are less frequent examples and resources in the literature of how to deal with challenging colleagues and emotional tension within a team – especially using an interprofessional approach (Young & Turner 2009). Skills for Health has in recent years improved their material to support health employers in the UK by providing a Core Skills Framework learning portfolio, which also includes key principles of conflict resolution (e.g. NHS Core Skills Framework learning portfolio 2013).

Effective communication and awareness of body language is very important when trying to resolve a conflict, or tensions, between people (Brent & Dent 2010). In order to help healthcare professionals, and those in a leading position in particular, to understand the relationship between emotional well-being and a team's ability to provide a high-quality service, the NHS Leadership Academy (2013) has developed a healthcare leadership model. This model outlines a number of key dimensions that describe to leaders what behaviours help in managing conflict. Where conflict is not dealt with appropriately, emotional stress is likely to build up, which can impact negatively on staff health and performance and this, in turn, can affect care delivery and safety (Maben *et al.* 2012).

One initiative that followed in the wake of the Francis report was the rolling out of the Schwartz Center Rounds (http://www.theschwartzcenter.org/) for staff, as a way to share difficult emotions that can occur for professionals during their working life. These Rounds have been successfully piloted in the UK (Goodrich 2011) and shown to be effective in helping professionals manage their own emotional well-being so that they can provide compassionate care for others.

Although the NHS Institute for Innovation and Improvement no longer exists, their Quality and Service Improvement Tools can still be accessed and used by both students and staff to practise ways of communicating around emotive topics (e.g. NHS Institute for Innovation and Improvement 2010). Some of these are very easy to use and can also act as a trigger for discussions related to interprofessional communication, such as the use of common language and issues around confidentiality.

Common language and consistency in the interpretation of confidentiality

A person who needs help from the police as well as social and health services may assume that all these different professionals understand each other, speak the same language and share relevant information. However, these groups use different language, models of care and interpretations of how they manage confidentiality across agencies (Police [Conduct] Regulations 2004; British Association of Social Workers 2008; General Medical Council 2009, 2013; Munro 2011). Confidentiality is a means to protect the individual, but it can also hinder care delivery (British Association of Social Workers 2008) and at worst cause harm (Munro 2011).

Multiagency safeguarding hubs (Home Office 2013) have been initiated across the UK to address concerns around the safety of children and vulnerable people in order to initiate early interventions. Professionals with concerns can contact the team, who will then share and analyse information and act accordingly. Early evidence suggests that these meetings are successful and the Home Office (2014) has recently published a report to share the findings from this way of working. One of the many key components that have been reported as important in sharing multiagency models is the need to overcome the culture differences between the professions by using a common language.

Acronyms and jargon are commonly used within each profession, and such language is developed throughout students' education. Learning to communicate in small interprofessional groups from the outset with the support of a trained facilitator gives students the chance to explore and reflect on how they come across when communicating with students from other courses in a safe environment (Freeman *et al.* 2010). As they progress in their courses, such opportunities can also help students learn to articulate their current understanding of their future roles and responsibilities as they develop their professional and interprofessional identities (Murdoch-Eaton & Roberts 2009), thus enabling them to build respect for what each profession brings to the care delivery process.

Respect towards, and trust in, the abilities of other professions

If health and social care students are educated in silos throughout their courses at university, they may graduate with a limited understanding of the abilities of each other's professions. Further to students being kept apart, students will also be subjected to varying philosophical approaches to education (Fitzsimmons & White 1997) and submerged with different ideological worldviews (Apker 2012).

Limited knowledge and understanding of what each profession contributes to care can breed negative attitudes that can inhibit communication and impact negatively on care delivery, as discussed by Hawkes and colleagues (2013). Findings presented in this paper show that students develop positive attitudes towards their professions as they participate in interprofessional learning and thus learn more about their different abilities. This way of working together may encourage future communication and thus enhance collaboration, leading to real benefits to care delivery. Indeed, it is stated – in a publication by the Centre for Workforce Intelligence (2013) – that team building promotes respect towards, and trust in, the abilities of other professions, which in turn empowers professionals to engage with each other. A main challenge is remaining, however, and that is finding the time for professionals to actively participate in such activities.

Time

The under-investment of time for professionals to get together to reflect on and discuss their current practice has long been reported as an issue due to their workload (Hornby & Atkins 2000). Since it is now recognised that patient safety depends on both individual and team working between professionals (UK Foundation Programme Curriculum 2012), protected time needs to be set aside for professionals to learn and work together. When they do, significant progress can be made that benefits both staff and service users (Watts *et al.* 2007; Watkin *et al.* 2009).

Further to the busy workload in practice, educators also struggle to find slots in the curricula for students from different professions to come together – especially if the numbers of professions and students are high (Barr & Low 2013). Making time for these meetings is the first step, but face-to-face encounters are not enough (Carpenter & Dickinson 2011). According to these authors there are other ingredients necessary for successful interaction and dialogue, such as:

• participants having equal opportunities to contribute views;
• working towards a common goal or vision;
• institutional support;
• opportunities to discuss similarities and differences;
• positive expectations and
• perception of members of other professions as representatives for that group.

With these parameters in place and with the support of a trained facilitator (Freeman *et al.* 2010), safe opportunities for education and training can take place to practise interprofessional communication.

Concluding remarks

Following a number of incidents where care has been less than optimal, and in some cases disastrous, the pressure is now on to improve quality of care by optimising available resources (Centre for Workforce Intelligence 2013; Francis 2013). Effective collaboration between professionals with excellent interprofessional communication skills is an essential component of this process.

The challenges listed in this chapter are not exhaustive but highlight important aspects of interprofessional communication that educators need to be aware of as they facilitate students and professionals during their education and training. Opportunities to learn and work with others, together with timely and constructive feedback, will help learners reflect on their development and how they manage these challenges from the outset and throughout their careers.

References

Apker, J. (2012) *Communication in Health Organizations* Polity Press, Cambridge.
Bachman, C., Abramovitch, H., Barbu, C.G., Cavaco, A.M., Elorza, R.D., Haak, R., Loureioro, E., Ratajska, A., Silverman, J., Winterburn, S. & Rosenbaum, M. (2013) A European consensus on learning objectives for a core communication curriculum in health care professions. *Patient Education and Counseling*, 93, 18–26.
Barr, H. & Low, L. (2013) *Introducing Interprofessional Education*. Centre for the Advancement of Interprofessional Education, Fareham, UK [WWW document]. URL http://caipe.org.uk/silo/files/introducing-interprofessional-education.pdf.
Belbin. (2013) *Method, Reliability & Validity, Statistics & Research: A Comprehensive Review of Belbin Team Roles* [WWW document]. URL http://www.belbin.com/content/page/5599/BELBIN (uk)-2013-A%20Comprehensive%20Review.pdf [accessed on 3 November 2014].
Berwick, D. (2013) *A Promise to Learn – a Commitment to Act*. Improving the Safety of Patients in England. National Advisory Group on the Safety of Patients in England [WWW document. URL https://www.gov.uk/government/uploads/system/uploads/attachment_data/file/226703/Berwick_Report.pdf.
Brent, M. & Dent, E.F. (2010) *The Leader's Guide to Influence*, Prentice Hall, Upper Saddle River, NJ.
British Association of Social Workers. (2008) *The Code of Ethics for Social Work – Statement of Principles* [WWW document]. URL https://www.basw.co.uk/codeofethics/.
Carpenter, J. & Dickinson, C. (2011) 'Contact is not enough': A social psychological perspective on interprofessional education. In: A. Kitto, J. Chesters, J. Thistlethwaite & S. Reeves (eds), *Sociology of Interprofessional Health Care Practice*, pp. 55–68, Nova Science Publishers, New York.
Centre for the Advancement of Interprofessional Education. (2002) *Defining IPE* [WWW document]. URL http://caipe.org.uk/resources/defining-ipe/ [accessed on 3 November 2014].
Centre for Workforce Intelligence. (2013) *Think Integration, Think Workforce: Three Steps to Workforce Integration* [WWW document]. URL http://www.cfwi.org.uk/publications/think-integration-think-workforce-three-steps-to-workforce-integration-1/@@publication-detail.
Champagne, D.W. & Hogan, R.C. (1979) *Supervisory and Management Skills: A Competency Based Training Program for Middle Managers of Educational Systems*. Privately published book.
Collins, M. & Lindqvist, S. (2013) Interprofessional practice and rank dynamics: Evolving effective team collaboration through emotional, social, occupational and spiritual intelligences. In: P. Canvenagh, S. Leinster, & S. Miles (eds), *The Changing Roles of Doctors*. Radcliffe Publishing, London.
Department of Health. (2001) *Working Together – Learning Together. A Framework for Lifelong Learning for the NHS London* [WWW document]. URL http://webarchive.nationalarchives.gov.uk/20130107105354/http://www.dh.gov.uk/prod_consum_dh/groups/dh_digitalassets/@dh/@en/documents/digitalasset/dh_4058896.pdf.
Department of Health. (2008) *High Quality Care for All*. NHS Next Stage Review Final Report. Presented to Parliament by the Secretary of State for Health by Command of Her Majesty. Command paper CM 7432.
Department of Health. (2011). *Health and Social Care Bill* [WWW document]. URL http://webarchive.nationalarchives.gov.uk/20130805112926/http://healthandcare.dh.gov.uk/bill/.
de Vries, E. N., Prins, H. A., Crolla, R.M.P.H., den Outer, A. J., van Andel, G., van Helden, S. H., Schlack, W.S., van Putten, A., Gouma, D.J., Dijkgraaf, M.G.W., Smorenburg, S.M. & Boermeester, M.A. (2010) Effect of a comprehensive surgical safety system on patient outcomes. *New England Journal of Medicine*, 363,1928–1937.
Fill, M. (2009) *Marketing Communications: Interactivity, Communities and Content*. Pearson Education Limited, Harlow, UK.
Fitzsimmons, P. & White, T. (1997) Crossing boundaries. Communication between professional groups. *Journal of Mangement in Medicine*, 11 (no. 2), 96–101.
Francis, R. (2013). *The Mid Staffordshire NHS Foundation Trust Public Inquiry*. An independent report into the care provided by Mid Staffordshire NHS Foundation Trust between January 2005 and March 2009 [WWW document]. URL http://www.midstaffspublicinquiry.com/ [accessed on 3 November 2014].
Freeman. S., Wright A. & Lindqvist, S. (2010) Facilitator training for educators involved in interprofessional learning. *Journal of Interprofessional Care*, 24 (no. 4), 375–385.

Frenk. J., Chen, L., Bhutta, Z.A., Cohen, J., Crisp, N., Evans, E., Fineberg, H., Garcia, P., Ke, Y., Kelley, P., Kistnasamy, B., Meleis, A., Naylor, D., Pablos-Medez, A., Reddy, S., Scrimshaw, S., Sepulveda, J., Serwadda, D. & Zurayk, H. (2010) Health professionals for a new century: Transforming education to strengthen health systems in an interdependent world. *Lancet*, 376 (no. 9756), 1923–1958.

General Medical Council. (2009) *Confidentiality*. General Medical Council, London.

General Medical Council. GMC (2009) *Tomorrow's Doctors: Outcome and Standards for Undergraduate Medical Education*. General Medical Council, London.

General Medical Council. (2013) *Good Medical Practice*. General Medical Council, London.

Goleman, D. (1995) *Emotional Intelligence*. Bantam Books, New York.

Goodrich, J. (2011) *Schwartz Center Rounds – Evaluation of UK Pilots*. The Kings Fund, London.

Gordon, F. (2009) Interprofessional capability as an aim of student learning. In: P. Bluteau & A. Jackson (eds), *Interprofessional Education – Making It Happen*. Palgrave Macmillan, Houndmills, UK.

Gordon, S., Mendenhall, M. & O'Connor, B. (2012) *Beyond the Checklist: What Else Health Care Can Learn from Aviation Teamwork and Safety. The Culture and Politics of Health Care Work*. Cornell University Press, Ithaca, NY.

Hammick, M., Freeth, D., Koppel, I., Reeves, S. & Barr, H. (2007) A best evidence systematic review of interprofessional education. *Medical Teacher*, 29, 735–751.

Haringey Council Local Safeguarding Children Board. (2009) *An Executive Summary of the Serious Case Review 'Baby Peter'* [WWW document]. UFL http://www.haringeylscb.org/executive_sum mary_peter_final.pdf [accessed on 3 November 2014].

Harmer, M. (2005). *Independent Review on the care given to Mrs Elaine Bromiley on 29 March 2005* [WWW document]. URL http://www.chfg.org/wp-content/uploads/2010/11/ElaineBromiley AnonymousReport.pdf.

Hawkes, G., Nunney, I. & Lindqvist, S. (2013) Caring for attitudes as a means of caring for patients – improving medical, pharmacy and nursing students' attitudes to each other's professions by engaging them in interprofessional learning. *Medical Teacher*, 35 (no. 7), e1302–1308.

Health and Care Professions Council. (2014) *Standards of Education and Training* [WWW document]. URL http://www.hpc-uk.org/assets/documents/1000295EStandardsofeducationandtraining-from September2009.pdf.

Home Office. (2013) *Multi-Agency Working and Information Sharing Project Early Findings* [WWW document]. URL https://www.gov.uk/government/uploads/system/uploads/attachment_data/ file/225012/MASH_Product.pdf [accessed on 3 November 2014].

Home Office. (2014) *Multi Agency Working and Information Sharing Project Final Report* [WWW document]. URL https://www.gov.uk/government/uploads/system/uploads/attachment_data/ file/338875/MASH.pdf [accessed on 3 November 2014].

Hornby, S. & Atkins, J. (2000) *Collaborative Care*, second edn. Blackwell Science, Alden Press, Oxford, UK.

Humphrey, R.H., Pollack, J.M. & Hawver, T. (2008) Leading with emotional labour. *Journal of Managerial Psychology*, 23 (no. 2), 151–168.

Kennedy, I., Howard, R., Jarman, B. & Maclean, M. (2001) *Learning from Bristol: The Report of the Public Inquiry into Children's Heart Surgery at the Bristol Royal Infirmary 1984–1995*. Command paper CM 5207.

Kurtz, S.M., Silverman, J.D. & Draper, J. (1998) *Teaching and Learning Communication Skills in Medicine*. Radcliffe Medical Press, Oxford.

Laming, Lord. (2003) *The Victoria Climbié Inquiry Report*. House of Commons, London [WWW document]. http://www.publications.parliament.uk/pa/cm200203/cmselect/cmhealth/570/570.pdf.

Lindqvist, S., Duncan, A., Shepstone, L., Watts, F. & Pearce, S. (2005) Development of the attitudes to health professionals questionnaire (AHPQ): A measure to assess interprofessional attitudes. *Journal of Interprofessional Care*, 19 (no. 3), 269–279.

Maben, J., Adams, M., Peccei, R., Murrells, T. & Robert, G. (2012) 'Poppets and parcels': The links between staff experience of work and acutely ill older peoples' experience of hospital care. *International Journal of Older People Nursing*, 7, 83–94.

McLaughlin, H. (2012) Keeping inter-professional practice honest. In: B. Littlechild & R. Smith (eds), *A Handbook for Interprofessional Practice in the Human Services: Learning to Work Together*, pp 50–61. Pearson Press, Harlow, UK.

Mizrahi, T. & Abramson, S.J. (2000) Social work and physician collaboration: Perspectives on a shared case. *Social Work in Health Care*, 31 (no. 3), 1–24.

Munro, E. (2011) *The Munro Review of Child Protection: Final Report. A Child-Centred System* [WWW document]. URL https://www.gov.uk/government/publications/munro-review-of-child-pro tection-final-report-a-child-centred-system [accessed on 3 November 2014].

Murdoch-Eaton, D.G. & Roberts, T.E. (2009) The doctor. In: M. Doel & S.M. Shardlow (eds), *Educating Professionals – Practice Learning in Health and Social Care*. Ashgate Publishing, Farnham, UK.

NHS Core Skills Framework learning portfolio. (2013) *Conflict Resolution* [WWW document]. URL http://www.cmtpct.nhs.uk/north-west-core-skills/resources/Conflict_Resolution_Reader_ Feb_2013.pdf [accessed 3 November 2014].

NHS Institute for Innovation and Improvement. (2010). *Quality and Service Improvement Tools. Conflict resolution* [WWW document]. URL http://www.institute.nhs.uk/quality_and_service_ improvement_tools/quality_and_service_improvement_tools/human_dimensions_-_managing_ conflict.html [accessed on 3 November 2014].

NHS Leadership Academy. (2011). *Clinical Leadership Competency Framework* [WWW document]. URL http://www.leadershipacademy.nhs.uk/wp-content/uploads/2012/11/NHSLeadership- Leadership-Framework-Clinical-Leadership-Competency-Framework-CLCF.pdf [accessed on 3 November 2014].

NHS Leadership Academy. (2013). *Healthcare Leadership Model* [WWW document]. URL https:// www.leadershipacademy.nhs.uk/wp-content/uploads/2013/10/NHSLeadership- LeadershipModel-10-Print.pdf [accessed on 3 November 2014].

Nursing and Midwifery Council. (2008). *The Code: Standards of Conduct, Performance and Ethics for Nurses and Midwives* [WWW document]. URL http://www.nmc-uk.org/Documents/Standards/ nmcTheCodeStandardsofConductPerformanceAndEthicsForNursesAndMidwives_ LargePrintVersion.PDF.

Paley, J. (2002) Caring as a slave morality: Nietzschean themes in nursing ethics. *Journal of Advanced Nursing*, 40 (no. 1), 25–35.

Patient Safety First Campaign. (2009) *The 'How to Guide' for Implementing Human Factors in Healthcare* [WWW document]. URL http://www.institute.nhs.uk/safer_care/general/human_ factors.html [accessed on 3 November 2014].

Police (Conduct) Regulations. 2004. URL http://www.nypolfed.org.uk/assets/uploads/PDFs/ discipline3.pdf.

Reeves, I., Lewin, S., Espin, S. & Zwarenstein, M. (2010a) *Interprofessional Teamwork for Health and Social Care*. Wiley-Blackwell, Chichester, UK.

Reeves, S., MacMillan, K. & Soeren, M. (2010b) Leadership of interprofessional health and social care teams: A socio-historical analysis. *Journal of Nursing Management*, 18, 258–264.

Silverman, J., Kurtz, S.M. & Draper, J. (2005) *Skills for Communicating with Patients*, second edn. Oxford Radcliffe, Oxford, UK.

UK Foundation Programme Curriculum. (2012, updated 2014). URL http://www.foundationpro gramme.nhs.uk/pages/home.

Watkin, A., Lindqvist, S., Black, J. & Watts, F. (2009) Report on the implementation and evalua- tion of an interprofessional learning programme for inter-agency child protection teams. *Child Abuse Review*, 18,151–167.

Watts, F., Lindqvist, S., Pearce, S., Drachler, M. & Richardson, B. (2007) Introducing a post-registration interprofessional learning programme for healthcare teams. *Medical Teacher*, 20, 443–449.

World Health Organization. (2009) *Implementation Manual WHO Surgical Safety Checklist* [WWW document]. URL http://whqlibdoc.who.int/publications/2009/9789241598590_eng.pdf [accessed on 3 November 2014].

World Health Organization. (2010) *Framework for Action on Interprofessional Education & Collaborative Practice* [WWW document]. World Health Organization, Geneva. URL http://www.who.int/ hrh/resources/framework_action/en/index.html [accessed on 3 November 2014].

Young, A. & Turner, J. (2009) Developing interprofessional training for conflict resolution – a scoping audit and training pilot. *Mental Health Review Journal*, 14 (no. 1), 4–11.

PART 3
Learning, Teaching and Assessment

Section Lead Editor: Jo Brown

CHAPTER 26

Introduction to Learning, Teaching and Assessment

Jo Brown

St George's University of London, London, UK

Thirty years ago in the UK clinical communication was seen as something that was learned during the traditional apprenticeship model by 'osmosis', or by simply observing the practice of a doctor – commonly referred to as 'sitting by Nellie'. Clinical communication as a subject was seen as intrinsic to the personality of the medical student or doctor and not as something that could be taught or learned. In this section we shall look at how the thinking around clinical communication has changed and how the teaching and learning of it came to become a distinct part of medical education, taught as part of the core curriculum of every medical school in the UK today. We will investigate the primary disciplinary origins of this education to understand how we have got to where we are today and will look at the pedagogy of education in general, its influence on medical education in particular, charting the shifts and changes that led to the emergence of a modern system of medical education.

We begin with the fascinating history of the rise of clinical communication as an increasingly formalised subject that is set against the backdrop of historical and political change in the UK, where the role of the doctor changes and where new skills and attributes are needed for the consultation and beyond.

We move on to explore the seminal models of learning that have informed and influenced clinical communication, most notably behaviourism, and look at important learning paradigms such as constructivism and experiential learning that have paved the way for how the subject is taught and learned today.

The workplace learning chapter signals a change in theoretical thinking and the emergence of situated learning as a new way of understanding how students learn to become expert as professionals, moving us on to look at workplace learning theory as an attempt to overcome the theory/practice gap in clinical communication education. This is followed by a look at the power of transformative educational pedagogy and the primary importance of critical reflection and feedback to the development of professional clinical practice.

We end the section with an overview of assessment, which some would say drives learning in the subject and certainly informs the notion of competence in clinical communication. We end with the assessment of performance and, most importantly, how clinical communication is assessed in the authentic clinical workplace.

Clinical Communication in Medicine, First Edition. Edited by Jo Brown, Lorraine M. Noble,
Alexia Papageorgiou and Jane Kidd.
© 2016 John Wiley & Sons, Ltd. Published 2016 by John Wiley & Sons, Ltd.

CHAPTER 27

The History of Clinical Communication Teaching

Victoria Bates[1], Jonathan Reinarz[2] and Connie Wiskin[2]

[1]*University of Bristol, Bristol, UK*
[2]*University of Birmingham, Birmingham, UK*

While clinical communication as a specific clinical skillset, or discipline, is culturally associated with contemporary times, the role of communication in medical history has a rich and colourful past. In past centuries, medicine was often described as more of an art than a science, which aligns with the current understanding of there being more to effective clinical practice than a purely biomedical model. With few 'proven' cures before 1900, a rounded approach to medical practice was necessary. Practitioners were not notably versed in the humanities – such as the 'art' of communication – in the way that we understand such terms today, but consideration of communication is not exclusive to recent times. Since the Hippocratic era, it has been recognised that medical encounters require the doctor and the patient to hear each other and achieve 'a common view of what matters and what should be done' (Reiser 1993, p. 272). The implication was that dialogue – in some form – was anticipated. Medical practitioners recognised that careful communication improved clinical interviews, but the profession took longer to fully appreciate the relationship between communication and patient satisfaction, recall of advice or adherence. Empathy and interest in patients undoubtedly existed prior to the modern age, and we should not underestimate the undocumented contribution of individual doctors. However, human factors were noticeably overtaken by a 'rush to science', particularly during and after the Second World War. Concerns about the 'dehumanisation' of biomedicine were expressed in both professional and cultural depictions of medical practice. In conjunction with the need to satisfy an increasingly wide range of patients under universal healthcare (the new National Health Service [NHS]), the later twentieth century witnessed a more formalised push to improve medical communication both in clinical practice and education. As with many historical developments, we learn from the past to inform the future, and both positive and more challenging cultural messages have played their part in driving change.

Before 1800, communication with patients was recognised as essential to compiling a good case history. Before the rise of scientific medicine with its new institutional structures and arsenal of diagnostic technology, including germ and cell theories, it was largely up to the *patient* to specify a malady. Without taking an oral history, the practitioner could not otherwise access this information. At this time doctors regularly deferred to patients who directed clinical encounters by describing their unique

Clinical Communication in Medicine, First Edition. Edited by Jo Brown, Lorraine M. Noble, Alexia Papageorgiou and Jane Kidd.
© 2016 John Wiley & Sons, Ltd. Published 2016 by John Wiley & Sons, Ltd.

complaints and changing symptoms in the context of a holistic humoral tradition (Jewson 1976). Good doctors were therefore by association good listeners, and patients, who 'called the shots' by virtue of their superior economic power and social status, required them to be good communicators. Most doctors modelled themselves on seniors they encountered during lengthy practical apprenticeships, so modes of responding to patients, along with any prevailing oratorical deficiencies, were often inherited from a single instructor (Lane 1985, p. 99). Arguably such imitative learning continues today. Indeed, the 2010 Francis inquiry report puts emphasis on role modelling and challenging negative examples that align entirely with historic experience (Mid Staffordshire NHS Foundation Trust Public Inquiry 2010, pp. 78, 80).

In the 1800s, greater numbers of doctors began to train in newly established medical schools, where lectures could be delivered by instructors who did not always take naturally to the lectern (Bonner 2000, p. 133). Some gained reputations as 'great' teachers in spite of an absence of pedagogical training. Most students simply aspired to become 'gentlemen scholars', assisted by the classical learning that occupied lectures almost as frequently as the investigative sciences. Previously trained by way of apprenticeship, surgeons also entered the emerging medical colleges and shed their craft backgrounds, mastering texts and a scientifically informed medical language. The professional bodies that governed medical practice thereafter noted deficiencies of unlicensed 'quack' competitors, which included mispronunciations, inability to speak Latin and unfamiliarity with orthodox theory. Orthodox medical practitioners, on the other hand, were routinely challenged as having 'blinded the sick with science' (Pelling 1995, p. 262). Less formal training did not preclude practitioners from developing good communication skills. In fact, many alternative healers operating on medicine's fringes may have effectively conversed with ordinary members of the public, due to their greater familiarity with a population largely excluded from formal education. Nevertheless, orthodox medical practitioners, valued too for their personal attention and bedside manner, more often attained strong social positions and were highly regarded within communities.

Many treatments on offer a century or more ago lacked efficacy in terms of clinical outcome and much seemed to be gained from practitioners maximising their pastoral roles in communities. Physicians and clergymen had traditionally trained alongside each other at universities, where theology and medicine were linked. In the 18th century, the medical doctorate gradually became distinct and the public increasingly turned to doctors in times of illness. Although there were few 'magic bullet' treatments with certain outcomes, there was considerable public demand for the sympathetic relationship offered by physicians, especially at the end of life. However, the lowest social classes were less likely to enjoy an empathic relationship with their doctor than the upper classes, on whose payments practitioners relied. Prior to an NHS in the UK, physicians, for example, infrequently visited the hospital wards that they voluntarily served, thus it was more usually porters and nurses who consoled or assisted families in times of hardship (Lewis 2007, pp. 20–26). Additionally, surgeons rarely consulted colleagues or performed operations with the full consent of patients (Stanley 2003, p. 200). Nevertheless, the enduring positive stereotype of the 'country practitioner' reminded many doctors that they were expected to function as men (in the days before female inclusion) and not just as scientists (Burnham 1982, p. 1476). As a result, good communication skills were valued, if not always in evidence.

In the 20th century, the entry of women and more working-class students into medical schools introduced new types of practitioners to hospitals and communities.

While resistance to female practitioners was evident, some being denied lectures on subjects deemed too 'sensitive' by male lecturers, they found favour among a broad spectrum of patients. Like their male colleagues from lower-class backgrounds, they were successful in overcoming differences that had formerly inhibited communication between many male practitioners and their patients. Gender differences between practitioners and patients likely affected the length, consultation content and structure of medical visits, as confirmed by more recent research into clinical communication (Roter *et al.* 1991). Evidence suggests early women doctors were actively sought out by females who would otherwise have remained untreated. Female general practitioners regularly offered longer hours, often in efforts to ease the burdens of work and poverty that frequently retarded recovery (Roberts 1993, p. 149).

In the wake of growing medical and surgical success, the public became increasingly enamoured with modern medicine and began to demand and expect uniformly trained practitioners. Hospital care expanded and was regarded as a necessity by all classes. There is some evidence, however, that the profession at this time was more driven by financial interest than more altruistic pursuits such as increasing access to services by organisational means (Burnham 1982, p. 1475; Porter 1995, p. 3). The communication skills of practitioners were employed, for example, to disseminate their latest research findings or promote their own professional interests (Burnham 1982, p. 1475). Medical education remained directive and dominated by an authoritative, didactic style that was historically and culturally characterised by the 'ritual humiliation' of students, aspects which endured in popular culture, and reports of other insensitivities rather than by lessons on doctor–patient relations (Waddington 2002). The hierarchical structure engendered formidable barriers to improvements in clinical communication, as it was not regarded as a curriculum priority or a trainable discipline. Doctors were either 'natural communicators' or people with less interpersonal skill tolerated for any social inadequacy on account of their medical talent. As new knowledge allowed practitioners to tackle infectious diseases with greater efficacy, and surgeons scaled enhanced reputational heights based on clinical results, many practitioners appeared content to let medicine speak for itself. Recollections of poor approaches and practices, like other difficult or unpalatable periods of history, should be considered in the context of the era and are important precisely because they provide a catalyst for change.

Change came after the Second World War, when clinical communication became part of a wider agenda to '(re)humanise' medical care. Misuse of medical and scientific knowledge during the war – most famously the experiments conducted at concentration camps and the bomb at Hiroshima – highlighted the potential dangers of scientific advancement when divorced from concern about the well-being of people. New medical technologies, specialties and treatments also fuelled concerns about knowledge overload in undergraduate education, at the perceived expense of the human aspects of medicine (General Medical Council 1957, pp. 10, 13). A number of key thinkers also highlighted the importance of using communication skills to counter-balance this apparent growing emphasis on reductionist biomedicine. One of the most influential thinkers in this regard was psychoanalyst Michael Balint (1896–1970), who wrote *The Doctor, His Patient and the Illness* (Balint 1957) in the context of Britain's new NHS.

This promotion of a more humanistic form of clinical communication was part of wider critiques of the medical profession, as promoted by authors including René Dubos (1959), Henry Miller (1973) and Thomas McKeown (1976) (on the contemporary influence of these texts, see Reynolds & Tansey 2007, p. xxi; Balint's work also influenced wider culture, such as the work of John Berger – see Whitehead 2014).

They discussed communication as part of a growing interrogation of human relationships and the empowerment of marginalised voices in wider society. In this framework, improved clinical communication was not only important in the individual clinical encounter but also facilitated wider medical engagement with behavioural and social sciences. Medical sociological works highlighting the roles taken in doctor–patient relationships and the importance of communication for insights into the 'biopsychosocial' rather than purely physical aspects of illness proliferated (e.g. see Bloom 1963; Robinson 1973; Engel 1977; on the sick role, see Burnham 2012).

In the 1970s, philosopher and priest Ivan Illich (1926–2002) further emphasised the societal importance of medical communication in *Medical Nemesis* (Illich 1975). In *Complaints against Doctors* (1973), policy analyst Rudolf Klein also suggested that much reported dissatisfaction with doctors could be avoided by improving communication between patients and practitioners (Klein 1973, p. 113). In line with such critiques of medicine from beyond the establishment, clinical communication became increasingly interwoven with the growing field of medical ethics. Recalling his influential series of Reith Lectures on medical ethics in the UK, *Unmasking Medicine* (1980), Ian Kennedy notes that a primary theme was how 'patients were neither heard nor listened to, to the degree which may be appropriate in a modern civilized society' (Reynolds & Tansey 2007, p. 46).

Communicating 'bad news' was central to such debates about the moral aspects of clinical communication. Under the paternalistic model of medical care, medical practitioners had commonly withheld terminal diagnoses from their patients. From the mid-20th century onwards, 'truth-telling' became a greater part of medical communication. Key thinkers such as Susan Sontag (1933–2004), in her seminal text *Illness as Metaphor* (1978), argued that the clinical reliance on metaphor operated to create a sense of shame around illnesses such as cancer and promoted a more direct form of doctor–patient relationship (Sontag 1978). As Cicely Saunders also noted in the 1970s, as part of her pioneering work on hospice care, 'skill is no substitute for sharing and understanding' for a patient with a terminal illness (Saunders 2006, p. 126; the quote is taken from 'A Place to Die', first published in *Crux* [1973–1974]).

In the UK, the nascent NHS created a range of new challenges associated with doctor–patient and intraprofessional communication. In the 1950s, there were an estimated 3,000 doctors who came to the UK from overseas to work and, despite their clear importance for the survival of the NHS, the rise of migrant practitioners and patients started to become a matter of concern among contemporaries (Esmail 2007). In the 1960s and 1970s, the *BMJ* regularly printed correspondence about perceived clinical communication problems, both cultural and linguistic, even though contemporary studies indicated that only a minority of doctors qualified overseas had such problems. Irrespective of the validity of these concerns, they served to shape attitudes towards clinical communication and fuelled growing calls for professional training provision in communication for doctors who had not graduated in the UK. Adequate provision of training opportunity in 'nonclinical' competencies – as aligned with NHS expectations – for international medical graduates remains highly topical at the time of writing.

When there was no longer a need to preach the value of doctor–patient communication, practitioners and authors turned to questions such as patient compliance and effective communication models. Influential publications such as those of David Pendleton and Philip Ley had been years in fruition, therefore were only a part of a longer story of changing attitudes to clinical practice (Pendleton & Hasler 1983; Ley 1988; for other influential literature on communication models, see Byrne & Long 1976). However, they remained significant in using health psychology to consider *how* communication could be taught and implemented. Such models fed into an existing interest in such education in the USA where, by the end of the 1970s, surveys indicated that an estimated 67–96% of medical schools provided education in interpersonal skills as part of the medical curriculum (Wakeford 1983, p. 237). In the UK the General Medical Council officially highlighted communication skills in its 1980 recommendations on medical education, and by 1989 nearly all UK medical schools provided some such education, mostly in departments of general practice (General Medical Council 1980; Whitehouse 1991, p. 311).

Some of these educational courses had basic and functional objectives, such as learning to take medical histories. Many were 'skills based', or course add-ons, but others had more 'humanistic' attitudinal objectives that included relationship building and sensitivity (Whitehouse 1991, pp. 313–314). In the 1990s, medical education in clinical communication increasingly focused on issues of compassion and empathy, backed by the General Medical Council's *Tomorrow's Doctors* (General Medical Council 1993). Schools turned increasingly towards interactive methods such as role play and developed assessments that involved simulated patient encounters, incorporated into existing or developing Objective Structured Clinical Examinations (OSCEs) (Harden *et al.* 1975). Although OSCEs usually assessed communication only as part of 'history taking', they represented a growing emphasis on the importance of 'good' communication. OSCEs marked a difference from early courses in communication skills that were not assessed in any formal way. This form of assessment dominates medical education to this day.

Conclusion

A classical university education produced many literate and enlightened medical 'gentlemen' in the 18th and 19th centuries. However, physicians did not really consciously develop their recognised penchant for polite conversation into explicit, professionalised 'clinical communication' at this time, except perhaps when dealing with more culturally synonymous genteel patient consumers. In the late 20th century, however, the emphasis changed. Increasingly formal education in communication became a focus of efforts to 'rehumanise' medicine in order to counterbalance the apparently reductionist biomedical model and to make space for the patient in the clinical encounter, as a previously marginalised voice. A notion of the community and professional team superseded the individual 'gentleman doctor', while equality replaced deference as the ideal doctor–patient relationship. The introduction of new technologies has provided new diagnostic methods, but there has been no substitute for communication between doctor and patient. Medical communication has changed form and purpose over the last 200 years but has been an ever-present aspect of the clinical encounter and remains so to this very day.

Acknowledgements

The authors are grateful to Professor John Skelton for his comments on an earlier draft of this chapter and to the Wellcome Trust for funding some of the research on which this chapter is based.

References

Balint, M. (1957) *The Doctor, His Patient and the Illness.* Tavistock, London.

Bloom, S.W. (1963) *The Doctor and His Patient: A Sociological Interpretation.* Sage, New York.

Bonner, T.N. (2000) *Becoming a Physician: Medical Education in Britain, France, Germany, and the United States, 1750–1945.* Johns Hopkins University Press, Baltimore.

Burnham, J.C. (1982) American medicine's golden age: What happened to it?' *Science*, 215 (no. 4539), 1474–1479.

Burnham, J.C. (2012) The death of the sick role. *Social History of Medicine*, 25 (no. 4), 761–776.

Byrne, P.S. & Long, B.E.L. (1976) *Doctors Talking to Patients: A Study of the Verbal Behaviour of General Practitioners Consulting in Their Surgeries.* HMSO, London.

Engel, G.L. (1977) The need for a new medical model: A challenge for biomedicine. *Science*, 196 (no. 4286), 129–136.

Esmail, A. (2007) Asian doctors in the NHS: Service and betrayal. *British Journal of General Practice*, 57 (no. 543), 827–834.

General Medical Council. (1957) *Recommendations as to the Medical Curriculum.* General Medical Council, London.

General Medical Council. (1980) *Recommendations on Basic Medical Education.* General Medical Council, London.

General Medical Council (1993) *Tomorrow's Doctors.* General Medical Council, London

Harden, R.M., Stevenson, M., Downie, W.W. & Wilson, G.M. (1975) Assessment of clinical competence using objective structured examination. *British Medical Journal*, 1, 447–451.

Illich, I. (1975) *Medical Nemesis: The Expropriation of Health.* Calder & Boyars, London.

Jewson, N. (1976) The disappearance of the sick man from medical cosmology, 1770–1870. *Sociology*, 10 (no. 2), 225–244.

Klein, R. (1973) *Complaints against Doctors: A Study in Professional Accountability.* Charles Knight, London.

Lane, J. (1985) The role of apprenticeship in eighteenth-century medical education in England. In: W.F. Bynum & R. Porter (eds), *William Hunter and the Eighteenth-Century Medical World.* Cambridge University Press, Cambridge.

Lewis, M.J. (2007) *Medicine and Care of the Dying: A Modern History.* Oxford University Press, Oxford.

Ley, P. (1988) *Communicating with Patients: Improving Communication, Satisfaction and Compliance.* Chapman & Hall, London.

Mid Staffordshire NHS Foundation Trust Public Inquiry. (2010) Executive Summary [WWW document]. URL http://www.midstaffspublicinquiry.com/sites/default/files/report/Executive%20summary.pdf [accessed on 27 May 2014].

Pelling, M. (1995) Knowledge common and acquired: The education of unlicensed medical practitioners in early modern London. In: V. Nutton & R. Porter (eds), *The History of Medical Education in Britain.* Rodopi, Amsterdam.

Pendleton, D. & Hasler, J. (eds) (1983) *Doctor-Patient Communication.* Academic Press, London.

Porter, R. (1995) *Disease, Medicine and Society in England, 1550–1860.* Cambridge University Press, Cambridge.

Reiser, S. (1993) Technology and the use of the senses in twentieth-century medicine. In: W.F. Bynum & R. Porter (eds), *Medicine and the Five Senses.* Cambridge University Press, Cambridge.

Reynolds, L.A. & Tansey, E.M. (eds) (2007), *Medical Ethics Education in Britain, 1963–1993.* Wellcome Trust Centre for the History of Medicine, London.

Roberts, S. (1993) *Sophia Jex-Blake: A Woman Pioneer in Nineteenth-Century Medical Reform.* Routledge, New York.

Robinson, D. (1973) *Patients, Practitioners and Medical Care: Aspects of Medical Sociology.* Heinemann Medical, London.

Roter, D., Lipkin, M., Jr & Korsgaard, A. (1991) Sex differences in patients' and physicians' communication during primary care medical visits. *Medical Care*, 29 (no. 11), 1083–1093.

Saunders, C. (2006) *Cicely Saunders: Selected Writings 1958–2004.* Oxford University Press, Oxford.

Sontag, S. (1978) *Illness as Metaphor.* Farrar, Straus and Giroux, New York.

Stanley, P. (2003) *For Fear of Pain: British Surgery, 1790–1850.* Rodopi, Amsterdam.

Waddington, K. (2002) Mayhem and medical students: Image, conduct and control in the Victorian and Edwardian London teaching hospital. *Social History of Medicine*, 15 (no. 1), 45–64.

Wakeford, R. (1983) Communication skills training in United Kingdom medical schools. In D. Pendleton & J. Hasler (eds), *Doctor-Patient Communication*. Academic Press, London.

Whitehead, A. (2014) The medical humanities: A literary perspective. In: V. Bates, A. Bleakley & S. Goodman (eds), *Medicine, Health and the Arts: Approaches to the Medical Humanities*. Routledge, London.

Whitehouse, C.R. (1991) The teaching of communication skills in United Kingdom medical schools. *Medical Education*, 25 (no. 4), 311–318.

Models of Learning

CHAPTER 28

Behaviourism as a Way of Learning

Jo Brown

St George's University of London, London, UK

Historical context

Behaviourism is a popular learning theory that when used in an educational context proposes that physical actions such as thinking, acting and feeling can be regarded as *behaviours* in a teaching and learning setting. Behaviourism proposes that *'Learning should be understood and explained in terms of what is directly observable'* (Hager 2011).

Behaviourism has been a major influence on medical education as a whole, and clinical communication education in particular, in recent decades. It originated in the early 20th century from the work of Thorndike (Thorndike & Woodworth 1901), an influential behavioural psychologist, who introduced the notion of 'transfer' of knowledge from one context to another and suggested that there is a Law of Effects (Thorndike 1932) whereby behaviours that are rewarded with good consequences are likely to be repeated by learners; for example, the diligent learner is rewarded by the praise of the teacher. Skills learning can be traced back to this early work and the proposal that Identical Elements – for example, where *'Lower level skills are taught before the higher level skills that include them'* (Tuomi-Grohn & Engestrom 2003) – are the vehicle of transfer between the original site of learning (the classroom) and the transfer situation (the clinical environment) (Brown 2010). Behaviourism, and therefore transfer, understand and explain learning as something that is held in the mind of the individual learner, which is a container for knowledge and skills, and propose that knowledge is a type of 'substance' that can therefore be moved around (Hager & Hodkinson 2009).

The transfer metaphor is an important one in education, as it has been developed and influenced as it has evolved in the various schools of thought about learning, ranging from cognitive (mind-centred) views of transfer and metacognition (Sternberg 1990) through to situated views (where learning takes place in a particular context or group) (Lave & Wenger 1991; Greeno *et al.* 1993). These different understandings of transfer as the vehicle for moving knowledge around have variously described it as happening between tasks (behaviourism) – for example, where a learner is able to learn a task in the classroom and transfer it to the clinical workplace – or in the mind of the individual learner (cognitive learning theories), where knowledge is learned in

Clinical Communication in Medicine, First Edition. Edited by Jo Brown, Lorraine M. Noble, Alexia Papageorgiou and Jane Kidd.
© 2016 John Wiley & Sons, Ltd. Published 2016 by John Wiley & Sons, Ltd.

the classroom, stored in the learner's mind and then transferred to the clinical workplace through memory and recall. More recently transfer has been proposed to happen through group learning processes in professional workplace contexts that are culturally influenced (situated learning) (Lave & Wenger 1991).

Hager and Hodkinson (2009) in a useful summary of debates about learning and transfer argue that in behaviourism the learning of 'skills' works in the same way; for example, their transfer is independent of the learner or the context, resulting in the ability of the learner to move a skill from place to place. An important point here is that behaviourism through its belief in transfer accepts learning as being independent of any context, and this influential understanding of how learning is moved around has enabled the front loading of knowledge and skills education to the early years of the medical curriculum in many subjects.

Learning by simulation – for example, learning by doing in a simulated setting by trying out situations and receiving feedback on performance – partially emerged from the behaviourism stable and partially from models of skills learning, particularly from the early work of Bandura (1965) and his four-stage training framework that called for the learner to pay attention to what is going on around them in the learning environment, to remember what has happened, to be physically competent to carry out skills and finally to be motivated to learn. Bandura also recognised the efficacy of modelling correct behaviours and skills to students. Building on this, Dreyfus and Dreyfus (1986) developed a staged model of skills learning that resulted in the learner acquiring gradual expertise by going through the stages of Novice, Advanced Beginner, Competent, Proficient and finally Expert. A model commonly used today is Miller's Pyramid of Assessment, which provides a framework for assessing skills competence (Ramani & Leinster 2008). All of these models rely on transfer as the vehicle of moving learning through time and space.

As part of ongoing educational research, learning theorists explored reflection as a tool for learning. An important milestone for reflection in medical education was Schon's (1991) seminal work *The Reflective Practitioner* in which learning was categorised as something that happened in an authentic practice context, where learners could reflect upon their experiences and actions and learn from these. Reflection had an impact on medical education and became a significant way of learning and developing professional practice for doctors and students alike. Reflection as a medium for learning is dealt with in more depth in chapters 31 and 32. Reflection certainly links learning with an authentic context but continues to locate learning solely in the mind of the learner and still requires transfer to enable what has been learned to be transferred to practice.

Current practice

A major achievement for clinical communication as a subject is that it has now come of age and is taught, learned and assessed as part of the core curriculum of all medical schools in the UK (Hargie *et al.* 2010). Most medical schools now use simulation with real or simulated patients as part of this learning (Hargie *et al.* 2010). However, in a change to earlier practice this formal education is now often timetabled to the early years of the medical curriculum (Hargie *et al.* 2010) to a time before students have much experience of working with patients or being in the clinical environment. This 'front loading' of teaching and learning (Evans *et al.* 2011) becomes possible when transfer of knowledge and skills provides the pedagogical approach to teaching and learning (Brown 2012a). Silverman *et al.* (2005) propose that as clinical communication is part of all medical practice, this should also be reflected in teaching by having a clinical communication curriculum that runs through all years of the medical course.

In over 70% of UK medical schools (Hargie *et al.* 2010) the dominant conceptual framework for teaching and learning clinical communication is the colloquially named Calgary-Cambridge model developed by Kurtz, Silverman and Draper in their seminal work *Teaching and Learning Communication Skills in Medicine* (Kurtz *et al.* 2005). This framework, amongst others, offers an integrated and evidence-based guide that intentionally deconstructs clinical communication learning into a series of learned skills that are developed in simulated settings where students learn experientially to develop skills and competence through practise and feedback. Its origins are behaviourist and as a framework it focuses on skills that, in this context, mean the implicit practical application of the knowledge and attitudes held by a learner, which is in keeping with the behaviourist belief that learning is directly observable. This systematic method of learning has led Hargie *et al.* (2010) to conclude that '*there is overwhelming evidence that, when used in a systematic, co-ordinated and informed fashion, communication skills training is indeed an effective training medium*'. However, in line with its behaviourist pedagogy, when simulation based, it relies on the transfer metaphor to allow learners to move their learning from classroom to clinical practice.

Of course, not all clinical communication education is timetabled as a separate activity or placed in early years education, as it often forms part of integrated teaching in other subjects and is part of teaching and learning in the clinical workplace. When used in the workplace it introduces the dimension of 'context' to learning and therefore the recognition of learning theories that have emerged from the disciplines of sociology and cultural studies, which propose that context, and the social interactions within it, provide the conditions for learning to take place. This of course gives a nod to the past in medical education, which relied heavily on the apprenticeship model of learning (Kurtz *et al.* 2005). There is now a growing recognition that major aspects of professional education can *only* be learned in the workplace (Hager 2011).

Situated learning pointed to a new direction in learning that acknowledged the context. In their influential book *Situated Learning: Legitimate Peripheral Participation* Lave and Wenger (1991) presented a theory of learning that outlined the processes a novice learner goes through to become a full member of a community of practice (Wenger 1998). They proposed that learning is dependent on the learning context and the social relations that take place within it. Learning is therefore something that takes place *outside* of the individual and happens within a network of social relations in the clinical context. The behaviourist metaphor of transfer does not fit here as learning is viewed as something that is shifting and changing and not 'fixed' in nature as it is constructed and reconstructed within a situated group, for example, a group of medical students, qualified doctors or other health professionals learning in the clinical workplace (Brown 2012b).

Behaviourism and simulation have therefore been influential paradigms that have shaped the teaching and learning of clinical communication to be systematic, consistent and assessable. Today in medical education these learning pedagogies are accepted as being effective and evidence based, but both rely on the notion of transfer to explain how students learn.

Future directions

But where is the teaching and learning of clinical communication heading? Will behaviourism and simulation continue to be the methods of choice? Will they continue to anchor clinical communication to classroom learning, and what happens if we look beyond the transfer metaphor to embrace more holistic learning frameworks?

The literature gives a clear steer. Bligh and Bleakley (2006) suggest that learning by simulation alone can become 'self-referential' and may result in a simulation of *learning* only and not of real-life situations; for example, it can simulate a learning exercise that is not part of real life. They suggest that simulation is a good prelude to learning in the workplace, but that effective interaction between simulation and workplace learning can increase the power of both. Next, Vygotsky (1963) famously offers us his 'Zone of Proximal Development' to explain the psychological space learners inhabit when they have developed a range of skills they can use with assistance but that cannot yet be used independently, which seems to ably describe the place that medical students reach when they transition into the clinical workplace. Last, Michael Eraut (2007) reminds us that *'Formal learning contributes most when it is both relevant and well timed, but still needs further workplace learning before it can be used to best effect'.*

So, perhaps we should accept that simulation, with its behaviourist origins, works well as a preparation for working with real patients in real clinical situations, but should we also accept that formal clinical communication education should run throughout the undergraduate curriculum, and beyond, to scaffold students throughout their learning? And should we accept that clinical communication education delivered or co-delivered by medical school teachers could also happen formally in the clinical workplace, as well as the classroom, to develop authentic, but evidence-based, clinical practice? In other words, should teachers not only facilitate in the medical school but also follow their learners into the clinical workplace to offer support (Silverman & Wood 2004)?

This latest thinking may point us towards workplace learning theories, which have grown in response to concerns that formal courses of professional education that appear at the beginning of a course of study no longer fit the learner for practice in the real workplace world (Hager 2011). Although no one definition unites them, in broad terms they are (adapted from Evans *et al.* [2011])

> about the relationship that exists between the individual learner and the group processes that are situated in the workplace. Workplace learning looks at how the individual, social and cultural processes of working affect learning in the workplace context.

Building on this definition, in chapter 29 we shall explore the origins and pedagogy of workplace learning in more detail and look at a model for its practical application to clinical communication education in the future.

References

Bandura, A. (1965) Behavior modification through modeling procedures. In: L. Krasner & L.P. Ullman (eds), *Research in Behavior Modification*, 310–340. Holt, New York.

Bligh, J. & Bleakley, A. (2006) Distributing menus to hungry learners: Can learning by simulation become simulation of learning? *Medical Teacher*, 28 (no. 7), 606–613.

Brown, J. (2010) Transferring clinical communication skills from the classroom to the clinical environment: Perceptions of a group of medical students in the United Kingdom. *Academic Medicine*, 85 (no. 6), 1052–1059.

Brown, J. (2012a) Perspective: Clinical communication education in the United kingdom: Some fresh insights. *Academic Medicine,* 87 (no. 8), 1101–1104.

Brown, J. (2012b) *Through the looking glass: Clinical communication in the clinical workplace.* EdD Thesis, Institute of Education, University of London

Dreyfus, H.L. & Dreyfus, S.E. (1986) *Mind over Machine: The Power of Human Intuition and Expertise in the Era of the Computer.* Free Press, New York.

Eraut, M. (2007) Learning from other people in the workplace. *Oxford Review of Education,* 33 (no. 4), 403–422.

Evans, K., Guile, D. & Harris, J. (2011) Rethinking work-based learning: For education professionals and professionals who educate. In: M. Malloch, L. Cairns, K. Evans & B. O'Connor, *The SAGE Handbook of Workplace Learning.* SAGE, Thousand Oaks, CA.

Greeno, J., Moore, J.L. & Smith, D.R. (1993) *Transfer of situated learning. In: Transfer on Trial: Intelligence, Cognition and Instruction.* Ablex, Norwood, NJ.

Hager, P. (2011) Theories of workplace learning. In: M. Malloch, L. Cairns, K. Evans & B. O'Connor, *The SAGE Handbook of Workplace Learning.* SAGE, Thousand Oaks, CA.

Hager, P. & Hodkinson, P. (2009) Moving beyond the metaphor of transfer of learning. *British Educational Research Journal,* 35 (no. 4), 619–638.

Hargie, O., Boohan, M. McCoy, M. & Murphy, P. (2010) Current trends in communication skills training in UK schools of medicine. *Medical Teacher,* 32(5): 385–391.

Kurtz, S.M., Silverman, J.D. & Draper, J. (2005) *Teaching and Learning Communication Skills in Medicine,* second edn. Radcliffe, Oxford.

Lave, J. & Wenger, E. (1991) *Situated Learning: Legitimate Peripheral Participation.* Cambridge University Press, Cambridge, UK.

Ramani, S. & Leinster, S. (2008) AMEE Guide no. 34: Teaching in the clinical environment. *Medical Teacher,* 30 (no. 4), 347–364.

Schon, D.A. (1991) *The Reflective Practitioner: How Professionals Think in Action.* Basic Books, New York.

Silverman, J. & Wood, D.F. (2004) New approaches to learning clinical skills. *Medical Education,* 38 (no. 10), 1021–1023.

Silverman, J.D., Kurtz, A.M. & Draper, J. (2005) *Skills for Communicating with Patients,* second edn. Radcliffe, Oxford.

Sternberg, R.J. (1990) Metamorphs of Mind: Conceptions of the Nature of Intelligence. Cambridge University Press, Cambridge, UK.

Thorndike, E.L. (1932) *The Fundamentals of Learning.* Teachers College Press, New Yorkl

Thorndike, E.L. & Woodworth, R.S. (1901) The influence of improvement in one mental function upon the efficiency of other functions. *Psychological Review,* 8, 247–261.

Tuomi-Grohn, T. & Engestrom, Y. (2003) Conceptualising transfer: From standard notions to developmental perspectives. In: *Between School and Work: New Perspectives on Transfer and Boundary Crossing. Advances in Learning & Instruction Series.* Pergamon, Oxford, UK.

Vygotsky, L.S. (1963) Learning and mental development at school age. In: *Educational Psychology in the USSR,* B. Simon, 21–34. Routledge & Kegan Paul, London.

Wenger, E. (1998) *Communities of Practice: Learning, Meaning, and Identity.* Cambridge University Press, Cambridge, UK.

CHAPTER 29

Situated and Work-Based Learning

Jo Brown

St George's University of London, London, UK

Historical context

Theories about how humans learn go back to the ancient Greek philosophers (Russ-Eft 2011), and yet today we are still unable to agree about how it actually happens! We know that professional or vocational education historically took place in the workplace as part of an apprenticeship model. But over time, and with the changing views of society about education in the UK, particularly galvanised by the Industrial Revolution, education became increasingly formalised and then removed from the workplace to places of learning such as universities. Universities took over the provision of education from the professions and changed our understanding of the term 'apprenticeship' to mean the '*off the job*' training that apprentices receive elsewhere (Hager 2011).

We have already seen in chapter 28 how behaviourism and simulation have been the pedagogical choices for teaching and learning clinical communication in recent years and, that in response to a public demand for more skilled doctors (Brown 2008), delivering medical education and therefore clinical communication education in a university medical school setting has resulted in many positive educational developments that fit students for practice in the modern world. But use of this pedagogy in a university setting has also resulted in a dissonance between the *types* of knowledge that medical educators now work with. To explain this dissonance we must acknowledge that all knowledge has a context in which it was originally created (Evans *et al.* 2011), and clinical communication knowledge in the medical school context is 'codified' knowledge taken from knowledge not necessarily specific to medicine but drawn from a mixed behavioural/social science/biomedical disciplinary base (Eraut 2004; Schaap *et al.* 2012), which before the publication of this book was not clearly linked to its origins. Codified knowledge comes from academic disciplines, usually in published form; for example, the knowledge that is contained in books, journals, literature and so forth. In contrast to this, 'situated' knowledge is that used in the workplace and constructed for the practical requirements of the service and is based on pragmatic working practices. Situated knowledge is rarely published in the academic sense. Barnett (2006) suggests that the kind of situated knowledge that is used in the workplace to get the job done often doesn't relate well with codified academic knowledge that needs to some extent to

Clinical Communication in Medicine, First Edition. Edited by Jo Brown, Lorraine M. Noble, Alexia Papageorgiou and Jane Kidd.

be independent of a context in order to be generally useful. Layton (1993) further comments that '*The problems which people construct from their experiences do not map neatly on to existing scientific disciplines and pedagogical organisations of knowledge*'.

A practical representation of this knowledge dissonance is given by Benbassat and Baumal (2008), who observe that in the early years of medical education students are taught clinical communication in the main by behavioural scientists, but that many clinical teachers who teach them in the clinical workplace are not expert in this field and therefore there is no continuity between these teaching domains for students. It should be noted, though, that in the UK many doctors are key innovators in the clinical communication field. Konkola *et al.* (2007) reinforce this knowledge dissonance by reporting that in occupational therapy educational settings university teachers and clinical teachers do not share goals for learning and so learning becomes fragmented for students. Evans *et al.* (2010) share this view and comment that in nurse education the lack of shared learning goals between teachers results in '*Students having to learn within a disintegrated learning context in which opposing values of learning exist*'.

So, situating medical education into universities and clinical communication education partly into the early years of the curriculum, may mean that in the medical education of today we should be exploring new teaching and learning methodologies to address any schism in knowledge types that exist and that may lead to conflicts in the student learning experience.

Current practice

Theories of workplace learning have become popular in the last 20 years because of two important changes in society. First, education is no longer seen as something that is confined to youth and the achievement of qualifications, as we now recognise that most adults in professions must be 'lifelong' learners who need to update their knowledge and skills on a regular basis throughout professional life. Second, knowledge and skills are themselves constantly changing in a complex professional life and require the learner to adapt to rapid change in a flexible way. Given these societal drivers, the workplace becomes the natural place for learning that is context specific and deals with a high degree of situated knowledge (Illeris 2011a; 2011b). The literature is also clear that the workplace has a profound effect on student learning (Williams *et al.* 2001; Silverman & Wood 2004; Eraut 2007), and in an interesting article written by medical students themselves (Malhotra *et al.* 2009), they recommend that '*an important step in improving future doctors' communication skills is to integrate communication teaching into every clinical course*'.

We have already seen a definition of workplace learning in chapter 28 that defines it as (adapted from Evans *et al.* [2011]):

> about the relationship that exists between the individual learner and the group processes that are situated in the workplace. Workplace learning looks at how the individual, social and cultural processes of working affect learning in the workplace context.

Workplace learning theories offer medical educators a rich conceptualisation of how learning takes place in the authentic and complex clinical workplace (Brown 2012).

Many divergent workplace learning theories exist, and it would not be possible to precis them in this short chapter. However, against this rich backdrop the theoretical construct of 'recontextualisation' stands out as an interesting and practical way to examine the changing nature of knowledge itself and therefore how it is learned. Developed by Evans, Guile and Harris (2008), this framework aims to inject '*Fresh thinking*' into the challenge of integrating theory and practice in work-based learning. Recontextualisation moves beyond the behaviourist metaphor of transfer to suggest that knowledge and concepts change as they are made teachable and become learnable by students who will make sense of them and eventually apply them to their practice (Allan *et al.* 2014). Taylor *et al.* (2010) suggest that '*the knowledge transfer problem in work-based learning programmes can be better understood when thinking breaks free of the transfer metaphor and is reframed according to a process model framework for recontextualisation*'. This theoretical framework suggests that the process of recontextualisation is a whole body response to learning that changes learners as individuals, as well as the context (workplace) within which they operate and ultimately the knowledge itself. It links the individual learner with the context and the group within which he or she learns, as learning is not independent of the learner, or of the context, or of the culture in which learning takes place, but requires all three to be complete.

To understand how knowledge is shaped and changed, four kinds of recontextualisation are important in this framework (adapted from Evans *et al.* [2008]):

- Content Recontextualisation – knowledge in the programme design environment – i.e. medical school teachers identify codified knowledge from its primary disciplinary sources (e.g. from books, publications and literature) and select it for inclusion in the Clinical Communication curriculum. They decide what it is important for students to learn and how much of it should be included in the curriculum. Clinical Communication knowledge is therefore selected and adapted for use in the medical school. We have seen how formative the Calgary- Cambridge guide (Kurtz, Silverman *et al.* 2005) has been to this selection as has the UK Consensus Statement (von Fragstein, Silverman *et al.* 2008), both of which outline the content of the curriculum.
- Pedagogic Recontextualisation - knowledge in the teaching and facilitation environment, i.e. the codified knowledge that has been selected is contextualised to the curriculum and medical school teachers design teaching methods to deliver it to students, e.g. they decide how and where it will be taught and learned in the curriculum. The Calgary-Cambridge guide has also been formative to this process, which in most medical schools involves systematic experiential learning and simulation as the pedagogy of choice.
- Workplace Recontextualisation – knowledge in the workplace environment, i.e. students learn situated knowledge from clinical teachers by a mixture of modelling, mentorship, observation, teaching and feedback in the clinical workplace. Clinical placements facilitate students to recontextualise and modify their Clinical Communication knowledge, attitudes and skills (learned in part in the simulated, medical school environment) into the authentic clinical workplace, mediated by workplace culture and practices.
- Learner Recontextualisation – what learners make of these processes, i.e. how medical students formulate personal strategies to bring together all forms of learned knowledge, skills and attitudes and recontextualise them to create new Clinical Communication knowledge, skills and insights into the workplace and assimilate these into their emergent clinical practice and professional identity.

To support the recontextualisation framework, Evans *et al.* (2008) propose that seven 'Principles of Recontextualisation' are needed in order that chains can be forged between the domains of recontextualisation that can bring together and connect knowledge. Learners create these chains across all contexts to allow them to draw together subject-based and work-based knowledge and skills:

1 *Partnerships and links must exist between medical school and the clinical workplace.* These links are important to allow recontextualisation to take place. Partnership allows 'cultural synchronicity' between medical school and clinical workplace. This could be achieved by setting up inclusive steering groups to decide what goes into the clinical communication curriculum and to design teaching, learning and assessment activities that are compatible with the clinical workplace. Illeris (2011a, 2011b) suggests that without cooperation of this kind, medical students may have to create the learning context for themselves.

2 *Gradual release of knowledge and responsibility must flow from medical school and clinical workplace teachers to students.* Medical students progress through a curriculum in clinical communication that starts with theory and simulation and moves to practise with real patients in the clinical workplace under the supervision of clinical teachers, therefore becoming increasingly complex as the range of tasks the students are asked to perform becomes more sophisticated. Evans *et al.* (2008) suggest that this gradual release of knowledge allows learners to develop their theoretical knowledge alongside their clinical practice knowledge. However, in clinical communication curricula that may be front loaded to the early years of the curriculum, this may not allow formal teaching and learning to be placed alongside emergent clinical practise in the more senior years of the curriculum to scaffold learning. This may therefore interfere with 'gradual release' of knowledge.

3 *Learning conversations must take place between teachers and students.* Learning conversations are those that are facilitated by teachers who recognise the knowledge a student has acquired and who then question them about this to develop that knowledge. Facilitated small group teaching, bedside teaching and ward round teaching with patients are opportunities for this and can be effective at facilitating students to develop their knowledge, skills and attitudes at the appropriate point of practice and could be seen as an example of learning in the 'Zone of Proximal Development' (Vygotsky 1963), or learning at a critical time of development for students, which was outlined in chapter 28.

4 *Medical students must utilise workplace clinical resources.* Being able to make use of clinical workplace resources is an important learning tool for students. Students must be able to access hospital intranet facilities, patient records, test results, clinical equipment and clinical protocols during clinical placements. During ward rounds students see patient records being used, tests carried out or ordered and discharge plans made. Students must have good access to a variety of learning resources and situations, as Beckett and Hager (2002) suggest these are the most significant factors in effective workplace learning.

5 *Sharing clinical communication problems between medical school and clinical workplace.* When a clinical communication problem is encountered in the clinical workplace or in the medical school classroom, how is it resolved? Cross-fertilisation between these two domains would be an excellent way to develop and share practice. Evans *et al.* (2008) and Van Oers (1998) suggest that working together on such problems develops the understanding of all teachers and gives medical school teachers insight into the clinical communication challenges of the clinical workplace and clinical teachers access to evidence-based theory and practice. Illeris (2011a) suggests these two domains should '*see each other as partners in a common project*'.

6 *Senior doctors act as knowledge brokers for students.* Senior doctors from the clinical workplace bring real-world perspectives to learning that can bridge medical school and clinical workplace and provide authenticity. They are able to mediate between the worlds of theory and practice by giving real-world examples and 'war stories' and by having shared a common training experience. Certainly students are keen to hear from qualified doctors, and their knowledge and experience is highly valued.

7 *Shared and integrated accreditation of students must exist.* In medicine shared accreditation between medical school and vocational licensing body, for example, the General Medical Council in the UK, has already been achieved and is important. Medicine has been integrated into the higher education system and graduates receive a MB BS or equivalent on graduation, at which time they are granted provisional inclusion onto the general medical register, subject to successful completion of foundation training and assessment. Interestingly, in the accreditation setting medical school and clinical teachers work together to devise accreditation methods (written and practical exams) and co-examine candidates. Accreditation is therefore a good example of collaborative practice.

Recontextualisation is offered here as a framework to explore and understand how learning takes place across the educational continuum as well as in the clinical workplace, as this continuum and integration into the workplace is perhaps the direction that clinical communication education should take in the future.

Future directions

The literature directs us to expand our thinking beyond behaviourism and simulated learning in clinical communication education to explore theories of workplace learning that examine the relationship between working and learning in an attempt to bridge the practice/theory gap in the workplace setting (Evans *et al.* 2011). Should we now perhaps move beyond behaviourism and also from the notion of clinical communication as '*skills*' based only (Salmon & Young 2011), to a richer conceptualisation of how clinical communication knowledge is developed and used in clinical practice?

The teaching and learning of clinical communication must surely span the whole curriculum so that in addition to giving students basic skills in preparation for working with patients, it is able to support and develop students during the important developmental clinical years to enable them to embed appropriate knowledge, skills and attitudes into their emerging clinical practice. Heaven *et al.* (2006) suggest that to bring this about teachers must support and supervise students on the wards, clinics and surgeries, and Silverman and Wood (2004) agree that teachers should not only facilitate learning in the medical school classroom but follow learners into the clinical world to offer support. Could medical school teachers therefore facilitate learning in the clinical workplace, working with patients in an authentic context, and thus linking their codified knowledge with the situated knowledge of the workplace, particularly in the later curriculum years? Could medical school teachers and clinical teachers co-facilitate clinical communication learning at the bedside?

The clinical workplace is the context that allows development and emergence of new knowledge, skills and attitudes that are linked to a real-world perspective and will be the everyday workplace of medical students both in the clinical years of the curriculum and at postqualification. This is not to suggest a return to the apprenticeship model, or that specialist medical school teachers should not teach the subject, or that the clinical workplace does not need to embrace a range of theoretical inputs to ensure that students develop holistically into capable and patient-centred doctors. But, formal clinical communication education in later years does need to focus on the clinical workplace and perhaps use workplace learning theory as a new lens with which to see how knowledge is used, moved around and changed by students to transform their learning and development.

To end this chapter, a word about thinking beyond formal undergraduate education to look at postgraduate/continuing education. The quest for developing excellent clinical communication does not end at qualification, and we know already the impact that qualified doctors have on the education of medical students. It is therefore logical to extend this kind of education into the postgraduate domain to provide a continuum of development that follows the principles of lifelong professional learning for doctors. Provision of this kind of learning is patchy and little literature about it exists in the UK, but could it usefully be an extension of undergraduate teaching and learning for the future?

References

Allan, H.T., Magnusson, C. *et al.* (2014) People, liminal spaces and experience:Understanding recontextualisation of knowledge for newly qualified nurses. *Nurse Education Today*, 35 (no. 2), e78–e83.

Barnett, M. (2006) *Vocational Knowledge and Vocational Pedagogy in Knowledge, Curriculum & Qualifications for South African Further Education*. Human Science Research Council, Cape Town, South Africa.

Beckett, D. & Hager, P.J. (2002) *Life, Work and Learning: Practice in Postmodernity*. Routledge, London.

Benbassat, J. & Baumal, R. (2008) A proposal for overcoming problems in teaching interviewing skills to medical students. *Advances in Health Sciences Education*, 14 (no. 3), 441–450.

Brown, J. (2008) How clinical communication has become a core part of medical education in the UK. *Medical Education*, 42 (no. 3), 271–278.

Brown, J. (2012) Through the looking glass: Clinical communication in the clinical workplace. EdD Thesis, Institute of Education, University of London.

Eraut, M. (2004) Transfer of knowledge between education and workplace settings. In: H. Rainbird, A. Fuller and A. Munro (eds), *Workplace Learning in Context*. Routledge, London.

Eraut, M. (2007) Learning from other people in the workplace. *Oxford Review of Education*, 33 (no. 4), 403–422.

Evans, K., Guile, D. & Harris, J. (2008). *Putting Knowledge to Work*. Teaching & Learning Research Briefing. Institute of Education, London.

Evans, K., D. Guile, Harris, J. & Allan, H. (2010). Putting knowledge to work: A new approach. *Nurse Education Today*, 30 (no. 3), 245–251.

Evans, K., Guile, D. & Harris, J. *et al.* (2011). *Rethinking work-based learning: For education professionals and professionals who educate*. In: M. Malloch, L. Cairns, K. Evans & B. O'Connor, *The SAGE Handbook of Workplace Learning*. SAGE, Thousand Oaks, CA.

Hager, P. (2011) Theories of workplace learning. In: M. Malloch, L. Cairns, K. Evans & B. O'Connor, *The SAGE Handbook of Workplace Learning*. SAGE, Thousand Oaks, CA.

Heaven, C., Clegg, J. & Maguire P. (2006) Transfer of communication skills training from workshop to workplace: The impact of clinical supervision. *Patient Education and Counseling*, 60 (no. 3), 313–325.

Illeris, K. (2011a) *The Fundamentals of Workplace Learning: Understanding How People Learn in Working Life*. Routledge, London.

Illeris, K. (2011b) Workplaces and learning. In: M. Malloch, L. Cairns, K. Evans & B. O'Connor, *The SAGE Handbook of Workplace Learning*. SAGE, Thousand Oaks, CA.

Konkola, R., Tuomi-Grohn, T., Lambert, P. & Ludvigsen, S. (2007) Promoting learning and transfer between school and work. *Journal of Education and Work*, 20 (no. 3), 211–228.

Kurtz, S.M., Silverman, J.D. & Draper, J. (2005) *Teaching and Learning Communication Skills in Medicine*, second edn. Radcliffe Medical, Oxford, UK.

Layton, D. (1993) Technology's challenge to science education. In: *Knowledge, Curriculum and Qualifications for South African Further Education* p. 147. Human Science Research Council, Cape Town, South Africa.

Malhotra, A., Gregory, I., Darvill, E., Goble, E., Pryce-Roberts, A., Lundbert, K. Konradsen, S. & Hafstad, H. (2009) Mind the gap: Learners' perspectives on what they learn in communication compared to how they and others behave in the real world. *Patient Education and Counseling*, 76 (no. 3), 385–390.

Russ-Eft, D. (2011) *Towards a meta-theory of learning and performance*. In: M. Malloch, L. Cairns, K. Evans & B. O'Connor, *The SAGE Handbook of Workplace Learning*. SAGE, Thousand Oaks, CA.

Salmon, P. & Young, B. (2011) Creativity in clinical communication: From communication skills to skilled communication. *Medical Education*, 45 (no. 3), 217–226.

Schaap, H., Baartman, L. & de Bruijn, E. (2012) Students' learning processes during school-based learning and workplace learning in vocational education: A review. *Vocations and Learning*, 5, 99–117.

Silverman, J. & Wood, D.F. (2004) New approaches to learning clinical skills. *Medical Education*, 38 (no. 10), 1021–1023.

Taylor, M., Evans, K. & Pinsent-Johnson, C. (2010) Work-based learning in Canada and the United Kingdom: A framework for understanding knowledge transfer for workers with low skills and higher skills. *Research in Post-Compulsory Education* 15 (no. 4), 347–361.

Van Oers, B. (1998) The fallacy of decontextualisation. *Mind, Culture and Activity*, 5 (no. 2), 143–152.

von Fragstein, M., Silverman, J., Cushing, A., Quilligan, S., Salisbury, Wiskin, C. & UK Council for Clinical Communication Skills Teaching in Undergraduate Medical Education. (2008) UK consensus statement on the content of communication curricula in undergraduate medical education. *Medical Education*, 42 (no. 11), 1100–1107.

Vygotsky, L.S. (1963) Learning and mental development at school age. In: Educational Psychology in the USSR, B. Simon, 21–34. Routledge & Kegan Paul. London.

Williams, C., Cantillon, P. & Mochrane, M. (2001) The doctor–patient relationship: From undergraduate assumptions to pre-registration reality. *Medical Education*, 35 (no. 8), 743–747.

CHAPTER 30

Experiential Learning

Jan van Dalen

Maastricht University, Maastricht, the Netherlands

Historical context

Until the 1970s communication skills had not received any systematic attention in medical education. Communication was not recognized as a field in which improvement was needed. Medical students as well as physicians were supposed to know how to communicate, just like physicians were supposed to know how to teach.

Barbara Korsch *et al.* (1968) were the first to reveal that these assumptions were not fully justified. They revealed dissatisfaction with the quality of communication in healthcare, and increasingly patients and the public became aware that there was a strong need for improvement.

The reaction in medical schools was to add communication skills training to the undergraduate curriculum. This training had to be negotiated and communication course organisers were challenged to prove that what they did had value. In the present day this has fortunately resulted in a compelling body of research that provides a deep understanding of what needs to be taught and learned and why (Silverman *et al.* 2013).

The type of communication skills training that was supported by the strongest scientific justification was directed at acquiring certain behaviours. In Chapter 28 we saw that these training objectives were based on a behaviouristic approach to learning (Ormrod 2012) (see Box 30.1).

This type of training works. Students learn when they are trained, judging from improved results throughout the years of training (van Dalen *et al.* 1998; 2002). Behaviouristic training is nowadays to be found in many medical schools around the world.

During the past five decades we have learned much more about how people learn, how new knowledge and skills are stored in our memories and under which conditions we can best recall them. We know the importance of three conditions for learning: elaboration, context and collaboration. *Elaboration* refers to the linking of new knowledge and skills to what we already know. This has been found to anchor the new knowledge and skills better in memory. *Context* adds relevance to the learning; learners will realise they need the new knowledge and skills in order to address patient problems. Learning preferably occurs in a surrounding that resembles the environment where the new knowledge and skills are needed. This facilitates retrieval when we need it. *Collaboration* allows the learner to weigh arguments and balance different

Clinical Communication in Medicine, First Edition. Edited by Jo Brown, Lorraine M. Noble,
Alexia Papageorgiou and Jane Kidd.

Box 30.1 Behaviouristic approach to training.

In this educational pedagogy examples of a basic skill (like 'asking open questions') are given and we expect learners to follow that model. Feedback is directed at how well the model is followed. We then assess whether learners can adequately demonstrate asking open questions in a test situation (e.g. OSCE), and when they can we judge that their communication skills are good enough.

viewpoints, which leads to more realistic awareness of society and different cultures. The term used in cognitive psychology for this approach to learning is 'constructivism' (Ormrod 2012, and see chapter 32). Recognition of the benefits of constructivism for learning has had enormous impact on the way medical schools organise their curricula. The caption used for this new organisation was problem-based learning, and it has gained acceptance on a global scale.

However, when we look at the training of skills, and in particular communication skills, they continue to be taught and learned using the principles of behaviourism, even in medical schools with an otherwise constructivistic approach to learning.

Current practice

If communication skills training that is based on the principles of behaviourism works, then is there even a problem?

I think there is, and that there are four problems, actually.

Motivation
It is the task of learners in medicine to develop and maintain high-quality communication. Teachers, course directors and infrastructure are usually available to assist learners in this process. Yet learners may not all be motivated and may not recognise the need for continued attention to this important aspect of good healthcare practice. They have been communicating all their lives before they even entered medical school and they probably have had no complaints about their communication, so why devote additional time and attention to this topic in an already crowded curriculum?

The answer has to do with awareness. Some students may have a naive attitude in which they see themselves as good communicators. This lack of awareness is described as 'unconsciously incompetent' (see Box 30.2).

This shouldn't be taken too literally as they are far from incompetent, but rather they don't know what they don't know. Learning takes learners through the consecutive phases of becoming 'consciously incompetent' (knowing what you don't know), moving gradually to 'consciously competent' (knowing what you do know) and finally reaching the stage of being 'unconsciously competent' (being less aware of what you do know). That final stage is also called being an expert and is said to be reached after some 10 years of experience (Ericsson *et al.* 2006).

The best driving force for effective and deep learning is the learner's motivation (Maehr & Mayer 1997). Preferably coming from within (e.g. wanting to become an even better communicator), but external motivation (wanting to pass the test, avoiding making a fool of yourself or being at a loss for words) also works. So,

Box 30.2 Stages in learning (attributed to Maslow 1954).

1 Unconsciously incompetent (high confidence, possibly false)
2 Consciously incompetent (low confidence)
3 Consciously competent (low to medium confidence)
4 Unconsciously competent (high confidence, justified)

when learners have a lack of insight into the need to improve their communication, we cannot count on their motivation. This can be solved in several ways. One solution would be to wait until they actually run into communication difficulties and then help them recognize this, analyse and reflect on the difficulty and then practice with a remedy. An alternative has been used at some medical schools (van Dalen *et al.* 1999; van Dalen 2013): organise early experiences in the curriculum that help students recognise the subtleties in professional communication. In these circumstances it is also helpful to know that we learn most in situations that have the strongest resemblance to reality (Ormrod 2012). The patient's voice, as an authentic stimulus, has great authority and is more influential than the teachers' (van Dalen *et al.* 1999).

Repeated practice

Kolb (1984) has described the way learning takes place. In his famous 'learning cycle' he describes how concrete experiences (inductively) lead to potential theories, which are (deductively) tested in new situations. This process is repeated regularly. It presupposes that the learner is actively involved in an experience, reflects on the experience, analyses the experience and uses the new ideas gained from the experience. It is this cyclical characteristic that helps any new information and skills to be stored in the memory and be retrieved when needed.

Unlike most other clinical skills, learners have vast experience of communication before they enter medical school. They may not be able to analyse their ability, nor may they be able to select alternatives in an evidence-based manner, but they are flexible communicators. Consequently, training in communication skills should benefit from these previous experiences to help develop analytical abilities and provide new experiences with which to experiment and build new behaviours. Yet training that uses behaviouristic principles is mostly prospective, aimed at improving future communication behaviour. Additionally, in communication learning it is not enough to practise just once, even when the learners are observed and receive feedback on their skills. This confrontation is instructive, but it also reinforces what learners do not do well. As suggested by Salmon and Young (2011), reflection should be included, and alternatives should be generated. Van den Eertwegh has revealed that the development of communicative ability proceeds from 'applying new behaviour' to a process of internalisation and personalisation, in which the alternative communication becomes more authentic. To allow this to happen, alternatives for the early, intuitive approach to communication should be tried out and experimented with (van den Eertwegh *et al.* 2014). This process must be repeated so that learners get the opportunity to evaluate the effect of any new behaviour. Only then can the cyclical process intended by Kolb be completed, and only then will it lead to an extension of the communication repertoire of the learner.

Reductionism and holism

Communication should be assessed in medical schools (Silverman *et al.* 2013). Learners should receive feedback about how well they do in a given situation, in comparison to what is expected of them (Kurtz *et al.* 1998). The hidden additional message that assessment of communication gives to students is that the medical school takes communication seriously, which is important for their extrinsic motivation (Posner & Rudnitsky 2006).

The instruments with which students are assessed (OSCE) are very well aligned with the way the training takes place, as they should be (van der Vleuten 1996). Attention is paid to describing the basic communication skills that are expected, and the background as to why they are important. Yet when we observe our students in practical examinations like an OSCE, we see them behave in quite artificial ways, in order to meet what they interpret as the *demands* of the instrument (see Box 30.3 for an illustration).

Assessment is a strong force to drive students' learning, and the instrument that reduces good communication to measurable entities may turn out to be the 'tail wagging the dog' (van der Vleuten 1996), unfortunately in a less desired direction. Hence the debate in the communication literature that started with Salmon and Young's (2011) plea for attention to skilled communication, rather than to communication skills. Training should be less exclusively directed at the acquisition of skills and additionally to the development of creativity.

Transfer

The fourth problem can be seen by teachers in medical schools who teach across different phases of the curriculum. Empathy tends to decline across the duration of the medical course (Neumann *et al.* 2011). Students who were able to communicate in a patient-centered way in preclinical training demonstrate less of that ability during the clinical phase of their study (Spencer 2004; Hojat *et al.* 2004; 2009; Neumann *et al.* 2011). The average duration of patients' first utterance before they were interrupted by their doctor has increased from 18 seconds in 1984 (Beckman & Frankel 1984) to 23 seconds in 1999 (Marvel *et al.* 1999), an increase of a glorious 5 seconds after 15 years of training. Participants in the Dutch 3-year vocational training for general practitioners started at a lower level of communication skills than the basic physicians who had graduated after 6 years of medical training. The general practitioners in training did not achieve an increase throughout their training programme (Kramer *et al.*

Box 30.3 A counter-productive test item.

We know that it is relevant to elicit the patient's agenda for the consultation. One particular telling piece of information is 'what it was that made the patient decide to consult the doctor; what tilted the balance?' So, when developing an OSCE station we created an item that attempted to measure whether the student addressed this topic. This item was illustrated by the question 'why did you come today?' intended as an example. Students, like all other efficient people, memorise these items, or, rather, the illustrative examples and remember that they must ask: 'why did you come today?' So during the OSCE they all ask this question, assuming that they increase their mark this way. Occasionally this question is actually phrased in such a way that the standardised patient hears: 'why did you wait so long?' and feels lectured and reacts defensively. Here the use of the instrument is counter-productive to what we wanted to achieve.

2004). Transfer of communication is problematic, be it from the preclinical to the clinical phase of the curriculum, from the clinical phase to being a junior doctor, or even from junior doctor to registrar. A recent review by van den Eertwegh *et al.* (2012) addressed this issue and pointed out that what we learn and how we address patients is largely influenced by the context in which we learn and work. The role models, and the 'communication-mindedness' of the workplace, as well as the physical resources available (cameras, supervision) are hugely different across various workplaces (van Weel-Baumgarten *et al.* 2012; van den Eertwegh *et al.* 2014). Consequently, taking these differences into account, the results in patient satisfaction and other outcomes of communication vary accordingly.

So, although students do acquire and maintain their communication competence, the four problems (motivation, repetition, reduction and lack of transfer) are far from solved and need educators' attention.

Future directions

The problems described above call for a more and more constructivistic and holistic approach to training, assessment and integration of communication teaching in all phases of the curriculum.

The debate in the literature about 'skilled communicators' versus 'communication skills' seems to have polarised somewhat. Interestingly enough we train students in how to address differences of opinion in others, but when we engage in a debate ourselves, about an issue that is dear to our hearts, it is not easy to practise what we preach. The two viewpoints should be seen as extremes on a continuum. It seems likely that a good 'communication curriculum' would benefit from the representation of both positions, the skills as well as the humanity, the craft as well as the harmony. Just like musicians need to do exercises to improve their technique and listen and perform to develop their interpretation of the musical score, or a car driver must learn how to handle the car technically as well as survive in traffic, learners should practise their basic skills and apply them in a wide variety of situations in the context of the doctor–patient encounter.

An example of such an approach could be to consider training along a longitudinal continuum, with regular meetings between students and teacher in which students alternate between learning their basic communication skills in a training session (with role plays and other exercises) and practise in a more complex environment with simulated patients and (later) with real patients. Such practise should be filmed, because of the instructive nature of watching one's own behavior (Kurtz *et al.* 1998; Dent & Harden 2009). The recordings should be reviewed with (simulated) patients, peers and a teacher (see Box 30.4 for an illustration).

In such a longitudinal communication curriculum, the group of students and the teacher will get to know each other over time. When they see each other's performance throughout the year their judgement will not suffer from an occasional incident but will rely on a more stable longitudinal overview (van der Vleuten & Schuwirth 2005). Feedback can gradually evolve from addressing the *process* of communication ('sufficient reflections of emotions') to feedback about the *product* (exchange of relevant information, patient satisfaction, patient feeling enabled and/or a resulting agreement between patient and student) (van der Vleuten & Schuwirth 2005; Schuwirth & van der Vleuten 2006).

Box 30.4 An alternative: Constructivistic training format.

> Groups of 10 students meet regularly, with a teacher, during a year-long training programme. In between meetings they record simulated patient encounters, review the recordings, provide analyses and feedback to their own and each other's consultations. In the group sessions comments are discussed and alternatives tried out in exercises and role plays. Feedback and attempts to try out alternatives result in learning goals for the next simulated patient encounter and, later, for the next year.
>
> Simulated patient scenarios require students to do whole (modest) clinical clerkings, including physical examination and negotiating the optimal help with the patient. Later on such training will evolve into recording and reviewing real patient encounters. Reviews will be guided by the students' own learning goals.
>
> Since students are required to demonstrate their best approach, they will soon see that different students show different 'best ways', with varying patient satisfaction. They develop alternatives for their intuitive way of communicating and become motivated to pay attention to doctor–patient communication (van Dalen 2013).

Such an educational continuum is optimal when embedded and integrated in the rest of the curriculum (Posner & Rudnitsky 2006). It requires proper integration in the curriculum: taking into account what subject matter has preceded the training and what will follow, as well as what goes on around the time of training. Course directors of communication skills training must therefore resist the temptation to work in isolation. Communication training should address topics that students have studied and should be relevant in the current context of their working environment (preclinical, clinical, etc.) (Posner & Rudnitsky 2006). Such courses should maximally employ the patient's voice (or the simulated patient's voice), since that has more authority than the teacher's (Silverman *et al.* 2013). Moreover, teachers should help learners to reflect on their experiences and to draw (deduce) learning objectives for the next practise session.

Such a programme is not cheap. Yet it has been adopted in medical schools that choose to invest resources in the improvement of the communication between future doctors and their patients. Moreover, such programmes have been realised in medical schools in various parts of the world. It is helpful to consider the advantages of improved communication in healthcare (increased patient satisfaction, improved health outcomes and a reduction in time needed to understand patients and tailor help). Considering what is at stake, this investment is a small price to pay.

References

Beckman, H.B. & Frankel. R.M. (1984) The effect of physician behavior on the collection of data. *Annals of Internal Medicine*, 101, 692–696.
Dent, J.A. & Harden, R.M. (2009) *A Practical Guide for Medical Teachers*. Churchill Livingstone, London.
Ericsson, A.K., Charness, N., Feltovich, P. & Hoffman, R.R. (2006) *Cambridge Handbook on Expertise and Expert Performance*. Cambridge University Press, Cambridge, UK.
Hojat, M., Mangione, S., Nasca, T.J., Rattner, S., Erdmann, J.B., Gonnella, J.S. & Magee, M. (2004) An empirical study of decline in empathy in medical school. *Medical Education*, 38, 934–941.
Hojat, M., Vergare, M.J., Maxwell, K., Brainard, G., Herrine, S.K., Isenberg, G.A., Veloski, J. & Gonnella, J.S. (2009) The devil is in the third year: A longitudinal study of erosion of empathy in medical school. *Academic Medicine*, 84 (no. 9), 1182–1191.
Kolb, D.A. (1984) *Experiential Learning*. Prentice Hall, Upper Saddle River, NJ.

Korsch, B.M., Gozzi, E.K. & Francis, V. (1968) Gaps in doctor-patient communication. *Pediatrics*, 42 (no. 5), 855–871.

Kramer, A.W.M., Düsman, H., Tan, L.H.C., Jansen, J.J.M., Grol, R.P.T.M. & van der Vleuten, C.P.M. (2004) Acquisition of communication skills in postgraduate training for general practice. *Medical Education*, 38 (no. 2), 158–167.

Kurtz, S., Silverman, J. & Draper, J. (1998) *Teaching and learning communication skills in medicine*. Radcliffe Medical Press, Oxon, UK.

Maehr, M.L. & Mayer, H.A. (1997) Understanding motivation and schooling: Where we've been, where we are and where we need to go. *Educational Psychology Review*, 9, 371–409.

Marvel, M.K., Epstein, R.M., Flowers, K. & Beckman, H.B. (1999) Soliciting the patient's agenda. Have we improved? *JAMA*, 281 (no. 3), 283–287.

Maslow, A.H. (1954) *Motivation and Personality*. Harper & Brothers, New York.

Neumann, M., Edelhäuser, F., Tauschel, D., Fischer, M.R., Wirtz, M., Woopen, C., Haramati, A. & Scheffer, C. (2011) Empathy decline and its reasons: A systematic review of studies with medical students and residents. *Academic Medicine*, 86 (no. 8), 996–1009.

Ormrod, J.E. (2012) *Human Learning*, sixth edn. Pearson, London.

Posner, G.J. & Rudnitsky, A.N. (2006) *Course Design: A Guide to Curriculum Development for Teachers*. Pearson, London.

Salmon, P. & Young, B. (2011) Creativity in clinical communication: From communication skills to skilled communication. *Medical Education*, 45 (no. 3), 217–226.

Schuwirth, L. & van der Vleuten, C.P.M. (2006) A plea for new psychometric model in educational assessment. *Medical Education*, 40, 296–300.

Silverman, J., Kurtz, S. & Draper, J. (2013) *Skills for Communicating with Patients*. Radcliffe Medical Press, Oxon, UK.

Spencer, J. (2004) Decline in empathy in medical education: How can we stop the rot? *Medical Education*, 38 (no. 9), 916–918.

van Dalen, J. (2013) Communication skills in context: Trends and perspectives. *Patient Education and Counseling*, 92, 292–295.

van Dalen, J., Prince, C.J.A.H., Scherpbier, A.J.J.A. & van der Vleuten, C.P.M. (1998) Evaluating communication skills. *Advances in Health Sciences Education*, 3, 187–195.

van Dalen, J., van Hout, J.C.H.M., Wolfhagen, H.A.P., Scherpbier, A.J.J.A. & van der Vleuten, C.P.M. (1999) Factors influencing the effectiveness of communication skills training: Programme contents outweigh teachers' skills. *Medical Teacher*, 21 (no. 3), 308–310.

van Dalen, J., Kerkhofs, E., van Knippenberg-van den Berg, B.W., van den Hout, H.A., Scherpbier, A.J.J.A. & van der Vleuten, C.P.M. (2002) Longitudinal and concentrated communication skills programmes compared: Two Dutch medical schools compared. *Advances in Health Sciences Education*, 7, 29–40.

van den Eertwegh, V., van Dulmen, S., van Dalen, J., Scherpbier, A.J.J.A. & van der Vleuten, C.P.M. (2012) Learning in context: Identifying gaps in research on the transfer of medical communication skills to the clinical workplace. *Patient Education and Counseling*, 90 (no. 2), 184–192. 2012.

van den Eertwegh, V., van Dalen, J., van Dulmen, S., van der Vleuten, C. & Scherpbier, A. (2014) Residents' perceived barriers to communication skills learning: Comparing two medical working contexts in postgraduate training. *Patient Education and Counseling*, 95 (no. 1), 91–97.

van der Vleuten, C.P.M. & Schuwirth, L.W.T. (2005) Assessing professional competence: From methods to programmes. *Medical Education*, 39 (no. 3), 309–317.

van der Vleuten, C.P.M. (1996) The assessment of professional competence: Developments, research and practical implications. *Advances in Health Sciences Education*, 1, 41–67.

van Weel-Baumgarten, E., Bolhuis, S., Rosenbaum, M. & Silverman, J. (2012) Bridging the gap: How is integrating communication skills with medical content throughout the curriculum valued by students? *Patient Education and Counseling*, 90 (no. 2), 177–183.

CHAPTER 31

Transformative Learning and High-Fidelity Simulation

Wesley Scott-Smith

Brighton and Sussex Medical School, East Sussex, UK

Historical context

Transformative and reflective learning are closely aligned in their historical development, combining fundamental ideas within educational theory. When expressed through a variety of simulated learning activities these theories enable us to challenge underlying ideas about clinical practice, creating a reflective discourse that enables reconstruction of various experiences to guide future practice, placing *constructivism* at the centre of this process – that is, that learners 'construe, validate, and reformulate the meaning of their experience' (Cranton 1994).

The educational theories providing the foundation for the spectrum of simulation activities include the concepts of *behaviourism* and *constructivism*. The former is generally reflected in the adoption of automated behaviour exemplified by basic life support training; however, constructivism explores how learners understand and construct their views of the world, facilitated through critical reflective practice (see chapter 32). It relates to the changing thoughts, attitudes and views illustrated by learners during exposure to real clinical practice as well as simulation-based activities. These attributes reflect the development of complex professional activities and specifically the role of clinical reasoning in the development of professional expertise and competence (Eraut 1994).

Undergraduate portfolios seek to encourage an ethos of critical reflective practice as a lifelong skill, with the hope that it will reduce errors in clinical practice and improve patient safety, particularly as flawed cognition accounts for most of the diagnostic errors in practice (Graber 2005; Mamede *et al.* 2008). The concepts of *cognitivism* and *social constructivism* are crucial in formulating ideas and learning from simulation, specifically how new experiences are *assimilated* and *accommodated* into new knowledge and social understanding. These notions illustrate a more complex understanding of various concepts and how they can be integrated into current thoughts that advance the learner's professional expertise.

This has considerable resonance with the gradual development of 'Illness Scripts' in medicine; that is, a complex representation of a single disease symbolised by symptoms, physical signs, pathophysiological features, epidemiological factors, investigations, treatment and management (Feltovich & Barrows 1984), For example, each time learners are exposed to a new patient with a specific disease, they assimilate the case

Clinical Communication in Medicine, First Edition. Edited by Jo Brown, Lorraine M. Noble, Alexia Papageorgiou and Jane Kidd.

into their prior understanding of the disease and in time will recognise not only the prototypical presentation but the atypical features of the disease. Moreover, the cognitive apprenticeship is firmly based upon experiential learning within a community of practice described as *situated learning* (Kolb 1984; Lave & Wenger 1991), which contributes towards learning through a variety of authentic settings.

Simulation-based medical education

Simulation-based activities provide the setting for learning specific technical skills, assessing competencies and analysing tasks that may entail any combination of *cognitive, psychomotor* or *attitudinal domains*, illustrated in the typology below in Table 31.1 (Decker *et al.* 2008).

Historically, simulation-based activities in many domains have primarily addressed technical competencies through a behaviouristic approach, making them easier to assess and provide greater transparency in the public domain. This belies the complexity of medical expertise, particularly decision making and problem solving, with a tendency towards adopting a reductionist approach in medical education (Maudsley & Strivens 2000).

Simulation is gradually being used to explore the complexities of clinical reasoning from the twin paradigms of information processing and judgement theory recognised under the term *'Dual Process Theory'* (Norman & Eva 2010; Pelaccia *et al.* 2011). This theory proposes that clinical reasoning is a combination of analytic and nonanalytic reasoning within multiple levels in the decision-making space, dictated by the context of the problem and the experience of the clinician.

Simulated experiences that approximate closely to real clinical practice with authentic decision making, such as the use of simulated patients in developing communications skills, for example, reflect features of high-fidelity simulation that garner a range of scenarios linked to educational goals in the curriculum. These opportunities create a safe environment in which to err but also allow deliberate practice using

Table 31.1 A typology of simulation-based education (adapted from Decker *et al.* 2008).

Tool	Descriptor
Partial task trainers (low-tech simulators)	Replica models or manikins used to learn and practice simple procedures
Peer-to-peer learning	Peer collaboration used to develop skills e.g. physical assessment
Screen-based computer simulations	Program to acquire knowledge, assess competency, and provide feedback on knowledge and critical thinking e.g. driving test simulation
Virtual reality	Computer-generated environment with multiple sensory systems via sophisticated training systems promoting authenticity
Haptic systems	A simulator that combines real-world and virtual reality exercises
Standardised patients (simulated patients and real patients)	Role playing in simulation using actors or students paid to portray a patient in a realistic manner
Full-scale simulation (medium to high fidelity)	Simulation involving a full-body manikin with programmable physiological responses to practitioner actions

learning strategies to suit individualised needs. Simulation-based activities ultimately reduce the risk to patients by exploring features of clinical practice through the creation of a controlled environment where mistakes can be made and learnt from, but they also provide standards with learning outcomes for governance and accountability issues and furthermore can compensate for reduced learning opportunities in practice (Maran & Glavin 2003; Ker & Bradley 2007).

Reviews of high-fidelity studies focus heavily upon the value of feedback in promoting and shaping learning alongside such concepts as deliberate practice and immersion in curricular outcomes that facilitate learning at increasing levels of difficulty (Ericsson 2004; McGaghie *et al.* 2010). Qualities of high-fidelity simulation include a close approximation to clinical practice, the simulation should be set within a controlled environment, and that it captures clinical variation (Issenberg *et al.* 2005).

Current practice: Feedback and cognitive processes in simulation

Feedback is often viewed as an 'extrinsic process' imparted by a trainer or facilitator who has the expertise to deliver constructive feedback using trusted guidelines such as *agenda-led, outcome-based analysis* ('ALOBA') or Pendleton's rules (Pendleton *et al.* 1984; Kurtz *et al.* 2005). Studies seeking to uncover cognitive attributes through simulation are better served through reflective discussions using generic prompts with the learner; for example, '*What were you thinking at this point'?* or '*How did this factor affect your decision making'?* Critical reflection may also be provoked through the *intrinsic conversation* embedded in the experience; that is, the internal conversation that the participant has with him or herself about what happened and why (Laurillard 1997). This may include reflection upon action, seeing ways of doing things differently, analysis of decision making, changing behaviour and reconsidering attitudes. These all provide impetus towards reconstructing practice for the learner (Mezirow 1991).

Transformative learning can be facilitated through either form of feedback and/or reflection, using personal experiences or vicarious learning through observation of others. High-fidelity simulations using standardised patients or human patient simulators with filmed performance for subsequent reflective discussion provide an additional opportunity to 'mull over' the consequences of actions and thoughts, sometimes using delayed reflection to maximise learning outcomes. The benefits of using videotapes of interviewing behaviour amongst qualified doctors were recognised in the 1970s (Adler *et al.* 1970), and not only can such filmed material be used in reflective discussions on decision making, but it can also provide an occasion to address issues of performance anxiety and distress over perceived mistakes. However, it must be acknowledged that performance may vary with the *cognitive load* created by the simulation activity, and this may inhibit learning by overloading working memory and sometimes by heightening emotional aspects of the interaction (Sweller 1988; Fraser *et al.* 2012).

Adaptive cognitive processes are employed by learners exposed to simulation activities, particularly those associated with the more significant transitions in the 'medical continuum'; for example, the transition from 'preclinical' or classroom-based learning to 'clinical rotations' on the wards, which are accompanied by a greater expectation of autonomous learning and 'stand-alone practice' (Teunissen & Westerman 2011). The adaptive processes of *assimilation* and *accommodation* of experiences into future practice can be illustrated through reflective discussions following high-fidelity simulation using simulated patients. Carefully facilitated discussions can tease out important strands from the intrinsic conversation going on in the learner's mind about performance and changing behaviour. Important features of communication skills and data gathering can emerge during such discussions, which evidence critical reflection upon knowledge organisation from the medical consultations, that is, how the learner copes with and thinks about organising the flood of data from a patient during a consultation. The examples below are taken from a reflexive discussion between a researcher and third-year medical students following a filmed consultation with a simulated patient (Scott-Smith 2013).

The first student is reflecting upon watching her data-gathering skills and the use of heuristics on screen, specifically the SOCRATES mnemonic to guide questioning about a patient's experience of pain (site, onset, character, radiation, associated factors, timing, exacerbating factors, severity);

> *(a) They (mnemonics) organise my mind a bit, hopefully not miss out things! I suppose there is so much information coming at you at once you want to organise it a little and take it one at a time…cover all the posts and I find it helps with structure.*

Similarly when the second student was asked what insight she had gained from watching film of herself taking a history, she replied:

> *(b) In the middle of interviewing there's lots of things going on in your mind, you think you have to get through everything else. I'm not that comfortable in front of patients to take a pause to gather my thoughts, I always feel I have to keep going and asking questions. Maybe if I took a few pauses…and tried to couple my ideas together.*

Both of these quotations illustrate not only constructive reflective analysis, but the last comment demonstrates transformative thought with a view to changing practice through chunking of ideas (ultimately leading to pattern recognition), in this case stepping back from the process of gathering information and pausing to collect ideas. In essence these are emergent features of higher cognitive aptitude and professional experience, which includes both consultation skills and clinical reasoning. These are recognised as features of developing metacognition, bringing concepts such as reasoning to the forefront of our consciousness, making decision making more explicit, and are sometimes described as the '*seventh sense*' (Nisbet & Schucksmith 1984).

Evidence of higher-level thought can also emerge through initiation of reflective discussions following simulation, for example, a consideration of the inference or related abstraction implied by a comment explained by *semantic theory* (Bordage & Lemieux 1991). Semantic qualifying statements provide intriguing evidence of how clinical features in the simulation are being interpreted or processed, demonstrated by example (c) below, where the student has recognised a 'tipping point' in the disease process, precipitating a medical consultation in a relapsing condition with worsening severity.

> *(c) This pain was a lot worse and milk wasn't making it better, and the pain wasn't going away after three days but getting worse after five days. I don't know how to describe it…pushing towards something bad happening, something had pushed her over the edge; some sort of significant problem had happened within her abdomen.*

This represents a change in disease acceleration recognised by the student through inferences within the simulation (illustrating greater depth in the appreciation and analysis of symptoms), encapsulated in the mind as part of an illness script for worsening dyspepsia. The last example below illustrates an emerging awareness of one of the commonest cognitive errors in clinical practice caused by premature diagnostic closure:

> (d) It's really important to keep an open mind. When you're doing things you need to have ideas rolling around but sometimes you run with one idea and it prevents you weighing up other options. It's important to keep a broad mind and weigh up the options properly.

Future directions

The increasing emphasis upon patient safety issues and the avoidance of diagnostic errors in clinical practice has propelled the study of cognition using high-fidelity simulation studies into the spotlight, with more significance upon exploring cognitive factors in medicine explicitly rather than pure technical competencies. Simulation-based strategies provide the learner with exposure to scenarios of increasing complexity in domains such as prescribing and decision making during ward rounds that could only have been learnt through assimilation 'on the job' previously. Technological advances such as virtual patients can augment the use of simulated patients in learning communication strategies during training with increasing complexity, enabling an opportunity for discourse on the higher cognitive skills involved in professional development, which include reflexivity and metacognition.

The more significant advantages conferred by practising skills through high-fidelity simulation relate to the transfer to practice, the highest level of the Kirkpatrick hierarchy (Kirkpatrick 1998). However, this is frequently translated through the concept of 'mastery of skills' using defined outcome criteria, whereas cognitive skills are much harder to assimilate and indeed measure. This is the challenge for simulation-based learning now and in the future; how do we facilitate the development of higher cognitive skills through the various modalities of simulation?

References

Adler, L.M., Ware, J.E. & Enelow, A.J. (1970) Changes in medicine interviewing style with two closed-circuit television techniques. *Journal of Medical Education*, 45, 21–28.
Bordage, G. & Lemieux, M. (1991) Semantic structures and diagnostic thinking of experts and novices. *Academic Medicine*, 66 (no. 9), S70–72.
Cranton, P. (1996) *Professional Development as Transformative Learning*. Jossey Bass, San Francisco, CA.
Decker, S., Sportsman, S., Puetz, L. & Billings, L. (2008) The evolution of simulation and its contribution to competency. *Journal of Continuing Education in Nursing*, 39 (no. 2), 74–80.
Eraut, M. (1994) *Developing Professional Knowledge and Competence*. Falmer Press, London.
Ericsson, K. (2004) Deliberate practice and the acquisition and maintenance of expert performance in medicine and related domains. *Academic Medicine*, 79 (Suppl. 10), 70–81.
Feltovich, P.J. & Barrows, H.S. (1984) Issues of generality in medical problem solving. In: H.G. Schmidt & M.L. De Volder (eds), *Tutorials in Problems Based Learning: A New Direction in Teaching Health Professionals*, pp. 128–142. Van Gorcum, Assen, the Netherlands.
Fraser, K., Ma, I., Baxter, H., Wright, B. & McLaughlin, J. (2012) Emotion, cognitive load and learning outcomes during simulation training. *Medical Education*, 46, 1055–1062.
Graber, M.L. (2005) Diagnostic error in internal medicine. *Archives of Internal Med*, 165, 1493–1499.

Issenberg, S.B., McGaghie, W.C., Petrusa, E.R., Gordon, D.L. & Scalese, R.J. (2005) Features and uses of high fidelity medical simulations that lead to effective learning: A BEME systematic review. *Medical Teacher*, 27 (no. 1), 10–28.

Ker, J. & Bradley, P. (2007) Simulation in medical education. In: *Understanding Medical Education*. Association for the Study of Medical Education, Edinburgh.

Kirkpatrick, D.L. (1998) *Evaluating Training Programmes*, second edn. Berrett-Koehler, San Francisco, CA.

Kolb, D. (1984) *Experiential Learning*. Prentice Hall, Englewood Cliffs, NJ.

Kurtz, S., Silverman, J. & Draper, J. (2005) *Teaching and Learning Communication in Medicine*. Radcliffe Publishing, Oxford, UK.

Laurillard, D. (1997) Learning formal representation through multimedia. In: N.F. Entwhistle (ed), *The Experience of Learning*, pp. 172–183). Scottish Academic Press, Edinburgh

Lave, J. & Wenger, E. (1991) Situated learning: Legitimate peripheral participation. In: J.S. Bowen (ed), *Learning in Doing. Cognitive and Computational Perspectives*. Cambridge University Press, Cambridge, UK.

Mamede, S., Schmidt, H. & Penaforte, J. (2008) Effects of reflective practice on the accuracy of medical diagnoses. *Medical Education*, 42, 468–475.

Maran, N.J. & Glavin, R.J. (2003) Low to high fidelity simulation – a continuum of medical education. *Medical Education*, 37 (Suppl. 1), 22–28.

Maudsley, J. & Strivens, G. (2000) 'Science', 'critical thinking' and 'competence' for *Tomorrow's Doctors*. A review of terms and concepts. *Medical Education*, 34, 53–60.

McGaghie, W.C., Issenberg, S.B., Petrusa, E.R. & Scalese, R.J. (2010) A critical review of simulation-based medical education research: 2003–2009. *Medical Education*, 44, 50–63.

Mezirow, J. (1991)*Transformative Dimensions of Adult Learning*. Jossey Bass, San Francisco, CA.

Nisbet, J. & Schucksmith, J. (1984)*The Seventh Sense: Reflections on Learning to Learn*. Scottish Council for Research in Education, Edinburgh.

Norman, G. & Eva, K.W. (2010) Diagnostic error and clinical reasoning. *Medical Education*, 44 (no. 1), 94–100.

Pelaccia, T., Tardif, J., Triby, E. & Charlin, B. (2011) An analysis of clinical reasoning through a recent and comprehensive approach: The dual-process theory. *Medical Education Online*, 16. doi:10.3402/meo.v16i0.5890.

Pendleton, D., Schofield, T., Tate, P. & Havelock, P. (1984) *The Consultation*. Oxford University Press, Oxford, UK.

Scott-Smith, W. (2013) Diagnostic reasoning in medical students using a simulated environment. EdD Thesis, University of Brighton, Brighton, UK.

Sweller, J. (1988) Cognitive load during problem solving: Effects upon learning. *Cognitive Science*, 12, 257–285.

Teunissen, P. & Westerman, M. (2011) Opportunity or threat: The ambiguity of the consequences of transitions in medical education. *Medical Education*, 45, 51–59.

CHAPTER 32

Reflective Practice

Sally Quilligan

School of Clinical Medicine, Cambridge, UK

Historical context

In 1933 the philosopher John Dewey proposed that practice could be enhanced if practitioners were able to learn from experience. He defined reflective thinking as 'active, persistent and careful consideration of any belief or supposed form of knowledge in the light of the grounds that support it and the further conclusion to which it tends' (Dewey 1933, p. 9). Writing extensively about reflective thought, Dewey highlighted that the ability of individuals to reflect is initiated only after they have identified a problem and recognised and accepted the uncertainty this generates (Tate & Sills 2004). Dewey (1933) focused specifically on the importance of systematically examining and questioning thinking for its underlying foundations and implications in order to search for possible explanations. More recently Dewey and Mezirow have extended this understanding to include emotions and the meaning making of the experience (Askeland & Fook 2009; Mann *et al.* 2009) and in doing so highlighted an important distinction between reflection and critical reflection.

Through his work with teacher education, Donald Schön presented the idea of the reflective practitioner (1991): someone who used reflection both to learn knowledge from experience and to resolve the complex and obscure problems of professional practice. Similarly, he identified that reflective learning included the handling of experience in different ways, reflecting both *in* and *on* action. Whilst he contends that practitioners draw on practical experience in a highly intuitive way, reflection is triggered when a situation requires further thought. Reflection *in* action refers to stopping, thinking and problem solving in the midst of activity – to a process of knowing in action. Alternatively, reflection *on* action is reserved for those nonroutine situations where the professional's reflection in action is inadequate to frame the problem; knowing through action (Schön 1991). In situations such as clinical communication teaching learners explore their understanding of their actions and experience, and the impact of these on themselves and others after the experience. Schön (1991) further added to our understanding of professional knowing and learning by categorising knowledge into two types: technical rationality and professional artistry. Technical rationality refers to the dominant scientific paradigm produced by research and 'knowing that' (the facts). Professional artistry is gleaned from knowledge largely emerging from professional practice and described as 'knowing how'. Tate suggests that it is professional artistry or intuitive knowledge that is developed through critical reflection (Tate & Sills 2004).

Clinical Communication in Medicine, First Edition. Edited by Jo Brown, Lorraine M. Noble,
Alexia Papageorgiou and Jane Kidd.
© 2016 John Wiley & Sons, Ltd. Published 2016 by John Wiley & Sons, Ltd.

Current practice

Whilst there is debate about what makes reflection critical, three definitions illustrate the nature of this activity and the way it is being conceptualised within this discussion.

First, Johns begins to signify the difference between reflection and critical reflection by highlighting both the complexity and difficulty that can be involved and the importance of personal experience being the object of reflection:

> A window through which the practitioner can view and focus self within the context of her own lived experiences in ways that enable her to confront, understand and work towards resolving the contradictions within her practice between what is desirable and actual practice.
>
> *(Johns 2000)*

Second, Fook and Gardner acknowledge that individual experience cannot be divorced from the social context. Thus, they articulate critical reflection as:

> a process of unsettling individual assumptions to bring about social changes. The assumptions may be individually held...but will involve some assumptions about social influences on personal lives.
>
> *(Fook and Gardner 2007)*

This definition prioritises the connection with critical social theory and the importance of analysing the power dynamics at work that frame the field of practice (Lyons 2009). Third, Mezirow, an educator and sociologist, signals the importance of reflection being at a deep level, which explores and evaluates hidden assumptions. He considers how such assumptions may be limiting ability to cope with diversity and uncertainty and to confront multiplicity within meaning making. He also points to the need for action to be taken in the light of the new understandings, when he describes critical reflection as:

> The process of becoming critically aware of how and why our presuppositions have come to constrain the way we perceive, understand and feel about our world; of reformulating these assumptions to permit a more inclusive, discriminating, permeable and integrative perspective; and of making decisions or otherwise acting on those new understandings.
>
> *(Mezirow 1990)*

Emphasising that a critical dimension of learning involves recognising and reassessing the structure of assumptions and expectations that frame our thinking, feeling and acting (Mezirow 2006), Mezirow describes these as a 'frame of reference'. Frames of reference can be transformed through critical reflection on the assumptions upon which our interpretations, beliefs and habits of mind or points of view are based. According to Mezirow, such assumptions may be epistemic, sociocultural or psychic (Mezirow 1990). Epistemic relates to understanding about the nature and use of knowledge; for example, a student may understand knowledge as fact and not believe that he or she is learning knowledge when observing a team. Sociocultural describes how socially dominant assumptions may be linked to power relations and inhibit actions (Mezirow 2000; Fook & Gardner 2007). For example, if a junior student attends a ward round and is not acknowledged by the team, the student may perceive that he or she is not wanted and feel unable to ask permission to participate. The understanding being that the assumptions of these networks and their associated ideologies need to be explored as part of critical reflection. Finally, psychic refers to the way individuals view themselves and may involve exploring the autobiographical context of a belief (Mezirow 1997).

Through these concepts Mezirow articulates critical reflection as critically questioning the content, process and premise on which the learner has defined a problem in order to make meaning or better understand the experience (Mezirow 1990). Each of the three components of reflection (content, process and premise) will result in changes in behaviour that reflect more fundamental changes in attitudes and beliefs. Analysis of content addresses analysis of the problem or situation. Process reflection involves analysing a range of potential strategies, exploring their suitability to address the situation and identifying alternative strategies that might be useable. However, premise reflection involves questioning the justification of the premise on which our beliefs have been constructed (that is, the taken-for-granted beliefs that people hold); this is much more challenging and not easy to achieve. Becoming aware of our assumptions is rarely achieved alone, and critical reflection is usually undertaken as part of a group activity.

Incorporating critical reflection into clinical communication skills teaching

Drawing upon Schön, Fook, Gardner and Mezirow, the steps outlined in Box 32.1 seem important.

Let's think of how this works in teaching. A novice learner is practising breaking bad news to a simulated patient. The session uses agenda-led outcome-based analysis (ALOBA), one of the feedback methods designed to ensure that feedback and reflection is underpinned by the personal goals of the learner (Kurtz *et al.* 2005). ALOBA begins with learners reflecting on and identifying the areas they want feedback on and what they are trying to achieve prior to seeing the patient. In this case: wanting to use a warning shot, to pick up on patient cues and sensitively deliver bad news. During the interaction they achieve the first point, but the news is delivered extremely quickly. After the interaction the learner again reflects with the group, explaining that they think they've confused the patient and needed to be clearer. At this point the learner is focusing on content reflection and encouraging the group to help with process reflection by suggesting alternative strategies. The facilitator now needs to move the group and learner towards premise reflection.

Box 32.1 Framework for critical reflection (Quilligan 2013).

1 Identifying and articulating an unsettling situation
2 Acknowledging and exploring emotions, such as fear, anger etc.
3 Identifying and critically assessing epistemic, sociocultural and psychic assumptions
  • Attending to connections between the personal experience and social or cultural influences
  • Exploring contextual awareness of one's own position, by articulating the impact of one's own behaviour and background
  • Considering other perspectives and what alternate views are missing from the account
4 Exploring new roles and possible actions
5 Planning a new course of action
6 Re-rehearsing

By encouraging descriptive feedback from the group members the facilitator raises awareness of assumptions that may shape behaviour. The group describes the nonverbal behaviour of the patient – he seemed to lose eye contact and become tearful, and the facilitator asks the patient to feed back how he was feeling. The patient says he felt 'overwhelmed and not able to take in the information'. A clip from the video is used to reflect in action on the patient's nonverbal response. Afterwards the facilitator, attempting to articulate the difficulties the scenario embodied and to acknowledge the emotional impact, asks the learner how he was feeling delivering the news.

Encouraging learners to identify and critically assess how their assumptions may have impacted on the interaction is important. The learners share thoughts about how their upbringing, prior experiences of receiving bad news and desire to remember the facts accurately may all have shaped their response. Once this is understood the learners are then in a position to explore alternate strategies and approaches with the group. Re-rehearsal may be key to the development of critical reflection. To be effective the learners need to have understood the previous assumptions they were making, had an opportunity to creatively explore and view the problem from different viewpoints and reflect again on what they are now trying to achieve. Re-rehearsal leads to further reflection by the group and learner and to gradual mastery of skills. Review of the video of both the initial interaction and re-rehearsal after the session allows for further reflection on action.

Through sharing experiences and challenging and learning from each other, these reflections and insights lead to decisions and action, achievement of goals and changes to immediate and future practice.

Future directions

As we look to the future, do we need to consider how to harness the power of critical reflection more effectively within our teaching?

Done well, communication teaching enables learners to critically reflect by looking at what they want to achieve, considering their emotions, assumptions, discussing alternative behaviours, helping them plan a new course of action that is flexible and reflects their personality and enables re-rehearsal. The incorporation of critical reflection is one of the great strengths of communication skills teaching, it is powerful and can produce transformational learning; that is learning that is sustained and changes us. The challenge is to ensure it is used systematically and consistently by learners. Early introduction of critical reflection initiates acceptance of an important ability for clinicians for continued lifelong learning, and we need to develop models to support understanding of critical reflection. Equally there are occasions when we don't seek the learner's agenda, use the video or offer re-rehearsal and we need to recognise that these are moments when we lose opportunities for critical reflection.

Perhaps when we suspect that the students' level of reflection is low, focusing only on the content, we may want to question whether our teaching methodologies enable us to highlight this to the learner and if so how we then move the student towards process and premise reflection. More importantly we need an approach that ensures that our teaching models the process and cultivates its use in learners both in the classroom and in clinical practice (Quilligan 2013). Engaging in critical reflection on the clinical context can begin in the classroom by ensuring we enable students at the end of a simulated teaching session to critically reflect on how they need to adapt what they've learnt to the clinical context. Equally, students need to be appropriately prepared to critically reflect on the clinical communication they observe in practice. Currently within clinical practice there are key moments that if critically reflected upon can produce powerful learning about clinical communication but that often go unnoticed. Our biggest challenge now is to support faculty and learners to find ways to see and critically reflect upon those moments.

References

Askeland, G.A. & Fook, J. (2009) Critical reflection in social work. *European Journal of Social Work*, 12, 287–292.
Dewey, J. (1933) *How We Think: A Restatement of Reflective Thinking to the Educative Process*. Houghton Mifflin, Boston, MA.
Fook, J. & Gardner, F. (2007) *Practising Critical Reflection: A Resource Handbook*. McGraw-Hill Education, Maidenhead, UK.
Johns, C. (2000) *Becoming a Reflective Practitioner*. Blackwell Science, London.
Kurtz, S.M., Silverman, J. & Draper, J. (2005) *Teaching and Learning Communication Skills in Medicine*. Radcliffe, Oxford, UK.
Lyons, N. (2009) *Handbook of Reflection and Reflective Inquiry: Mapping a Way of Knowing for Professional Reflective Inquiry*. Springer Verlag, New York.
Mann, K., Gordon, J. & Macleod, A. (2009) Reflection and reflective practice in health professions education: A systematic review. *Advances in Health Sciences Education*, 14, 595–621.
Mezirow, J. (1990) *Fostering Critical Reflection in Adulthood: A Guide to Transformative and Emancipatory Learning*. Jossey-Bass, San Francisco, CA.
Mezirow, J. (1997) Transformative learning: Theory to practice. *New Directions for Adult and Continuing Education*, 74, 5–12.
Mezirow, J. (2000) Learning to think like an adult. In: J. Mezirow (ed), *Learning as Transformation: Critical Perspectives on a Theory in Progress*. Jossey Bass, San Francisco, CA.
Mezirow, J. (2006) An overview on transformative learning. In: P. Sutherland & J. Crowther (eds), *Lifelong Learning: Concepts and Contexts*. Routledge, London
Quilligan, S. (2013) *Enabling fourth year student-doctors to learn through participation on ward rounds: An action research study*. EdD Thesis, Institute of Education, University of London.
Schön, D.A. (1991) *The Reflective Practitioner: How Professionals Think in Action*. Avebury, Aldershot, UK.
Tate, S. & Sills, M. (2004) *The Development of Critical Reflection in the Health Professions* (occasional paper). LTSN Centre for Health Sciences and Practice, London.

CHAPTER 33

Models of Feedback

Catherine J. Williamson[1], Jill Dales[2] and John Spencer[2]

[1]*Durham University, Stockton, UK*
[2]*Newcastle University, Newcastle, UK*

> Feedback is the lifeblood of learning and it must be kept flowing.
>
> *(Rowntree 1982)*

Historical context

What is feedback?

Feedback lies at the heart of teaching, learning and assessment and underpins many important developments in contemporary health profession education, such as workplace-based assessment, the move towards competency-based curricula, and appraisal, mentoring and coaching. Without feedback mistakes remain uncorrected, effective performance is not reinforced, and a false sense of competence may be conferred.

The concept of feedback as an informative process has been at the heart of the 'apprenticeship' model used for the development of workplace learning for millennia, apparently as far back as ancient Greece. Specific mention of a phenomenon known as 'feedback', however, only appeared in Western writing at the beginning of the 20th century with reference to electronic circuitry and biological systems (Thorndike 1918).

Feedback to support learning has theoretical underpinning from a range of theories including behaviourism, social learning, constructivism, experiential learning and motivational learning. Nonetheless the concept of feedback as a method of evaluating and improving performance within education, and specifically within medical education, appeared only relatively recently. Norbert Weiner describes how the concept of feedback was extended from electronic circuitry to the humanities:

> Feedback is the control of a system by reinserting into the system the results of its performance. If these results are merely used as numerical data for criticism of the system and its regulation, we have the simple feedback of the control engineer. If, however, the information which proceeds backwards from the performance is able to change the general method and pattern of the performance, we have a process which may very well be called learning.
>
> *(Norbert Weiner in Ende 1983, p. 777)*

Clinical Communication in Medicine, First Edition. Edited by Jo Brown, Lorraine M. Noble, Alexia Papageorgiou and Jane Kidd.
© 2016 John Wiley & Sons, Ltd. Published 2016 by John Wiley & Sons, Ltd.

Varying definitions of feedback have been proposed, highlighting differences in what authors regard as the key components and/or the purpose of feedback. For their pivotal literature review, Black and William proposed that, in the interests of simplicity, the term feedback be used *'to refer to any information that is provided to the performer of any action about that performance'* (Black & William 1998, p. 53). However, some authors argue that for feedback to exist there must also be evidence of comparison to a reference standard (Ramaprasad 1983; Sadler 1998), use of an external agent (Kluger & DeNisi 1996), receipt by the learner (Hattie & Jaeger 1998) or use to improve performance (Ramaprasad 1983).

Feedback has long been accepted as a core component of formative assessment, defined by Black and William as encompassing *'all those activities undertaken by teachers, and/or by their students, which provide information to be used as feedback to modify the teaching and learning activities in which they are engaged'* (Black & William 1998, pp. 7–8); they conclude that for formative assessment to exist feedback information has to be actually used by the recipient enacting one of a range of potential learning opportunities in response to information provided. Harlen and James concur with the notion of over-lapping concepts of feedback and formative assessment: *'Formative assessment, therefore, is essentially feedback both to the teacher and to the pupil about present understanding and skill development in order to determine the way forward'* (Harlen & James 1997, p. 369).

Does feedback work?

Feedback in education has been extensively studied and is arguably one of the better-evidenced areas of educational practice. For example, in a recent systematic review, Hattie and Timperley reported a synthesis of over 500 meta-analyses from the general educational literature in which over a hundred potential factors that might influence achievement were studied. The average effect size (a measure of the strength of an intervention) was 0.40; however, the effect size for feedback was 0.79, thereby rank-ing feedback among the top influences on achievement (Hattie & Timperley 2007). Nonetheless, they described considerable variation between studies, concluding that different types of feedback have different effectiveness.

In the context of clinical practice, Veloski *et al.* reviewed available evidence from 1966 to 2003 linking feedback with effect on physician performance; 74% of studies in which the independent effect of feedback was studied showed a positive effect on physician performance, rising to 77% of studies in which feedback was combined with other interventions, such as educational programmes, guidelines and reminders. They concluded that feedback can change clinical performance when it is systematically delivered from credible sources (Veloski *et al.* 2006).

However, feedback does not always have positive effects. For example, Kluger and DeNisi (1996) reviewed 131 papers and found that, although feedback had an overall significant effect on performance (average effect size 0.4), around two in every five effects were negative. They explain this by proposing four possible responses when an individual is presented with evidence of discrepancy between actual and desired levels of performance, that is, a 'feedback-standard discrepancy': first, behaviour may be changed to improve performance to better match the desired standard; second, the standard may be altered to match current behaviour (raised when positive feedback is received, thereby encouraging future improvement, but lowered when negative feed-back is received); third, the feedback itself may be rejected in an attempt to deny any discrepancy exists; finally, an individual might abandon the standard completely in an attempt to avoid the situation in future.

Obviously feedback information must be received and interpreted by the recipient before it can influence performance. Hattie and Jaeger commented that:

> Not all students receive the same information in the same way. Some students are more able to seek and assimilate feedback information, and these differences relate to the students' manner in which they process information relating to the self, that is to their beliefs about self or self-esteem.
>
> *(Hattie & Jaeger 1998, p. 116)*

Archer, in a review of the evidence of the effectiveness of feedback in health profession education, recommended that educators need to acknowledge the psychosocial needs of the recipient, while ensuring that the feedback provided is both honest and accurate. Feedback that threatens self-esteem is less effective, and negative feedback may be rejected, blamed on external factors or perceived as *'useless, burdensome, critical or controlling'*. He concluded that facilitation is central to feedback success in that it can take potentially damaging negative feedback and use it to create positive outcomes (Archer 2010, p. 105).

King discussed the tendency for educators to focus mainly on poorer aspects of performance rather than what was done well, thereby reducing the likelihood of repetition of poor performance but also potentially increasing anxiety and reducing the recipient's openness to further learning (King 1999). She described a range of possible defensive reactions including blaming, denial, rationalisation and anger:

> Here is the nub of the feedback challenge: how to draw trainees' attention to their less satisfactory aspects while maintaining or even increasing their desire to learn, improve, and seek further evaluation.
>
> *(King 1999, S2-7200)*

Current practice

Influences on feedback

In his review, Archer highlighted the many variables influencing feedback, including type, structure, format and timing; characteristics of the recipient; and impact.

Consideration must be given to whether feedback is to be directive or facilitatory (the latter approach being more appropriate for advanced learners), as well as to the specificity of feedback (neither too specific nor too general, or learning will be constrained); further, feedback information should not be too complex. Feedback may come from a range of sources, including patients, and in a variety of formats, although in communication teaching this will most often be face-to-face. Timing is important and may influence effectiveness; generally it seems that immediate feedback is the most effective in the context of skills training.

In terms of the recipient, reference has already been made to the variety of ways in which feedback is received, the need for emotional safety and support, and the likelihood that feedback that threatens self-esteem will generally be ineffective. Somewhat counter-intuitively, it has been shown that nonspecific and unconditional praise, however well intentioned, is not only unhelpful but may lead to worsening of performance (Butler 1987), and that giving grades can undo positive effects of feedback comments (Butler 1988).

One problem is that people may not recognise feedback from others. This may not seem a problem as a person's ability to self-assess is seen as fundamental to the success of feedback and most models purport to promote it. Yet, as Archer states, there is a dearth of evidence in support of the effectiveness or accuracy of self-assessment (Archer 2010). Indeed he argues that the unconscious self strives to protect us from anything that threatens self-esteem; we are also prone to attribute our behaviour to external forces. Furthermore, people whose performance is poor tend to overestimate their abilities, whereas those at the top of the range may underestimate, the so-called Kruger-Dunning effect (Kruger & Dunning 1999). Thus it is not helpful to pursue development of 'self-assessment' skills as a goal of feedback but instead we should nurture so-called 'self-directed assessment seeking' behaviour (Eva & Regehr 2008).

There are many potential barriers to providing feedback. First and foremost, delivering feedback constructively and consistently is not easy, especially in experiential (as opposed to classroom) settings and takes time. The fact that feedback may be more valuable to the learner than (yet) more teaching may not be appreciated by either party. Second, teachers may worry about upsetting learners or about the impact of 'negative' feedback on their relationship with them. Third, many teachers have had no training in giving feedback, thus avoid doing it, especially in challenging circumstances such as a learner with little insight (arguably a situation in which the need for honest, constructive feedback is at its greatest).

There is no doubt that feedback in health profession educational settings is complex, diverse and challenging. Notwithstanding the complexity, however, the core features of effective feedback distilled from the evidence are remarkably consistent. Effective feedback:

- focuses on the task and task performance;
- is specific, linked to personal goals and includes information about how to improve;
- is descriptive and nonevaluative;
- focuses on behaviour, not on personal attributes;
- does not threaten the recipient or undermine self-esteem and
- should be given in a context of trust and mutual respect.

Models of feedback

Perhaps the best-known approach to feedback is a model formalised by Pendleton and colleagues in the 1980s in the context of consultation skills training in general practice (Pendleton *et al.* 1984), which ultimately became known as 'Pendleton's rules'. The model intended to provide balance and safety to counteract the historical tendency for feedback to focus on negative aspects, often with little or no emotional support, turning it into a potentially destructive and de-motivating process. The aims of the approach are to encourage self-evaluation and, by focusing on positives first, to reinforce strengths and forestall a spiral of defensiveness.

The model was taken up widely, and with great zeal, in other areas of health professional education, notably undergraduate medical education. Problems with the model are well recognised, not least by Pendleton and colleagues, in that it can feel contrived and patronising and may be overly protective; the learner's agenda is discovered late in the process, such that he or she may not actually 'hear' the positives when they finally arrive; it uses time inefficiently; the learner's desire/need to discuss areas of weakness may be blocked; and it becomes repetitious and formulaic. As Pendleton observed, 'when the rules are used as laws rather than guidelines, they are inappropriately dogmatized' (Pendleton *et al.* 2003, p. 77). They recommended that their feedback principles should be treated as such and advocated 'directness and sensitivity' (Pendleton *et al.* 2003, p. 80) when providing feedback.

An alternative 'set of strategies for analyzing interviews and giving feedback which maximizes learning and safety in experiential sessions' was developed by the authors of the Calgary-Cambridge Guide to communication teaching (Kurtz *et al.* 2005, p. 113). Known as 'agenda-led outcome-based analysis' (ALOBA), it is complemented by an approach to providing descriptive, nonevaluative feedback, the so-called 'SET-GO' approach (i.e. what I **s**aw; what **e**lse did you see?; what do you **t**hink?; clarify **g**oal; and any **o**ffers as to how might get there?). ALOBA starts with the learner's agenda, which allows early identification of problems experienced by the learner and what help he or she would like from the facilitator and/or group. In theory this helps allay anxiety, reduces defensiveness and is arguably more time efficient. Feedback is focused on what outcomes the learner (and, in the context of a consultation, the patient) is (are) trying to achieve or would have liked to achieve, which encourages problem solving and promotes engagement and 'ownership'. This does not mean that strengths are not discussed and reinforced; indeed it is most important that feedback is balanced but without the slavish focus on 'the positives' characteristic of the sandwich models.

Another approach developed in the USA is the six-stepped Chicago model (Brukner *et al.* 1999). Like ALOBA, it starts with recapping aims and objectives the trainee is supposed to be pursuing. The other steps are to give feedback of a positive nature; ask trainee to appraise his or her own performance; give feedback focused on behaviour not personality, and on observation not opinion; give specific examples; and suggest areas for improvement.

Another general approach to giving feedback on clinical communication is to focus it on tasks or stages of the consultation. Frameworks, such as Pendleton's seven tasks (Pendleton *et al.* 1984), Neighbour's five stages – connect, summarise, handover, safety-net, housekeeping (Neighbour 2005) – and the Calgary-Cambridge framework (Silverman *et al.* 2005) have been used as a foundation for analysing the consultation for teaching, learning and assessment. For example, the Leicester Assessment Package, which is based in part on Pendleton's tasks, comprises a checklist that is used to deconstruct the consultation and the processes observed, with the aim of informing feedback and assessment (McKinley *et al.* 2000). It has been shown to be valid and to have acceptable reliability for use in summative assessment but is also a useful tool in giving feedback.

Whatever the differences in detail, using any of the above approaches requires a high level of facilitation skills (Kurtz *et al.* 2005). For example, attention must be paid to structuring the session appropriately, ensuring that the learner's agenda is as specific as possible, monitoring the emotional climate, and nurturing helpful and constructive discussion. The facilitator needs to be flexible in approach, and to be able to 'scaffold' learning accordingly, for example, using examples, putting things in context, asking questions and modelling behaviour.

Future directions

Given the complexity of feedback, there is clearly a need for more research, not least into what approach works best for whom and under what circumstances. Nonetheless there is consensus about the core principles of helpful feedback. Thus it has been argued there should be a shift towards maximising effectiveness of feedback through application of these principles, rather than simply giving more feedback (Hattie & Jaeger 1998; Hattie & Timperley 2007). Unfortunately, in the context of healthcare education, although clinical teachers think they give adequate feedback, this is not always the perception of learners (Liberman *et al.* 2005). Furthermore, feedback, including feedback during communication skills training, is usually episodic, a one-off or stand-alone event. However, many authors, for example, Evans (2013), talk about the importance of conceptualizing feedback as an ongoing and integrated process to support learning – this is captured in the concept of 'feed-forward' and 'feed-up'.

Patients' views are increasingly being sought in the context of service (National Health Service 2011), clinical practice (Chief Medical Officer for England 2008) and education (General Medical Council 2011). For example, the General Medical Council recommends that '*All…patients and carers who come into contact with the (medical) student should have an opportunity to provide constructive feedback about their performance*' (General Medical Council 2011, p. 9). Intuitively this can only be seen as a 'good thing', yet the evidence of the robustness of this approach is mixed. For example, Lyons *et al.*, in the context of a London medical school, piloted a questionnaire-based process for soliciting feedback from patients about encounters with undergraduate students. Although the feedback was about broader aspects of professional behaviour as well as communication, and was anonymous, they argued that it was practicable and acceptable (Lyons *et al.* 2009). On the other hand, Burford *et al.* explored the use of the Doctors' Interpersonal Skills Questionnaire for feedback to junior doctors in the northeast of England and concluded that, whereas the process was feasible, it must be sensitive to local circumstances, and questions of access, engagement and logistics need to be addressed (Burford *et al.* 2009). In light of the fact that patients seem generally less likely to be critical, rendering any feedback of limited utility, Wass and Archer were more sceptical: '*Current methodologies suggest they are either being asked the wrong questions or are not empowered to answer honestly*' (Wass & Archer 2010, p. 244). However, simulated patients have been shown to be able to give helpful feedback in the context of both teaching and assessment (Cleland *et al.* 2009), and although caution must be applied in interpreting research findings (Lane & Rollnick 2007), there is no reason to think that 'real' patients could not also be trained appropriately. There is obviously a need for more research in this area.

Several authors have argued convincingly for the need to create a learning environment within healthcare in which feedback-seeking behaviour is the norm and is encouraged with opportunities actively sought by learners, practitioners and teachers. As Archer put it: '*If the health professions are serious about effective feedback, an evidence-based cultural shift will also be required*' (Archer 2010, p. 106). This has wide-ranging implications, not least the need for training for both teachers and learners, not only in how to give effective feedback but also how to receive it.

References

Archer, J. (2010) State of the science in health professional education: Effective feedback. *Medical Education*, 44, 101–108.

Black, P. & William, D. (1998) Assessment and classroom teaching. *Assessment in Education*, 5, 7–73.

Brukner, H., Altkorn, D.L., Cook, S., *et al.* (1999) Giving effective feedback to medical students: A workshop for faculty and house staff. *Medical Teacher*, 21, 161–165.

Burford, B., Bedi, A., Morrow, G., Kergon, C., Illing, J., Livingston, M. & Greco, M. (2009) Collecting patient feedback in different clinical settings: Problems and solutions. *Clinical Teacher*, 6, 259–264.

Butler, R. (1987) Task-involving and ego-involving properties of evaluation: Effects on different feedback conditions on motivational perceptions interest and performance. *Journal of Educational Psychology*, 29 (no. 4), 474–483.

Butler, R. (1988) Enhancing and undermining intrinsic motivation; The effects of task-involving and ego-involving evaluation on interest and performance. *British Journal of Educational Psychology*, 58, 1–14.

Chief Medical Officer for England. (2008) *Medical Revalidation – Principles and Next Steps.* Department of Health, London [WWW document]. URL http://www.dh.gov.uk/publications (accessed on 12 February 2014).

Cleland, J.A., Keiko, A. & Rethans, J.-J. (2009) The use of simulated patients in medical education. AMEE Guide No 42. *Medical Teacher*, 31, 477–486.

Ende, J. (1983) Feedback in clinical medical education. *JAMA*, 250 (no. 6), 777–781.

Eva, K. & Regehr, G. (2008) 'I'll never play professional football' and other fallacies of self-assessment. *Journal of Continuing Education in the Health Professions*, 28, 14–19. doi:10.1002/chp.150.

Evans, C. (2013) Making sense of assessment feedback in Higher Education. *Review of Educational Research*, 83, 70–120.

General Medical Council. (2011) *Patient and Public Involvement in Undergraduate Medical Education. Advice Supplementary to Tomorrow's Doctors 2009* [WWW document]. URL http://www.gmc-uk.org/Patient_and_public_web.pdf_40939542.pdf (accessed on 12 February 2014).

Harlen, W. & James, M. (1997) Assessment and learning: Differences and relationships between formative and summative assessment. *Assessment in Education: Principles, Policy and Practice*, 4 (no. 3), 365–379.

Hattie, J. & Jaeger, R. (1998) Assessment and classroom learning: A deductive approach. *Assessment in Education: Principles, Policy and Practice*, 5 (no. 1), 111–122.

Hattie, J. & Timperley, H. (2007) The power of feedback. *Review of Educational Research*, 77, 81–112.

King, J. (1999) Giving feedback. *BMJ*, 318, S2-7200.

Kluger, A.N. & DeNisi, A. (1996) The effects of feedback interventions on performance. *Psychological Bulletin*, 119, 254–284.

Kruger, J. & Dunning, D. (1999) Unskilled and unaware of it: How difficulties in recognizing one's own incompetence lead to inflated self-assessments. *Journal of Personality and Social Psychology*, 77 (no. 6), 1121–1134.

Kurtz, S., Silverman, J. & Draper, J. (2005) *Teaching and Learning Communication Skills in Medicine*, second edn. Radcliffe Publishing, Oxford, UK.

Lane, C. & Rollnick, S. (2007) The use of simulated patients and role-play in communication skills training: A review of the literature to 2005. *Patient Education and Counseling*, 67, 13–20.

Liberman, A.S., Liberman, M., Steinert, Y., McLeod, P. & Meterissian, S. (2005) Surgery residents and attending surgeons have different perceptions of feedback. *Medical Teacher*, 27, 470–477.

Lyons, O., Willcock, H., Rees, J. & Archer, J. (2009) Patient feedback for medical students. *Clinical Teacher*, 6, 254–258.

McKinley, R.K., Fraser, R.C., Hasting, A.M. & van der Vleuten, C. (2000) Formative assessment of the consultation performance of medical students in the setting of general practice using a modified version of the Leicester Assessment Package. *Medical Education*, 34, 573–579.

Neighbour, R. (2005) *The Inner Consultation: How to Develop an Effective and Intuitive Consulting Style*, second edn. Radcliffe Medical Press, Oxford, UK.

National Health Service. (2011) *NHS Choices: Managing Patient Feedback* [WWW document]. URL http://www.nhs.uk/aboutNHSChoices/professionals/healthandcareprofessionals/your-pages/Pages/managingfeedback.aspx (accessed on 12 February 2014).

Pendleton, D., Schofield, T., Tate, P. & Havelock, P. (1984) *The Consultation: An Approach to Learning and Teaching.* Oxford University Press, Oxford, UK.

Pendleton, D., Schofield, T., Tate, P. & Havelock, P. (2003) *The New Consultation: Developing Doctor–Patient Communication.* Oxford University Press, Oxford, UK.

Ramaprasad, A. (1983) On the definition of feedback. *Behavioural Science*, 28, 4–13.

Rowntree, D. (1982) *Educational Technology in Curriculum Development*, second edn. Paul Chapman Publishing, London.

Sadler, D.R. (1998) Formative assessment: Revisiting the territory. *Assessment in Education: Principles, Policy and Practice*, 5 (no. 1), 77–84.

Silverman, J., Kurtz, S. & Draper, J. (2005) *Skills for Communicating with Patients*, second edn. Radcliffe Publishing, Oxford, UK.

Thorndike, E.L. (1918) The nature, purposes, and general methods of measurement of educational products. In: S.A. Courtis (ed), *The Measurement of Educational Products. 17th Yearbook of the National Society for the Study of Education Pt. 2*, pp. 16–24. Public School Publishing, Bloomington, IL.

Veloski, J., *et al.* (2006) Systematic review of the literature on assessment, feedback and physicians' clinical performance. BEME Guide no 7. *Medical Teacher*, 28 (no. 2), 117–128.

Wass, V. & Archer, J. (2010) Assessing learners. In: T. Dornan, K. Mann, A. Scherpbier & J. Spencer, *Medical Education: Theory and Practice*. Churchill Livingstone, Edinburgh.

The Assessment of Communication

CHAPTER 34

Introduction to Assessment in Communication

Jane Kidd

University Hospitals Coventry and Warwickshire NHS Trust, Coventry;
Institute of Medical and Biomedical Education, St George's University of London, London, UK

Historical context

The introduction of effective communication as a topic in both undergraduate and postgraduate health professional curricula resulted in a need to ensure effective assessment of the skills, attitudes and knowledge underpinning the required behaviours. Exploring the assessment of clinical communication calls upon drawing on evidence related to assessment of the broader topic of clinical skills.

As mentioned by John Skelton (chapter 7), Miller (1990) described assessment in the healthcare professions as having four levels:

- *knows* – where a candidate is required to demonstrate that he or she knows basic facts;
- *knows how* – which requires a candidate to apply the knowledge;
- *shows how* – where a candidate demonstrates what he or she is able to do in clinical practice (competence) and
- *does* – where a candidate demonstrates what he or she actually does in clinical practice (performance).

Knowledge about effective communication (the rationale, skills, models) could be assessed using methodologies familiar to examiners, for example, multiple choice questions (Scriven 1991; van Dalen *et al.* 2002), essay papers (Love *et al.* 1993), extended matching questions and short answer questions (Weinman 1984; ASME 2003; Schuwirth & van der Vleuten 2004a). However, many learning outcomes of communication curricula were phrased with the expectation that students 'demonstrated' that they were effective communicators, using appropriate skills to meet the needs of any particular consultation. While written knowledge tests can validate the importance of the subject to learners, they correlate poorly with the ability of the learner to use communication skills in practice (Kurtz *et al.* 2005). Assessment of effective communication required consideration of assessment tools that targeted the 'shows how' and 'does' levels of Miller's skills triangle (Norman 1985; Rethans *et al.* 1991; Boon & Stewart 1998).

To be educationally effective, any assessment tool has to be developed by blue-printing it against curricula learning outcomes to ensure that a whole range of outcomes are assessed during a course of study. At the same time, an assessment tool

Clinical Communication in Medicine, First Edition. Edited by Jo Brown, Lorraine M. Noble,
Alexia Papageorgiou and Jane Kidd.
© 2016 John Wiley & Sons, Ltd. Published 2016 by John Wiley & Sons, Ltd.

needs to have evidence of validity, reliability, acceptability and educational impact, which together with cost can be used to determine the utility of any assessment method (van der Vleuten 1996).

It was recognized that the use of the unobserved 'long case' in which students assessed a patient unobserved and were asked a series of questions about the patient was not sufficiently robust for assessment purposes (Hardy *et al.* 1998) with concerns expressed over its reliability (Swanson *et al.* 1995; Wass *et al.* 2001), the limited sample that was used and that different students saw different patients (Petrusa 2002).

A move was made to assess practical clinical skills with a wider range of tools including the Objective Structured Clinical Examination (OSCE) (Harden & Gleeson 1979) (see chapter 35), the Objective Structured Long Examination Record (OSLER) (Gleeson 1997), and the mini-clinical evaluation exercise (mini-CEX).

OSCEs consist of a series of timed stations, each one focused on a different task. Each station within an OSCE is developed to assess a range of learning outcomes including effective communication. Lay people are trained to play the part of a patient, to provide the same experience for everyone taking the assessment. The examiner or simulated patient uses a checklist of specific behaviours or a global rating form to evaluate the student's performance.

The OSLER was developed with a view to improving the objectivity, validity and reliability of the traditional long case. All candidates are observed by examiners working to a structured marking scheme that includes communication and the history-taking process.

The mini-CEX assesses short specific tasks within a patient encounter, including interviewing skills, humanistic qualities and counselling, during which the candidate is directly observed and rated.

Current practice

Effective communication as an outcome of undergraduate and postgraduate training is described by most regulatory bodies (Sutnick *et al.* 1993; Bataldean *et al.* 2002; Frank & Danoff 2007; General Medical Council 2009). This section will consider current practice in assessment of communication with attention to *why* it is assessed, *what* is assessed, *who* assesses, *when* assessments are made and *how* the assessment is made.

Why assess?

Assessment of competence in clinical communication has the same purpose as other assessments in medical education:

- to enhance the learning of all students by providing motivation and information on the direction for future learning;
- to identify those not yet ready to pass to the next stage of learning and
- to protect the public by identifying those who are not competent.

Assessment can be formative (assessment *for* learning) or summative (assessment *of* learning) (chapter 35). The purpose of any assessment will determine which instrument is selected, how the assessment is implemented, how scores are interpreted, the amount of faculty involvement required and how the results will be used.

Formative assessments are designed to allow learners to develop a sense of how well they are mastering the information and skills they have been taught, where their strengths and weaknesses lie and what elements could be improved (Friedman

Ben-David 2000). Formative assessments require time to provide feedback to the learner, as well as time for reflection by the learner (Schon 1991).

Summative assessments tend to be used to decide whether a learner is ready to progress. It has, however, been recognised that even with summative assessments, it is best practice to give feedback (Schuwirth & van der Vleuten 2004b).

What is assessed?

Effective communication contains three components: attitude, skills and knowledge (Levinson & Roter 1995; Kurtz *et al.* 2005). An assessment needs to reflect the learning that has taken place and to assess the learning outcomes that are *important* to assess as well as those that are *easy* to assess. Blueprinting the assessment against the curriculum learning outcomes helps with these tasks.

While it can be argued that attitudes may determine the extent to which an individual may be an effective communicator, the influence on effective communication behaviours is not well established. Levinson and Roter (1995) reported that the psychosocial beliefs of physicians correlated with their patient communication skills. The Communication Skills Attitude Scale (CSAS) (Rees *et al.* 2002) has been used to track the impact of teaching in the UK and Norway (Langille *et al.* 2001; Rees & Sheard 2003; Anvik *et al.* 2007; Anvik *et al.* 2008) but these studies have not reported on how the attitude to learning communication skills influences the use of the skills.

In respect of knowledge, an assessment placed in the early years of a curriculum might ask a student to list tasks or models of a consultation or skills for gathering information. During the later stages of the curriculum a written assessment might require a list of the skills that are required to be effective when working with a particular model of behaviour change or shared decision making.

Early in a curriculum a practical assessment of communication skills might expect students to demonstrate how they open a consultation, how they gather information, or how they close a consultation; during the intermediate years the practical assessment might include the ability of the student to share information with a patient or carer. Towards the final stage the communication task will be more complex and may include breaking bad news, telephone consultations with a consultant, communication in operating theatres, communication at handover and written communication (Boulet *et al.* 2004). At all stages, however, the assessment has to be designed to address both content (what information is gathered or given) and process (how it is gathered or given) (Kurtz *et al.* 2005).

Another decision in respect of what to assess is to determine to what extent the communication skills element of an assessment is integrated with other skill sets, such as conducting a physical examination or constructing clinical reasoning. With a spiral curriculum, it is possible to start with an assessment that focuses on basic communication skills, which are then revisited later in the curriculum when tasks may be integrated (Kurtz & Heaton 1987; Vu *et al.* 1992; Nestel *et al.* 2003; LeBlanc *et al.* 2009).

Who assesses?

Self and peer assessment may be of considerable value in formative assessment (Jolly *et al.* 1994; Zick *et al.* 2007). Due to the complexity of medical education assessment programmes, including the time commitment required to complete the task, a wide range of people are involved, including clinicians, basic scientists, peers, patients, simulated patients and other healthcare professionals (Cooper & Mira 1998; Boulet *et al.* 2002; Joshi *et al.* 2004; Whelan *et al.* 2005; Kurtz *et al.* 2005).

Joshi *et al.* (2004) reported a significant correlation between the scores of faculty and ancillary staff, with scores from peers correlating negatively with all other categories of evaluators and scores from patients not correlating with any of the other evaluators. Whelan *et al.* (2005) suggest that it is 'best to use the person who is most familiar with the domain being assessed'. This might mean that in an integrated assessment the simulated patient may be best placed to determine the effectiveness of some of the process skills such as building and maintaining a relationship, while a trained examiner can be expected to have the knowledge and skills to perform reliably on domains such as history taking and physical examination.

Examiner performance is enhanced when examiner training on the purpose of the examination is combined with a well-written OSCE mark sheet, a review of the checklist and global rating scales and what is expected of them in that particular examination (Martin *et al.* 1996).

The inclusion of patients in the assessment of effective communication, certainly at postgraduate level, has resulted in the development of psychometrically sound questionnaires to provide patient feedback to their doctors such as the Doctors' Interpersonal Skills Questionnaire (Greco *et al.* 2001, 2002), the American Board of Internal Medicine Patient Assessment for Continuous Professional Development (Lipner *et al.* 2002), the Patient Perception of Patient Centredness questionnaire (Stewart *et al.* 2000), and the Consumer Assessment of Healthcare Providers and Systems Hospital Survey (Weidmer *et al.* 2013; Consumer Assessment of Healthcare Providers and Systems n.d.) The evidence of the use of patient assessment of effective communication in undergraduate medical education is less well established.

When is communication assessed?

Some applicants to medical school are assessed on their cognition about aspects of effective clinical communication such as integrity, perspective taking and team involvement as part of the selection process for medical school in the United Kingdom Clinical Aptitude Test (UKCAT).

During undergraduate programmes students are likely to be assessed formatively whenever they have experiential sessions on effective communication. Makoul (2003) reviewed surveys conducted into communication skills training in the UK and USA and reported that 79% of the responding medical schools indicated that the primary teaching method was student interviews with simulated patients.

The timing of summative assessments of communication depends on the assessment plan for the programme. Medical schools approved by the General Medical Council in the UK include communication in their final assessment to demonstrate that candidates have met the outcomes described in *Tomorrow's Doctors* (General Medical Council 2009). In the USA the United States Medical Licensing Examination Step 2 Clinical Skills, used to license physicians, includes an assessment of communication competences with standardised patients rating communication and interpersonal skills.

To gain a place on the UK Foundation Programme medical school graduates complete a written situational judgement test (SJT) designed to assess professionalism and interpersonal skills. Two of the five sections explore patient focus and effective communication, allowing a candidate to demonstrate that he or she 'knows' how one should respond to a range of issues. The situational judgement test is additional to the educational performance measure (EPM) assessing clinical knowledge/academic ability.

Evidence of the psychometric properties of situational judgement tests and the competencies they are designed to measure is available (Lievens *et al.* 2008; Lievens 2013, 2014). Work is ongoing to establish the extent to which the situational judgement tests predict communication behaviours at a later stage (Edwards *et al.* 2014; Martin *et al.* 2014).

In the UK the Royal Colleges include assessment of effective communication as part of their membership examinations (see e.g. the Royal College of General Practitioners) and in the USA effective communication is included in the Maintenance of Certification assessment of the American Board of Medical Specialities (American Board of Medical Specialities).

How is communication assessed?

As described above there are a range of assessment instruments to test knowledge.

For practical elements there are also a range of assessment tools such as OSCE, OSLER and workplace-based assessments including mini-CEX and 360-degree appraisal (see chapter 36).

Direct observation as required by the structured long case (Norman 2002) or the mini-CEX (Norcini *et al.* 2003) allows an examiner to observe a candidate perform a focused history taking and physical examination over a predetermined number of minutes. The candidate then presents a diagnosis and a treatment plan and the assessor rates the trainee and may provide educational feedback. It can be argued that these structured direct observations focus on selective rather than habitual behaviours and that the process is relatively time consuming; however, feedback can be provided by credible experts (Epstein 2007).

The OSCE is described above and consideration has to be given to the number of stations required for an effective assessment. The number of stations in an OSCE varies between 10 and 20 and the time allocated to each station can vary between 5 and 10 minutes (Marks & Humphrey-Murto 2009).

Epstein (2007) identified that such OSCEs may seem artificial in respect of their timing and setting, that the use of checklists may penalise examinees who use shortcuts, and that they are expensive to run. However, he also identified that they can be tailored to educational goals, are reliable, with consistent case presentation and ratings, can be observed by faculty or standardized patients and are realistic.

In 1993 Reznick and colleagues determined that a minimum of 10 stations is necessary to achieve a reliability of 0.85 to 0.9 (Reznick *et al.* 1993). Further evidence around the number of stations required for a reliable assessment shows that better than average reliability is associated with a greater number of stations and a higher number of examiners per station (Petrusa 2002; Brannick *et al.* 2011). Brannick *et al.* (2011) also reported that interpersonal skills were evaluated less reliably across stations and more reliably within stations compared with clinical skills.

In the design of these assessment tools it is necessary to consider a number of elements. One consideration is the use of checklists or global rating scales (Reznick *et al.* 1998; Fink 2013). A checklist approach allows the assessor to record whether any one discrete skill has been observed. Thus a series of specific behaviours can be listed and the examiner can make a decision about whether the behavior was demonstrated or not. Global ratings allow for an element of judgement on behalf of the assessor. In practice both types of scales are often used in any one assessment. A checklist approach can inform specific and timely feedback to the learner, while the global approach is perceived as providing a more holistic approach to the assessment.

Table 34.1 Example of a behaviourally anchored global rating scale assessing the domain of initiating the consultation.

Satisfactory	Borderline satisfactory	Fail
• Greets the patient using patient's full name • Smiles • Checks what patient likes to be called • Picks up cues re shaking hands • Introduces self – full name • Explains role • Seeks consent • Starts with an open question	• Greets the patient using patient's full name • Introduces self – full name • Explains role • Seeks consent • Starts with an open question	• Greets patient by first name only • Introduces self – first name only • Tells patient what he/she intends to do • Starts with a closed question

Global rating scales may require an assessor to identify which point on a scale a candidate is perceived to be performing at. The scale may be evaluative (excellent, good, borderline, poor) or frequency based (never, sometimes, often) (Likert 1932). The number of points on the scale may vary based on the construct/domain being measured (Spector 1992). With the intention of making it easier to provide an accurate global rating of performance, some scales provide information on the specific examples of behaviour anchored to each point on the scale (Likert 1932; Smith & Kendall 1963). See Table 34.1 for an example. In this way a global rating of 'satisfactory' will have been informed by the candidate performing a series of observable skills.

Global ratings scales are difficult for examiners and learners to interpret and learn from and may be prone to errors of reliability due to cognitive biases in judgement and decision making (Gilovich et al. 2002; Hardman 2009). Tann et al. (1997) provided evidence that a holistic judgement is as reliable as a checklist that incorporated detailed behavioural items. Regehr et al. (1998) determined that for less-experienced observers, checklists provided clearer behavioural definitions that may improve reliability, while experts do as well or better using ratings that use criteria rather than checklists. This suggests that a checklist may be the preferred tool when faculty are learning to assess communication skills and that global ratings might be used when the medical communication expertise of the faculty is well developed. Hodges et al. (1999) determined that checklists did not differentiate as well as global scales between learners with increasing expertise.

Ensuring that all examiners are provided with extensive training on the use of the rating scales can minimise cognitive biases in judgements and decision making (Kogan et al. 2009). This level of training may also reduce the number of examiners required to produce a reliable score. Ziv et al. (1998) demonstrated that when simulated patients are provided with extensive training in the use of a global rating scale, and all examinees are observed under the same conditions, then 10 simulated patient raters are sufficient for a reliable score. Conversely, when assessments are taking place in real-life situations and examinees are exposed to examiners under different clinical environments, a higher number of raters is required to produce a reliable score.

Another way of conceptualising, investigating and designing reliable observations is to use generalizability theory (Cronbach et al. 1963; Brennan 1983). This statistical method looks at sources of variation that are potential sources of error (such as raters, forms, time, setting) to quantify the amount of error caused by each element and interactions of elements. These results can then be used in a decision study to examine how the generalisability coefficients would change under different consequences (number of raters, number of stations) and consequently determine the ideal conditions under which the measurements would be the most reliable.

Another consideration is the method used to set the standard for passing any assessment. A standard is the score on an assessment that will set the boundary between qualitatively different performance (e.g. pass/fail).

Livingston and Zieky (1982) describe four main categories of standard setting: *relative methods* where a standard is based on the performance of a group of examinees, *absolute methods* based on judgements about test questions (test-centred), *absolute methods* based on judgements about individual examinees (examinee-centred) and *compromise methods*. Berk (1986) and Cusimano (1996) provide reviews and detailed descriptions of these methods, with Cusimano concluding that there was no consensus regarding which method should be used for standard setting. In 2009, Marks and Humphrey-Murto advocated that standard setting should be criterion referenced to ensure candidates have a minimum acceptable level of competency and suggested that if clinician examiners are used then the modified borderline group method (Dauphinee *et al.* 1997a, 1997b) may be used to set a pass mark.

Whatever method of standard setting is used it is important that it produces results that are informed by expert judgement, that due diligence in its application can be shown, that it is supported by a body of research, and that it is easy to explain and implement, making it fit for purpose.

Future considerations

The information presented briefly here allows identification of a range of areas for future consideration.

How do attitudes to effective communication influence the behaviours demonstrated by students and practising physicians? To what extent will the international trend to focus on values influence those who enter the medical profession and the skills they develop?

With integrated assessments, what impact would there be on whether or not a candidate passes an individual OSCE station or a whole assessment if domains within an OSCE or within the communication field are weighted differently?

What is the potential impact of giving more weight to a patient perspective on the effective communication of a candidate and what would be the argument put forward for doing so? Patient questionnaires are currently in use in the postgraduate arena; can they be adapted for use in the undergraduate curricula?

What does the most recent evidence tell us about whether the behaviours we are currently measuring impact on patient outcomes beyond satisfaction with the consultation and concordance with medication?

Can we enhance our knowledge of the influence of gender, ethnicity and age on effective communication by exploring the impact of these demographic variables on the two individuals present in a consultation – the doctor and the patient?

As we think ahead, could we consider what might be available to us through the medium of virtual patients (web-based representations of clinical cases)? While virtual patient cases are already used to assess knowledge, can we develop a performance-based assessment that allows the virtual patient to respond in an interactive manner with a candidate and provide immediate feedback?

Currently the Medical Schools Council Assessment Alliance is developing written assessment items that each medical school in the UK can use to assess their students and then compare performance on comparable items (Medical Schools Council). Can an argument be made for the development of a number of communication skills assessments to be developed and used in the same way? On a small scale this would mirror a part of the United States Medical Licensing Examination (USMLE) and the assessment that has to be taken by all foreign graduates in order to practise in the USA.

Are there ways in which we can predict individuals who will struggle with this topic? If so what can we do to help them succeed? Are there any attributes that identify those who struggle, and would early identification allow such an individual access to appropriate support, learning and careers advice? Two papers on emotional intelligence and its ability to predict future academic performance provide contrasting results. Humphrey-Murto *et al.* (2014) using the Mayer-Salovey-Caruso Emotional Intelligence test, reported that emotional intelligence does not appear to reliably predict future academic performance, while Libbrecht *et al.* (2013), using the Situational Test of Emotional Understanding and the Situational Test of Emotional Management (MacCann & Roberts, 2008), reported that one of the dimensions of emotional intelligence, the ability to regulate emotions, predicted performance in courses on communication and interpersonal sensitivity over 3 years of medical school.

Finally, is there value in addressing effective communication as a core clinical skill in the revalidation process that is being rolled out across the UK for qualified doctors, looking for evidence of regular continual professional development in this field?

References

American Board of Medical Specialties. (n.d.) *Board Certification and Maintenance of Certification* [WWW document]. URL http://www.abms.org/board-certification/.

Anvik, T., Gude T., Grimstad, H., Baerheim, A., Fegner O.B., Hjortdahl, P., Holen, A., Risberg, T. & Vaglum, P. (2007) Assessing medical students' attitudes towards learning communication skills: Which components of attitude do we measure? *BMC Medical Education*, 7, 4.

Anvik, T., Grimstad, H., Baerheim, A., Bernt Fasmer, O., Gude, T., Hjortdahl, P., Holen, A., Risberg, T. & Vagulm, P. (2008) Medical students' cognitive and affective attitudes towards learning and using communication skills – a nationwide cross country study. *Medical Teacher*, 30 (no. 3), 272–279.

Association for the Study of Medical Education (ASME). (2003) *Tossing Salads Too: A Users' Guide to Medical Student Assessment*. ASME, Edinburgh.

Bataldean, P., Leach, D., Swiing, S., Dreyfus, H. & Dreyfus, S. (2002) General competencies and accreditation of graduate medical education. *Health Affairs*, 21 (no. 5), 103–111.

Berk, R.A. (1986) A consumer's guide to setting performance standards on criterion-reference tests. *Review of Educational Research*, 56, 137–172.

Boon, H. & Stewart, M. (1998) Patient–physician communication assessment instruments: 1986–1996 in review. *Patient Education and Counseling*, 35, 161–175.

Boulet, J.R., McKinley, D.W., Norcini, J.J. & Whelan, G.P. (2002) Assessing the comparability of standardized patient and physician evaluations of clinical skills. *Advances in Health Science Education*, 7, 85–97.

Boulet, J.R., Rebbechi, T.A., Denton, E.C., McKinley, D.W. & Whelan, G.P. (2004) Assessing the written communication skills of medical school graduates. *Advances in Health Science Education*, 9 (no. 1), 47–60.

Brannick, M.T., Erol-Korkmaz, H.T. & Prewett, M. (2011) A systematic review of the reliability of objective structured clinical examination scores. *Medical Education*, 45, 1181–1189.

Brennan, R.L. (1983) *Elements of Generalisability Theory*. American College Testing Program, Iowa City, IA.

Consumer Assessment of Healthcare Providers and Systems. (n.d.) *Surveys and Tools to Advance patient-Centred are* [WWW document]. URL www.cahps.ahrq.gov.

Cooper, C. & Mira, M. (1998) Who should assess medical students' communication skills: Their academic teachers or their patients? *Medical Education*, 32 (no. 4), 419–421.

Cronbach, L.J., Nageswari, R. & Gleser, G.C. (1963) Theory of generalizability: A liberation of reliability theory. *British Journal of Statistical Psychology*, 16, 137–163.

Cusimano, M.D. (1996) Standard setting in medical education. *Academic Medicine*, 71 (no. 10), S112–120.

Dauphinee, W.D., Blackmore, D.E., Smee, S.M., *et al.* (1997a) Optimizing the input of physician examiners in setting standards for a large scale OSCE. In: A.J.J.A. Scherpbier, C.P.M. van der Vleuten, J.J. Rethans, A.F.W. van der Steeg (eds). *Advances in Medical Education: Proceedings of the Seventh Ottawa International Conference in Medical Education and Assessment*, pp. 656–658. Springer, New York.

Dauphinee, W.D., Blackmore, D.E., Smee, S.M., *et al.* (1997b) Using the judgement of physician examiners in setting standards for a national multi-centre high stakes OSCE. *Advances in Health Sciences Education*, 2, 201–211.

Edwards, H., Patterson, F., Fitzpatrick, S. & Walker, K. (2014) Validation of the FY1 selection tools. Presented at INReSH, London, November 2014.

Epstein, R.M. (2007) Assessment in medical education. *New England Journal of Medicine*, 356, 387–396.

Fink, A. (2013) *How to Conduct Surveys: A Step by Step Guide*, fifth edn. Sage Publications, Thousand Oaks, CA.

Frank, J.R. & Danoff, D. (2007) The CanMEDS initiative: Implementing an outcome-based framework of physician competencies. *Medical Teacher*, 29 (no. 7), 642–647.

Friedman Ben-David, M. (2000) The role of assessment in expanding professional horizons. *Medical Teacher*, 22, 472–477.

General Medical Council. (2009) *Tomorrow's Doctors: Outcomes and Standards for Undergraduate Medical Education*. General Medical Council, London.

Gilovich, T., Griffin, D. & Kahneman, D. (2002) *Heuristics and Biases: The Psychology of Intuitive Judgment*. Cambridge University Press, Cambridge, UK.

Gleeson, F. (1997) AMEE Medical Education Guide No.9: Assessent of Clinical Competence Using the Objective Structured Long Examination Record (OSLER). *Medical Teacher*, 19, (no. 1), 7–14.

Greco, M., Brownlea, A. & McGovern, J. (2001) Impact of patient feedback on the interpersonal skills of general practice registrars: Results of a longitudinal study. *Medical Education*, 35, 748–756.

Greco, M., Spike, N., Powell, R. & Brownlea, A. (2002) Assessing communication skills of GP registrars: A comparison of patient and GP examiner ratings. *Medical Education*, 36, 366–376.

Harden, R.M. & Gleeson, F.A. (1979) Assessment of clinical competence using an objective structured clinical examination (OSCE). *Medical Education*, 13, 41–54.

Hardman, D. (2009) *Judgment and Decision Making: Psychological Perspectives*. Wiley-Blackwell, Hoboken, NJ.

Hardy, K.J., Demos, L.L. & McNeil, J.J. (1998) Undergraduate surgical examinations: An appraisal of the clinical orals. *Medical Education*, 32, 582–589.

Hodges, B., Regehr, G., McNaughton, N., Tiberius, R. & Hanson, M. (1999) OSCE checklists do not capture increasing levels of expertise. *Academic Medicine*, 74, 1129–1134.

Humphrey-Murto,, S., Leddy, J.J., Wood, T.J., Puddester, D. & Moineau, G. (2014) Does emotional intelligence at medical school admission predict future academic performance? *Academic Medicine*, 89 (no. 4), 638–643.

Jolly, B., Cushing, A. & Dacre, J. (1994) Reliability and validity of a patient-based workbook for assessment of clinical and communication skills. *Proceedings of the Sixth Ottawa Conference of Medical Education*, University of Toronto. Bookstore Custom Publishing, Toronto.

Joshi, R., Ling, F.W. & Jaeger, J. (2004) Assessment of a 360-degree instrument to evaluate residents' competency in interpersonal communication skills. *Academic Medicine*, 79 (no. 5), 458–463.

Kogan, J.R., Holmboe, E.S. & Hauer, K.E. (2009) Tools for direct observation and assessment of clinical skills in medical trainees: A systematic review. *JAMA*, 302 (no. 12), 1316–1326.

Kurtz, S.M. & Heaton, C.J. (1987) Co-ordinated clinical skills evaluation in the preclinical years: Helical progression makes sense. In: I.R. Hart & R.M. Hardin (eds), *Further Developments in Assessing Clinical Competence*. Heal Publications, Montreal.

Kurtz, S., Silverman, J. & Draper, J. (2005) *Teaching and Learning Communication Skills in Medicine*. Radcliffe Publishing, Oxon, UK.

Langille, D.B., Kaufman, D.M., Laidlaw, T.A., Sargeant, J. & Macleod, H. (2001) Faculty attitudes towards medical communication and their perceptions of students' communication skills training at Dalhousie University. *Medical Education*, 35 (no. 6), 548–554.

LeBlanc, V.R., Tabak, D., Kneebone, R., Nestel, D., NacRae, H. & Houlton, C. (2009) Psychometric properties of an integrated assessment of technical and communication skills. *American Journal of Surgery*, 197 (no. 1), 96–101.

Levinson, W. & Roter, D. (1995) Physicians psychosocial beliefs correlate with their patient communication skills. *Journal of General Internal Medicine*, 10, 375–379.

Libbrecht, N., Lievens, F., Carette, B. & Cote, S. (2013) Emotional intelligences predicts success in medical school. *Emotion*, 14 (no. 1), 64–73. doi:10.1037/a0034392.

Lievens, F. (2013) Adjusting medical school admissions: Assessing interpersonal skills using situational judgement tests. *Medical Education*, 47, 182–189.

Lievens, F. (2014) Long term use of situational judgement tests in medical school admission: Validity and coaching effects. Presented at INReSH, London, November 2014.

Lievens, F., Peeters, H. & Schollaert, E. (2008) Situational judgement tests: A review of recent research. *Personnel Review*, 37 (no. 4), 426–441.

Likert, R.A. (1932) A technique for the measurement of attitudes. *Archives of Psychology*, 140, 1–55.

Lipner, R.S., Blank, L.L., Leas, B.F. & Fortuna, G.S. (2002) The value of patient and peer ratings in re-certifications. *Academic Medicine*, 77 (10 Suppl.), S64–S66.

Livingston, S.A. & Zieky, M.J. (1982) *Passing Scores: A Manual for Setting Standards of Performance on Educational and Occupational Tests*. Educational Testing Service, Princeton, NJ.

Love, R., Newcombe, P., Schiller, J., Wilding, G. & Stone, H. (1993) A comparison of knowledge and communication skill evaluations by written essay and oral examinations in preclinical medical students. *Journal of Cancer Education*, 8, 123–128.

Makoul, G. (2003) Communication skills education in medical school and beyond. *JAMA*, 289 (no. 1), 93–94.

Marks, M. & Humphrey-Murto, S. (2009) Performance assessment. In: J.A. Dent & R.M. Harden (eds), *A Practical Guide for Medical Teachers*, third edn, pp. 333–340. Elsevier, Amsterdam.

Martin, J.A., Reznick, R.K., Rothman, A., *et al.* (1996) Who should rate candidates in an objective structured clinical examination? *Academic Medicine*, 71 (no. 2), 170–174.

Martin, S., Kerrin, M., Patterson, F. & Greatrix, R. (2014) Supporting the widening participation agenda in medical and dental admission selection in the UK: Early evidence from the SJT. Presented at INReSH, London, November 2014.

McCann, C. & Roberts, R.D. (2008) New paradigms for assessing emotional intelligences: Theory and data. *Emotion*, 8, 540–551.

Medical Schools Council. (n.d.) *Medical Schools Council Assessment Alliance* [WWW document]. URL http://www.medschools.ac.uk/MSCAA/Pages/default.aspx.

Miller, G.E. (1990) The assessment of clinical skills/competence/performance. *Academic Medicine*, 65 (no. 7), S63–67.

Nestel, D., Kidd, J. & Kneebone, R (2003) Communicating during procedures: Development of a rating scale. *Medical Education*, 37, 480–481.

Norcini, J.J. (2003) Setting standards on educational tests. *Medical Education*, 37, 464–469.

Norcini, J.J., Blank, L.L., Duffy, F.D. & Fortna, G.S. (2003) The mini-CEX: A method for assessing clinical skills. *Annals of Internal Medicine*, 138, 476–481.

Norman, G. (1985) Objective measurement of clinical performance. *Medical Education*, 19, 43–47.

Norman, G. (2002) The long case versus objective structured clinical examinations. *BMJ*, 324, 748–749.

Petrusa, E.R. (2002) Clinical performance assessments In: G.R. Norman, C.P.M. van der Vleuten & D.I. Newble (eds), *International Handbook of Research in Medical Education*, pp. 673–709. Kluwer, Dordrecht, the Netherlands.

Rees, C. & Sheard, C. (2003) Evaluating first year medical students' attitudes to learning communication skills before and after a communication skills course. *Medical Teacher*, 25 (no. 3), 302–307.

Rees, C., Sheard, C. & Davies, S. (2002) The development of a scale to measure medical students' attitudes towards communication skills learning: The Communication Skills Attitude Scale (CSAS). *Medical Education*, 36 (no. 2), 141–147.

Regehr, G., MacRae, H., Reznick, R.K. & Szalay, D. (1998) Comparing the psychometric properties of checklists and global rating scales for assessing performance on an OSCE-format examination. *Academic Medicine*, 73 (no. 9), 993–997.

Rethans, J.J., Sturman, F., Drop, R., van der Vleuten, C. & Hobus, P. (1991) Does competence of general practitioners predict their performance? Comparison between examination setting and actual practice. *BMJ*, 303, 1377–1380.

Reznick, R.K., Blackmore, D., Cohen, R., *et al.* (1993) An objective structured clinical examination for the licentiate of the Medical Council of Canada: From research to reality. *Academic Medicine*, 68 (Suppl.), S4–S6.

Reznick, R.K., Regehr, G., Yee, G., Rothman, A., Blackmore, D. & Dauphinee, D. (1998) High-stakes examinations: What do we know about measurement?: Process-rating forms versus task-specific checklists in an OSCE for medical licensure. *Academic Medicine*, 73 (no. 10), S97–99.

Royal College of General Practitioners. (n.d.) *MRCGP Examinations* [WWW document]. URL http://www.rcgp.org.uk/training-exams/mrcgp-exams-overview.aspx.

Schuwirth, L.W. & van der Vleuten, C.P. (2004a) Different written assessment methods: What can be said about their strengths and weaknesses? *Medical Education*, 38, 974–979.

Schuwirth, L.W. & van der Vleuten, C.P. (2004b) Merging views on assessment. *Medical Education*, 38, 1208–1210.

Schon, D.A. (1991) *The Reflective Practitioner: How Professionals Think in Action*. Basic Books, New York.

Scriven, M. (1991) *Evaluation Thesaurus*, fourth edn. Sage Publications, Newbury Park, CA.

Smith, P.C. & Kendall, L.M. (1963) Retranslation of expectations: An approach to the construction of unambiguous anchors to rating scales. *Journal of Applied Psychology*, 47, 149–155.

Spector, P. (1992) *Summated Rating Scale Construction*. Sage Publications, Newbury Park, CA.

Stewart, M., Brown, J.B., Donner, A., McWhinney, I.R., Oates, J., Weston, W.W. & Jordan, J. (2000) The impact of patient-centred care on outcomes. *Journal of Family Practice*, 49 (no. 9), 796–804.

Sutnick, A.I., Stillman, P.L., Norcini, J.J., Friedman, M., Regan, M.D., Willliams, R.G., Kachur, E.K., Haggerty, M.A. & Wilson, M.P. (1993) ECFMG assessment of clinical competence of graduates of foreign medical schools. *JAMA*, 27 (no. 9), 1041–1045.

Swanson, D.B., Norman, G.R. & Linn, R.L. (1995) Performance-based assessment: Lessons learnt from the health professions. *Educational Research*, 25 (no. 5), 5–11.

Tann, M., Amiel, G.E., Bitterman, A., Ber, R., & Cohen, R. (1997) Analysis of the use of global ratings by standardized patients and physicians. In: A.J.J.A. Scherpbier, C.P.M. van der Vleuten, J.J. Rethans, A.F.W. van der Steeg (eds). *Advances in Medical Education: Proceedings of the Seventh Ottawa International Conference in Medical Education and Assessment*. Springer, New York.

van Dalen, J., Kerkhofs, E., Vrwijnen, G.M., van Knippenberg-van den Berg, B.W., van den Hout, H.A., Scherpbier, A.J. & van der Vleuten, C.P. (2002) Predicting communications skills with a paper-and-pencil test. *Medical Education*, 36, 148–153.

van der Vleuten, C.P.M. (1996) The assessment of professional competence: Developments, research and practical implications. *Advances in Health Sciences Education*, 1, 41–67.

van der Vleuten, C.P.M. & Swanson, D.B. (1990) Assessment of clinical skills with standardised patients: State of the art. *Teaching and Learning in Medicine*, 22, 58–76.

Vu, N.V., Barrows, H., Marcy, M., Verhulst, S.J., Colliver, J.A. & Travis, T. (1992) Six years of comprehensive clinical performance-based assessment using standardized patients at the Southern Illinois University School of Medicine. *Academic Medicine*, 67, 42–50.

Wass, V., Jones, R. & van der Vleuten, C. (2001) Standardized or real patients to test clinical competence? The long case revisited. *Medical Education*, 35, 321–325,

Weidmer, B., Brah, C., Slaughter, M.E. & Hays, R.D. (2012) Development of items to assess patients' health literacy experiences at hospitals for the Consumer Assessment of Healthcare Providers and Systems (CAHPS) Hospital Survey. *Medical Care*, 50, S12–S21.

Weinman, J. (1984) A modified essay question evaluation of pre-clinical teaching of communication skills. *Medical Education*, 18, 164–167.

Whelan, G.P., Boulet, J.R., McKinley, D.W., Norcini, J.J., van Zanten, M., Hambleton, R.K., Burdick, W.P. & Peilzman, S.J. (2005) Scoring standardized patient examinations: Lessons learned from the development and administration of the ECFMG Clinical Skills Assessment. *Medical Teacher*, 27 (no. 3), 200–206.

Zick, A., Granieri, M. & Makoul, G. (2007) First-year medical students' assessment of their own communication skills: A video-based, open-ended approach. *Patient Education and Counseling*, 68 (no. 2), 161–166.

Ziv, A., Curtis, M. Burdick, W.P., *et al.* (1998) An holistic and behaviourally anchored measure of interpersonal skills; Issues of rater consistency. Proceedings of the Eighth International Ottawa Conference on Medical Education and Assessment.

CHAPTER 35

Assessing Performance

Connie Wiskin[1] and Janet Lefroy[2]

[1]*University of Birmingham, Birmingham, UK*
[2]*Keele University, Staffordshire, UK*

Assessment can be 'of learning' (summative) and 'for learning' (formative). Summative assessment of clinical communication – that is, deciding whether the learner is competent enough in consulting and other clinical communication contexts to progress – comprises an increasing proportion of a UK medical student's progression marks as he or she moves from first to final year and beyond. In qualifying, required competencies defined by the General Medical Council (2009) must be met. Each UK medical school, however, currently devises its own system of communication assessment, so emphasis and methodologies vary.

Formative assessment is a teaching method. There is, however, some truth in the claim that summative assessment also drives learning, although the drivers are complex (Muijtjens *et al.* 1998; MacLachlan 2006; Joughin 2010). Accepting that students will associate teaching with testing, it is prudent to refer to the same standards of competence and use similar assessment instruments in both formative and summative scenarios. To the learner summative (permitting/preventing progression) and formative (guiding/facilitating learning) contexts may well feel different, but there is methodological synchronicity. An obvious example is using a 'real-time' consultation with a simulated patient in both classroom teaching and progression assessments.

Students need to develop the confidence and ability to respond flexibly to both expected *and* unexpected workplace scenarios. This cautions against rote learning and 'teaching to the test' for managing complex interpersonal situations. However, synergy of methods and message in learning and assessment helps maturing students to benchmark their progress against required standards. There is the additional and somewhat under-used opportunity to turn summative assessment into a learning opportunity by routinely offering post-examination feedback.

In this chapter we will therefore consider communication assessment in summative, formative and combined circumstances. The future direction of assessment may be to reduce the differences between summative and formative.

It is not possible in a brief chapter to discuss all communication assessment methods. The UK Council for Clinical Communication in Undergraduate Medical Education's survey of UK medical schools, however, offers a comprehensive summary of currently employed systems of summative assessment, including methods and frequency (Laidlaw *et al.* 2014). In summative testing the Objective Structured Clinical Examination (OSCE) was the most frequently reported assessment – a pattern replicated in much Western literature, and beyond. We therefore focus primarily on the OSCE to acknowledge that it is

Clinical Communication in Medicine, First Edition. Edited by Jo Brown, Lorraine M. Noble,
Alexia Papageorgiou and Jane Kidd.
© 2016 John Wiley & Sons, Ltd. Published 2016 by John Wiley & Sons, Ltd.

by reputation the most prevalent and contextually valid summative approach for consulting performance. Points are included additionally at the end of each section relating to the formative position, in acknowledgement that summative and formative methods have a role to play in benchmarking performance.

The aim of this chapter is to encourage discussion, action and further engagement with the evidence base. The operational detail of how communication is assessed varies between institutions (Laidlaw *et al.* 2014) but should be underpinned by a set of fundamental principles. These are that clinical communication performance is assessed by 'actually doing' rather than by written statement of 'intention to do'; that observation of communication should be in a valid context; that differentiation between what is and is not an acceptable standard needs transparent criteria and that assessors should be trained in the criteria and qualified to make a judgement.

Historical context

Historically medical summative assessments were neither particularly 'objective' nor 'structured'. The OSCE's predecessor, the 'Clinical Examination' was, according to oral reports from the 1940s through to the 1960s, random. Short and long cases for clinical skills assessment depended on which hospitalised patients were available, *and well enough*, for inclusion, introducing an element of 'chance'. The system was informally reported as open to abuse, being too easily influenced by personal relationships. Individual clinical examiners wielded far more personal autonomy than today, as standardised marking schedules were rarely used.

The OSCE directly challenged such inconsistencies. Attributed to Harden as a result of his work in the mid-1970s (Harden *et al.* 1975), the OSCE is an interactive assessment in which the candidates move around a series of stations (booths) and at each one, under observation, perform a verbal or skill-based task. Harden recommended rotations of up to but not more than 20 students. The aim, he said, was that 'bias is removed as far as possible' given the three variables of patient, candidate and examiner. 'It is an approach' rather than 'a rigid prescription for examining'. The format of candidates rotating between tasks not only addressed the question of valid context but importantly offered standardization. This was not just as an operational function but to embed the concept of *fairness* (via objectivity, and similarity of opportunity to do well) to learners.

The OSCE developed thereafter a substantial history, easily confirmed by a rich and readily available literature. Much of this evidence concurs with the first principle above – that although many aspects of medical knowledge historically were (and remain) tested by written examination or multiple choice questions, validity concerns and cultural change over time have demanded more innovative tactics in relation to attributes that could not be meaningfully measured by written word or machine marked tests. In communication terms, a student's ability to, say, offer a comprehensible, sensitive and acceptable explanation simply does not correlate with his or her ability to select the 'correct' answer from a menu of options. The OSCE has made significant inroads into addressing this dis-harmony and has influenced the overall development of a more interactive approach to both the teaching and testing of communication. This trend was not peculiar to assessment. A tangible move towards patient-centred consulting has occurred in parallel since the 1960s (popularly attributed to Balint [1968]). In line, teaching methods evolved from the didactic to the experiential.

Across the Atlantic another champion of interactivity, Barrows, was developing a system of lay inclusion in medical education that would have far-reaching impact on the way OSCEs were developed and perceived (Barrows & Abrahamson 1964). Barrows and Abrahamson advocated the inclusion of 'patient representatives' in teaching and assessment, not only validating lay/actor inclusion methodologically but generating a comprehensive list of previously unrecognised opportunities for healthy individuals to authentically simulate clinical conditions. The first 'Standard Patient Program' in the USA was in the late 1960s, based on earlier 'Programmed Patient' work (Barrows & Abrahamson 1964). The term 'Standardized Patient' reflected the goal that all candidates attending an assessment would receive a consistent experience and hence be evaluated consistently. The abbreviation 'SP' – representing Standardized and/or Simulated Patient – has an extensive international literature of scholarly output and evaluation, which is easily accessed. The aspirations of early pioneers (Colliver, Vu, Tamblyn, Stillman, Bouhuijs, van der Vleuten, Cohen, Hodge, Turnbull, Newble and Swanson, among others) established the fundamental principles that underpin contemporary OSCE work. Modern interpretations have followed, but the bedrock of simulated patient use in the summative OSCE is this: candidates facing the same test must experience a psychometrically consistent assessment, with equal opportunity to perform well, facing staff trained to assess objectively, and simulated patients trained to respond authentically and flexibly in the moment, in line with educational objectives/expectations for that stage of candidate training.

The history of formative assessment of clinical communication assessment with constructive feedback in the classroom and in workplace-based assessment is covered in other chapters, but it is worth pointing out the related discovery that repetitive testing in itself (without feedback) helps learning. There is evidence that assessment (a) enhances effort and efficacy of studying, and (b) enhances retrieval of learning, especially by repetition (Larsen & Dornan 2013). This effect has been found to be independent of feedback.

Formative self-assessment of clinical communication has some history and typically uses video playback. This has been undertaken effectively, and self-awareness is known to be enhanced by immediate tutor feedback for comparison with self-assessment (Aspegren 1999; Zick *et al.* 2007). Self-assessment is a cornerstone of ongoing personal professional development (Nicol & Macfarlane 2006; Sargeant *et al.* 2010). It does tend to be unreliable but can be trained up by enhancing self-awareness (Eva & Regehr 2005).

Current practice

Contemporary impetus for innovation in assessment in the UK came in the General Medical Council's 1993 recommendation (General Medical Council 2003) to teach undergraduate communication skills and employ/extend small group teaching opportunities nationally. Medical schools around Britain were therefore encouraged to develop curricula and by extension to validate new assessment tools.

In summative testing, the OSCE remains dominant. Acceptability and level of application can be taken at this stage of the OSCE's history as a given. Below, therefore, we reflect on topical aspects of the OSCE in relation to clinical communication. These include issues of scoring responsibility, global (versus checklist) scoring, station numbers/duration ('testing time') and the trend for integration.

Scoring responsibility

When considering *who* should score, of ongoing interest is the representation of the 'patient's voice' as a measure of the quality of doctor–patient interactions in high-stakes assessments. Although the 'voice of biomedicine' and the 'voice of the life-world (personal truth)' (Michler 1983) are different, doctors are generally considered expert enough to take responsibility for assessing how well learners communicate, as evidenced by the responsibility given to them in the majority of assessments where communication is an item judged (Boulet *et al.* 1998). Doctors who are doing a task themselves day in day out should have 'expertise' at it, but this cannot be taken for granted, especially when many of today's assessors were not themselves taught patient-centred consulting. Furthermore, observing a consultation and speculating how the patient might feel is not the same as reacting firsthand to a doctor's professional style.

If learners are to be assessed on *overall* consulting ability it is arguable that observation by a clinician alone lacks an important dimension. The patient perspective can, and should, be meaningfully included in the assessment of interpersonal and other professional skills if we are to claim validity for assessments that reflect the remit of the qualified health professional (Wilkinson & Fontaine 2002).

In current practice the previously missed opportunity to include patient voices in student learning and assessment has been recognised. 'Doctors are experts, but so are patients', and individuals with illnesses are seen to have the potential to work effectively in educational partnership with clinicians (Wilson 1999). A more common inclusion – usually in the interests of consistency and comfort – is the simulated patient. The challenge 'but it's not the real thing' merits scant attention. It is precisely because it is simulated (therefore not actual) that it is educationally useful. Simulated patients offer case and character standardization, a concept key to 'fairness' in testing. The simulated patient can enable blueprinting of the clinical case and task to be assessed, can provide a more reliable assessment for a candidate cohort, and can be trained to assess and to give feedback. The latter leads us to simulated patient potential as scorers.

In assessment the institutional nervousness around inclusion of 'nonclinicians' in high stakes scoring that existed 20 years ago appears to have diminished at least in some organisations (Boulet *et al.* 1998). Commonality of understanding of domains is important and must relate to what can be reasonably expected of the learner at that stage of training (which is where assessor training comes in). However, it is also, arguably, acceptable to have different assessors looking for different things – a patient representative, for example, would be well placed to comment on 'building and maintaining the relationship', but any nonclinical assessor (patient or staff) would have difficulty making judgments about, for example, clinical reasoning. Work done to date shows psychometric consistency for simulated patient scorers in relevant domains, including high-stakes postgraduate examples (Boulet *et al.* 1998; Wiskin *et al.* 2013b).

Global scoring

OSCE global scoring aims for a more creative and relevant assessment (Hodges & McIlroy 2003). There is not room here for discussion, but the relationship between knowledge, communication and the uniqueness and fluidity of every interaction means that contemporary simulated patient stations usually resist the 'checklist' approach to scoring.

Global scoring avoids reducing communication to a list of 'skills' for assessment purposes. Skelton reminds us that 'To teach skills and only skills is too often to teach the banal, and always to teach restrictively – and it misunderstands the educational tradition', and few 'other skills in life are taught and tested as lists' (Skelton 2005). A skater, for example, might tell us that solely learning and repeating technical moves is not what makes an 'exceptional performance'. Interpretation, passion, quality of delivery, commitment, emotion and a range of other attributes contribute to the impact on others.

Measuring the impact of a student's style, including professional values, is not easy but is fundamental. This is a current prerogative, as evidenced by the 'Francis Report' (Francis 2013), urging 'a common culture of caring, commitment and compassion'. Communication by nature needs personal judgement, whoever is scoring. Associated risks are moderated by training all scorers to develop a shared understanding of the level of achievement sought and an appreciation that while there are many 'right' ways to communicate the one that matters is whether that style was 'right' for that patient.

Best practice is to approach communication scoring, global or otherwise, in the same way as other clinical competencies. Poor communication is dangerous. A candidate with an unsafe clinical technique would not be 'allowed to pass' because of perception that he or she was nervous that day ('and would probably be better unobserved'), nor would he or she be deprived of remediation because the assessor shied away from raising an 'awkward' issue ('I'll let that technique go, it's likely to be "cultural"').

Testing time
Work has been done on optimal station duration and number, with mixed outcomes (Wass *et al.* 2001). A common sense consensus is that the station length should reflect, as far as is possible, the consulting task at hand. To have an acceptable reliability (>0.7), total OSCE testing time has been calculated at between 2 and 12 hours depending on the breadth of competencies to be tested (Turner & Dankoski 2008). If longer (more integrated) consulting tasks are desirable, the minimum total testing time will lengthen, as task variation is an important component of OSCE validity.

Integration (in teaching and testing)
The argument for integrated testing (looking at the *whole* consultation, including aspects of professionalism and clinical/technical skill) in a clinical context is obvious (Epstein & Hundert 2002; van der Vleuten & Schuwirth 2005). Testing 'communication' on its own is a futile exercise, as all communication has a context. In an OSCE, communication is assessed during a defined task such as taking a focused history, explaining a test result appropriately, taking the patient's blood pressure, gaining consent and so on… Schools in the UK and internationally are finding creative ways of developing integrated assessments, where the student's ability to communicate effectively with the patient is scrutinised as *part of,* rather than separate from, the clinical task (Wiskin *et al.* 2013a). The proportion of the marks awarded for communication can vary according to the determined by the core outcome for the station.

Thinking of formative assessment, all UK medical schools currently use practice with feedback as a primary method of embedding clinical communication. Peer assessment helps students to learn from and reflect on interactions, both by observing impactful strategies and positive role models and by critiquing efforts by peers that proved less effective. Tutors will recognise this effect by comparing the first role play of a communication class to later attempts, where lessons have been learned and incorporated. However, sustainability outside the classroom (in this and other assessment contexts) merits more research attention.

Most schools explain assessment criteria for clinical communication to students in teaching. In doing so, they align their instruction with their summative assessment and avoid mythologies developing around how to 'pass' assessments. As an example, students approaching an integrated OSCE should understand that neither 'unsafe information communicated well' nor 'good information badly given' is acceptable.

Future directions

The relationship between the OSCE assessment of communication and professionalism is likely to strengthen going forward. Communication is so fundamental to the student's developing of an appropriate professional identity that it needs more explicit reference in assessment schedules. 'Professionalism', including demonstration of good values and attitudes, is already assessed in some OSCEs, often as part of the 'communication' requirement. The relationship between communication and professionalism is complex, needing further research and development to both facilitate students' understanding of what professionalism means and to improve lay and clinical assessor confidence in passing judgement on attributes that resist easy measurement.

Simulated patient scoring in OSCEs is standard practice in the USA, including in high-stakes assessments. This has developed in the UK and elsewhere, as simulated patient training has been shown to enable satisfactory reliability (Wiskin *et al.* 2003). A key point appears to be building on the historic point that simulated patients and clinical scorers offer differing perspectives rather than being 'interchangeable' (Finlay *et al.* 1995) and being more courageous about scoring beyond tokenism. Degrees of confidence in summative scoring by simulated patients are nationally variable, and a more systematic approach – sharing psychometric data and good experiences – is needed.

While the research base for improved psychometrics using global scoring is growing (Regehr *et al.* 1999; Wass *et al.* 2001; Crossley *et al.* 2002), there is room for evidence that holistic marking can be employed without bias, presented in a form acceptable to an audience conditioned toward reliability outcomes. Clinically anchored rating scales for OSCE global scores are being developed with the aim of reducing inter-rater variability in application of the grading scale (Crossley *et al.* 2011).

Assessment for learning is a future prerogative of the OSCE. National student exit surveys tell us that undergraduates want more individual feedback. Theoretically *all* candidates could learn from OSCE assessors' and teachers' observations, but these are often used only for remediation. Mobile tablet technology is one way forward and has enabled systems of scoring where audio feedback is captured by each assessor during marking time between candidates (Harrison *et al.* 2013). With cohort sizes of 400+ in some medical schools there is undoubtedly logistic challenge, but the educational community has responsibility to improve individual feedback opportunities and to embrace, rather than shy from, the challenge.

Another direction to take assessment for learning is the programmatic approach (van der Vleuten & Schuwirth 2005), in which multiple assessment points during the student's year are each used as the opportunity for feedback and remedial learning. Each individual assessment is low stakes but contributes to high-stakes decisions about progression. The approach has been developed since 2005 and now has quality criteria, learning activities, assessment activities and support activities based on a theory-driven framework of learner-centredness and reflection for deep learning (Dijkstra *et al.* 2010; van der Vleuten *et al.* 2012). Some schools have already implemented this approach (Dannefer & Henson 2007; Driessen *et al.* 2012). Key to the programmatic approach is the social interaction with a senior colleague who helps to scaffold the student's self-directed learning (Sargeant *et al.* 2008). The risk is that students regard their clinical supervisors as assessors rather than coaches. The programmatic approach to assessment is the ultimate merger of formative and summative assessment, and the pendulum may swing in that direction if the evidence from early adopting medical schools proves that it is effective.

References

Aspegren, K. (1999) BEME Guide No. 2: Teaching and learning communication skills in medicine - a review with quality grading of articles. *Medical Teacher*, 21 (no. 6), 563–570.

Balint, M. (1968) The Doctor, His Patient and the Illness. Pitman, London.

Barrows, H. & Abrahamson, S. (1964) The programmed patient: A technique for appraising student performance in clinical neurology. *Journal of Medical Education*, 39, 802–805.

Boulet, J.R., Ben-David, M.F., Ziv, A., Burdick, W.P., Curtis, M., Peitzman, S. *et al.* (1998) High-stakes examinations: What do we know about measurement? Using standardized patients to assess the interpersonal skills of physicians. *Academic Medicine*, 73 (no. 10), S94.

Crossley, J., Davies, H., Humphris, G. & Jolly, B. (2002) Generalisability: A key to unlock professional assessment. *Medical Education*, 36 (no. 10), 972–978.

Crossley, J., Johnson, G., Booth, J. & Wade, W. (2011) Good questions, good answers: Construct alignment improves the performance of workplace-based assessment scales. *Medical Education*, 45 (no. 6), 560–569.

Dannefer, E.F. & Henson, L.C. (2007) The portfolio approach to competency-based assessment at the Cleveland Clinic Lerner College of Medicine. *Academic Medicine* 82 (no. 5), 493–502.

Dijkstra, J., van der Vleuten, C.P.M. & Schuwirth, L.W.T. (2010) A new framework for designing programmes of assessment. *Advances in Health Sciences Education: Theory and Practice*, 15 (no. 3), 379–393.

Driessen, E.W., van Tartwijk, J., Govaerts, M., Teunissen, P. & van der Vleuten, C.P.M. (2012) The use of programmatic assessment in the clinical workplace: A Maastricht case report. *Medical Teacher*, 34 (no. 3), 226–231.

Epstein, R.M. & Hundert, E.M. (2002) Defining and assessing professional competence. *JAMA*, 287 (no. 2), 226–235.

Eva, K. & Regehr, G. (2005) Self-assessment in the health professions: A reformulation and research agenda. *Academic Medicine*, 80, 46.

Finlay, I.G., Stott, N.C.H. & Kinnersley, P. (1995) The assessment of communication skills in palliative medicine: A comparison of the scores of examiners and simulated patients. *Medical Education*, 29 (no. 6), 424–429.

Francis, R. (2013) *Report of the Mid Staffordshire NHS Foundation Trust Public Inquiry Executive Summary Report of the Mid Staffordshire NHS Foundation Trust Public Inquiry*. The Stationery Office, London.

General Medical Council. (2003) *Tomorrow's Doctors* [WWW document]. URL http://www.gmc-uk.org/education/undergraduate/undergraduate_policy/tomorrows_doctors.asp.

General Medical Council. (2009) *Tomorrow's Doctors*. General Medical Council, London.

Harden, R.M., Stevenson, M., Downie, W.W. & Wilson, G.M. (1975) Assessment of clinical competence using objective structured examination. *BMJ*, 1, 447–451.

Harrison, C.J., Könings, K.D., Molyneux, A., Schuwirth, L.W.T., Wass, V. & van der Vleuten, C.P.M. (2013) Web-based feedback after summative assessment: How do students engage? *Medical Education*, 47 (no. 7), 734–744.

Hodges, B. & McIlroy, J.H. (2003) Analytic global OSCE ratings are sensitive to level of training. *Medical Education*, 37 (no. 11), 1012–1016.

Joughin, G. (2010) The hidden curriculum revisited: A critical review of research into the influence of summative assessment on learning. *Assessment and Evaluation in Higher Education,* 35 (no. 3), 335–345.

Laidlaw, A., Salisbury, H., Doherty, E.M. & Wiskin, C. (2014) National survey of clinical communication assessment in medical education in the United Kingdom (UK). *BMC Medical Education,* 14, 10.

Larsen, D.P. & Dornan, T. (2013) Quizzes and conversations: Exploring the role of retrieval in medical education. *Medical Education,* 47 (no. 12), 1236–1241.

McLachlan, J.C. (2006) The relationship between assessment and learning. *Medical Education,* 40 (no. 8), 716–717.

Michler, E. (1983) *The Discourse of Medicine: Dialectics of Medical Interviews.* Ablex Publishing, Norwood, NJ.

Muijtens, A., Hoogenboom, R., Verwijnen, G. & van der Vleuten, C. (1998) Relative or absolute standards in assessing medical knowledge using progress tests. *Advances in Health Sciences Education,* 3 (no. 2), 81–87.

Nicol, D.J. & Macfarlane, D.D. (2006) Formative assessment and self-regulated learning: A model and seven principles of good feedback practice. *Studies in Higher Education,* 31 (no. 2), 199–218.

Regehr, G., Freeman, R., Hodges, B. & Russell, L. (1999) Assessing the generalizability of OSCE measures across content domains. *Academic Medicine,* 74 (no. 12), 1320–1322.

Sargeant, J., Mann, K., van der Vleuten, C. & Metsemakers, J. (2008) 'Directed' self-assessment: Practice and feedback within a social context. *Journal of Continuing Education in the Health Professions,* 28 (no. 1), 47–54.

Sargeant, J., Armson, H., Chesluk, B., Dornan, T., Eva, K., Holmboe, E., *et al.* (2010) The processes and dimensions of informed self-assessment: A conceptual model. *Academic Medicine,* 85 (no. 7), 1212.

Skelton, J. (2005) Everything you were always afraid to ask about communication skills. *British Journal of General Practice,* 55, 40–46.

Turner, J.L. & Dankoski, M.E. (2008) Objective structured clinical exams: A critical review. *Family Medicine,* 40 (no. 8), 574–578.

van der Vleuten, C.P.M. & Schuwirth, L.W.T. (2005) Assessing professional competence: From methods to programmes. *Medical Education,* 39 (no. 3), 309–317.

van der Vleuten, C.P.M., Schuwirth, L.W.T., Driessen, E.W., Dijkstra, J., Tigelaar, D., Baartman, L.K.J., *et al.* (2012) A model for programmatic assessment fit for purpose. *Medical Teacher,* 34 (no. 3), 205–214.

Wass, V., van der Vleuten, C., Shatzer, J. & Jones, R. (2001) Assessment of clinical competence. *Lancet,* 357, 945–949.

Wilkinson, T.J. & Fontaine, S. (2002) Patients' global ratings of student competence. Unreliable contamination or gold standard? *Medical Education,* 36 (no. 12), 1117–1121.

Wilson, J. (1999) Acknowledging the expertise of patients and their organizations. *BMJ,* 319, 771–774.

Wiskin, C., Allan, T.F. & Skelton, J.R. (2003) Hitting the mark: Negotiated marking and performance factors in the communication skills element of the VOICE examination. *Medical Education,* 37 (no. 1), 22–31.

Wiskin, C., Doherty, E.M., von Fragstein, M., Laidlaw, A. & Salisbury, H. (2013a) How do United Kingdom (UK) medical schools identify and support undergraduate medical students who 'fail' communication assessments? A national survey. *BMC Medical Education,* 13 (no. 1), 95.

Wiskin, C., Elley, K., Jones, E. & Duffy, J. (2013b) Clinician and simulated patient scoring – the psychometrics of a national programme recruiting dentists to DF1 training posts. *British Dental Journal,* 215, 125–130.

Zick, A., Granieri, M. & Makoul, G. (2007) First-year medical students' assessment of their own communication skills: A video-based, open-ended approach. *Patient Education and Counseling,* 68 (no. 2),161–166.

CHAPTER 36

Workplace-Based Assessment

Jane Kidd[1,2] and Janet Lefroy[3]

[1]*University Hospitals Coventry and Warwickshire NHS Trust, Coventry, UK*
[2]*Institute of Medical and Biomedical Education, St George's University of London, London, UK*
[3]*Keele University, Staffordshire, UK*

Historical context

For many years assessment in the medical profession was conducted by testing knowledge. More recently, tools were developed to assess skills, and competence-based assessments are now commonplace in medical school assessments and membership examinations.

With evidence that competence does not reliably predict performance (Rethans *et al.* 2002), an understanding developed of the need to assess clinical performance encompassing, among other elements, effective communication, interpersonal skills and professionalism (General Medical Council 2001) *in context*. Workplace-based assessments were the outcome of this development and aim to be an '*assessment of what doctors actually do in practice*' (Swanick & Chana 2009).

On-the-job workplace-based assessment instruments in common current use are the mini-clinical evaluation exercise (mini-CEX), the direct observation of procedural skills (DOPS), case-based discussion, also known as chart stimulated recall, and multisource feedback (MSF) (Norcini & Burch 2007). The direct observation tools are designed to assess single encounters and allow for immediate formative feedback, while the MSF approach allows observation of performance over time. The mini-CEX was developed in the USA as a tool to overcome some of the challenges posed by the traditional 'long case' assessment. The assessor observes the trainee's ability to undertake specific clinical tasks, discusses the case and gives structured feedback (Norcini *et al.* 2003; Norcini & Burch 2007).

DOPS (Wragg *et al.* 2003) requires the assessor to observe a procedure being carried out in the workplace and provide feedback on the trainee's performance.

Case-based discussion requires the trainee to use one of his or her written patient records to stimulate a discussion of and receive feedback on management, decision making and note keeping of the case with the assessor.

The MSF tools assess performance across a range of competencies and have been used outside healthcare systems for many years (Handy *et al.* 1996; Atwater & Waldman 1998; Ghorpade 2000). They draw on the literature of human resource management and leadership research (Hedge *et al.* 2001; Smither *et al.* 2005).

Clinical Communication in Medicine, First Edition. Edited by Jo Brown, Lorraine M. Noble,
Alexia Papageorgiou and Jane Kidd.
© 2016 John Wiley & Sons, Ltd. Published 2016 by John Wiley & Sons, Ltd.

A key element of the MSF approach is the self-assessment component, and a unique feature of this questionnaire-based method is that it is designed to provide the person being assessed with feedback on a range of competencies from individuals with whom they work. In a healthcare setting these individuals may include fellow doctors, nurses, allied health professionals, clerical and managerial staff and patients.

As Crossley (2011) has identified, *'the patient has a unique and important perspective on a clinician's performance as they are the experts on certain aspects of relational performance such as building trust and listening'*. This is particularly important if we are interested in effective communication, and of the workplace-based assessment tools identified, only the MSF instruments can incorporate input from patients.

Although it was back in the 1980s when patient feedback was first considered as a potential source of information for service improvement, drawing on job satisfaction (Lawlor 1973) and consumer survey literature (Pascoe 1983; Feletti *et al.* 1985; Matthews & Feinstein 1989; Baker 1990), it was not until the 2000s that the potential for patients to provide feedback for individual practitioners came into focus (Greco *et al.* 1998, 2001; Wensing *et al.* 2003).

Workplace-based assessment tools are designed to assess the performance of an individual across all relevant competencies as part of an integrated assessment (Kogan *et al.* 2009), but they do not focus on effective communication. This chapter will consider the tools as a whole, presenting information on the assessment of effective communication where it is available.

Current practice

'On-the-job' workplace-based assessment instruments were developed for assessing doctors and have since been adopted by medical schools, as there is some evidence for their validity, and they provide continuity of assessment to the student before and after becoming a doctor.

Those that explicitly include domains related to effective communication, and are widely used, are the mini-CEX, the DOPS (direct observation) and the MSF (multisource) instruments.

The mini-CEX modified for the National Health Service (NHS) in the UK contains seven domains, with the domains of 'communication skills' and 'professionalism' assessing effective communication with the patient (Table 36.1).

Table 36.1 The seven domains of the consultation assessed in the mini-CEX modified for the NHS in the UK.

Domain
1 History taking
2 Physical examination skills
3 Communication skills
4 Critical judgement
5 Professionalism
6 Organisation and efficiency
7 Overall clinical care

Table 36.2 The original 11 domains of the DOPS assessment tool.

Domain
1 Demonstrates understanding of indications, relevant anatomy, technique of procedure
2 Obtains informed consent
3 Demonstrates appropriate pre-procedure preparation
4 Demonstrates situation awareness
5 Aseptic technique
6 Technical ability
7 Seeks help where appropriate
8 Post-procedure management
9 Communication skills
10 Consideration for patient
11 Overall performance

The DOPS tool contains 11 domains relating to the performance of a clinical procedure (Table 36.2). The clinical communication domains assessed are:
• Obtains informed consent and
• Communication skills.
And communication may also be assessed under:
• Seeks help where appropriate;
• Consideration for patient and
• Post-procedure management
   Response scales for assessors in the NHS with both the mini-CEX and DOPS have been related to the expected competency level of the trainee doctor or medical student:
• Well above expectations;
• Above expectations;
• Meets expectations;
• Borderline;
• Below expectations or
• Well below expectations.
   In a recent development, the Royal College of General Practitioners (2014a) have amended the rating scale of the DOPS to:
• Insufficient evidence;
• Needs further development;
• Competent or
• Excellent,
with two comments boxes to identify what was performed well and areas for further development.
   A frequently used MSF tool is the Team Assessment of Behaviour (Whitehouse *et al.* 2005; Foundation Programme 2015). This tool assesses individuals across four domains, listing behaviours expected in each domain (Table 36.3).
   In this tool, effective communication with the patient is assessed in the first two domains and communication with colleagues is assessed in the third domain.
   Following the Donaldson report of 2006 (Donaldson 2006), feedback from patients has received a fresh impetus, with the General Medical Council (Campbell & Wright

Table **36.3** Domains of the team assessment of behaviour.

Domain
1 Maintaining trust/professional relationship with patients
2 Verbal communication skills
3 Team working/working with colleagues
4 Accessibility

2012) and the Royal College of General Practitioners (2014b) both having patient questionnaires as one element of their MSF tools.

The General Medical Council (2014) patient questionnaire explores the patient's perception of how 'good' the doctor was on a series of communication tasks as well as his or her level of agreement with statements about a doctor's professionalism.

The Royal College of General Practitioners Patient Satisfaction Questionnaire (Royal College of General Practitioners 2014b) asks patients to respond to 11 questions that explore perceptions of how well a doctor demonstrated effective communication throughout the consultation.

In a systematic review of 55 tools used for direct observation and assessment of the clinical skills of medical trainees, Kogan *et al.* (2009) reported that the mini-CEX had the strongest evidence of validity. Their review identified that most of the tools had been developed for the purpose of formative assessment. They reported that information that would assist an individual to assess the feasibility, validity and educational impact of the tools was infrequently reported.

Wilkinson *et al.* (2008), looking at Specialist Registrar training, and Davies *et al.* (2009), reporting on the initial evaluation of the foundation assessment programme, concluded that the mini-CEX, DOPS and MSF were feasible methods of assessment. Including the giving of feedback, the mini-CEX required 25 minutes, DOPS 15 minutes and MSF 7 minutes to complete per rater. Neither of the studies reported on the systems or time required to collate the results of the MSF and provide the feedback to the trainee. Wilkinson also reported that the methods provided reliable scores with appropriate sampling.

Miller (2010) reviewed studies of workplace-based assessment, concluding that there were few published studies exploring the impact on doctors' education and performance. From the 16 studies on doctors' performance, she concluded that MSF can lead to performance improvement, noting that individual differences, the context of the feedback and the presence of facilitation influence the response of trainees. Her findings are supported by the psychology literature (Smither *et al.* 2005).

The majority of literature on MSF tools in medical education is concerned with their reliability and validity (Wood *et al.* 2006), with less emphasis on the acceptability and educational impact.

Burford *et al.* (2010) compared users' attitudes to two MSF tools; the main difference between the tools being one provided textual feedback and the second numerical feedback. They reported that both tools were acceptable and perceived to be feasible by the users. They also reported a preference for textual feedback.

Violato *et al.* (2008) examined validity of MSF instruments for general practice and reported that there was evidence of construct validity and for stability over time. They also reported that there were some positive changes in performance over the 5 years of the study as rated by medical colleagues and co-workers, although this was not reported from the patient's perspective.

Effective communication is only ever one of the domains assessed in the workplace-based assessment process, and there is little literature on the extent to which behaviour change related to effective communication is achieved. A study by Brinkman and colleagues (2007) focused on the impact of MSF on communication skills and professional behaviour in paediatric residents. They reported that after 5 months the MSF group showed significant improvements in 'communicating effectively with the patient and family, timeliness of completing tasks and demonstrating responsibility and accountability'. These results were only apparent when rated by nursing staff, and, as the experimental group also participated in a tailored coaching session, it is not clear if the same performance improvements would have occurred without that intervention.

Future directions

Workplace-based assessment with feedback is considered potentially one of the most powerful interventions in medical education (Veloski *et al.* 2006; Norcini & Burch 2007; Norcini 2010).

The evidence to date suggests that these assessments have not yet met their potential as educational interventions.

Crossley and Jolly (2012) looked at some basic workplace-based assessment instrument design issues and suggested ways to optimize their validity and reliability. Their suggestions include: 'the response scales should be aligned to the reality map of the judges; judgements rather than objective observations should be sought; the assessment should focus on competencies that are central to the activity observed and the assessors who are best-placed to judge performance should be asked to participate.' Reviewing the tools currently used with these suggestions in mind may enhance their performance.

Increases in the effectiveness of the tools and assessment process in terms of behaviour change and enhancing patient outcomes may be forthcoming if:

* *The content of feedback is sufficient.* Current workplace assessments can result in a greater focus on assessment rather than feedback, with the design of the forms often contributing to limited feedback (Norcini & Burch 2007). For example, the assessor is expected to give one grade for the entirety of communication skills and is given little guidance about how to give helpful feedback in free text, so assessors may tick boxes and omit to write any free text or only provide a general comment. Faculty training and instruments are now being developed that address the need for more specific and detailed feedback and encourage the assessor to give more than a grade (McKinley *et al.* 2000; Lefroy *et al.* 2011). The recent changes to the scales on the assessment forms from the Royal College of General Practitioners (2014a) and the Joint Royal Colleges of Physicians Training Board (2014) reflect this.
* *The process of assessment and feedback is followed.* Feedback that is done as a dialogue between assessor and learner is most likely to motivate the learner to use the feedback constructively (VandeWalle *et al.* 2001; Archer 2010). This dialogue assists the assessor to tailor the feedback content to be optimal for the learner. Such dialogue would ideally precede any written feedback, but there should also be a second discussion after the trainee has reflected on the feedback, to establish what actions

will take be taken. Tutors are often discouraged from providing appropriate feedback because of time constraints, and the action planning stage of the feedback process is often lacking (Holmboe 2004).

- *The relationship with the assessor is one of trust.* Feedback in formative assessment is a social interaction. Feedback had a positive impact on physician performance in 74% of studies in a Best Evidence Medical Education systematic review (Veloski *et al.* 2006). This review identified that feedback was acceptable to the trainee and most effective when it was systematic and given over a period of time by an authoritative, credible source. This fits ideally with student workplace-based assessment in a clinical placement where there is time to develop a one-to-one relationship.

- *The recipient of the feedback is in an appropriate state of mind.* Self-regulation theories suggest that (medical) students may focus on improvement or preventing failure (Goevarts *et al.* 2007; Kluger & Van Djik 2010). Those who are in prevention focus and have passed an assessment may feel little incentive to make use of feedback that is available (Harrison *et al.* 2013). Providing a grade may draw attention away from feedback about the task. Assessing and giving feedback without the use of grades may be beneficial. The dilemma is that the self-regulatory focus of a trainee must include self-awareness relative to agreed standards, which implies grading. A study comparing workplace-based assessment with and without grades concluded that a more personalised approach to feedback would enable students not to have grades if they would be harmful and to make better use of their feedback if they did prefer to have grades (Lefroy *et al.*, 2015).

Future work will be required to conduct well-designed studies to explore how the specific domains related to effective communication within workplace-based assessment tools are perceived and influence behaviour.

The challenge will then be to explore the impact of these educational interventions delivered in complex learning environments on trainee behaviour and patient outcomes.

References

Archer, J.C. (2010) State of the science of health professional education: Effective feedback. *Medical Education*, 44 (no. 1), 101–108.

Atwater, L. & Waldman, D. (1998) Accountability in 360 degree feedback. *Human Resources Magazine*, 43 (no. 6), 96–102.

Baker, R. (1990) Development of a questionnaire to assess patients' satisfaction with consultation in general practice. *British Journal of General Practice*, 40, 487–490.

Brinkman, W.B., Geraghty, S.R., Lanphear, B.P., Khoury, J.C, Gonzalez del Rey, J.A. & Dewitt T.G. (2007) Effect of multisource feedback on resident communication skills and professionalism: A randomized controlled trail. *Archives of Pediatrics and Adolescent Medicine*, 161, 44–49.

Burford, B., Illing, J., Kergon, C., Morrow, G. & Livingston, M. (2010) User perceptions of multisource feedback tools for junior doctors. *Medical Education*, 44, 165–176.

Campbell, J. & Wright, C. (2012) *GMC Multi-Source Feedback Questionnaires: Interpreting and Handling Multisource Feedback Results: Guidance for Appraisers* [WWW document]. URL http://www.gmc-uk.org/Information_for_appraisers.pdf_48212170.pdf.

Crossley, J. (2011) Why patients' views matter: Assessing the patient perspective. In: D. Bhugra & A. Malik (eds), *Workplace-Based Assessments in Psychiatric Training*. Cambridge University Press, Cambridge, UK.

Crossley J. & Jolly, B. (2012) Making sense of work-based assessment; Ask the right questions, in the right way, about the right things, of the right people. *Medical Education*, 46, 28–37.

Davies, H., Archer, J., Southgate, L. & Norcini, J. (2009) Initial evaluation of the first year of the Foundation Assessment Programme. *Medical Education*, 43, 74–81.

Donaldson L. (2006) *Good Doctors, Safer Patients: Proposals to Strengthen the System to Assure and Improve the Performance of Doctors and to Protect the Safety of Patients*. Department of Health, London.

Feletti, G., Firman, D. & Sanson-Fisher, R. (1985) Patient satisfaction with primary care consultations. *Journal of Behavioral Medicine*, 9, 389–399.

Foundation Programme (2015) *FP Curriculum 2012: Frequency of Assessments and Guidance on SLEs* [WWW document]. URL http://www.foundationprogramme.nhs.uk/pages/foundation-doctors/training-and-assessment/fpcurriculum2012.

General Medical Council. (2001) *Good Medical Practice*. General Medical Council, London.

General Medical Council. (2014) *GMC Questionnaires and Resources* [WWW document]. URL http://www.gmc-uk.org/doctors/revalidation/colleague_patient_feedback_resources.asp.

Ghorpade, J. (2000) Managing five paradoxes of 360-degree feedback. *Academy of Management Executive*, 14, 140–150.

Goeverts, M., van der Vleuten, C., Schuwirth, L. & Muitjens, A. (2007) Broadening perspectives on clinical performance assessment: Rethinking the nature of in-training assessment. *Advances in Health Sciences Education*, 12, 239.

Greco, M., Francis, W., Buckley, J., Brownlea, A. & McGovern, J. (1998) Real-patient evaluation of communication skills teaching for GP registrars. *Family Practice*, 15, 51–57.

Greco, M., Brownlea, A. & McGovern, J. (2001) Impact of patient feedback on the interpersonal skills of general practice registrars: Results of a longitudinal study. *Medical Education*, 35, 748–756.

Handy, L., Devine, M. & Heath, L. (1996) *360 degree feedback: Unguided Missile or Powerful Weapon?* Ashridge Management Research Group, Berkhamsted, UK.

Harrison, C.J., Konings, K.D., Molyneux, A., Schuwirth, L.W.T., Wass, V., van der Vleuten, C.P.M. (2013) Web-based feedback after summative assessment: How do students engage? *Medical Education*, 47 (no. 7), 734–744

Hedge, J.W., Borman, W.C. & Birkeland, S.C. History and development of multisource feedback as a methodology. In: D.W. Bracken, C.W. Tilmmreck & A.H. Church (eds), *The Handbook of Multisource Feedback: The Comprehensive Resource for Designing and Implementing Multisource Feedback Processes*. Jossey-Bass, San Francisco, CA.

Holmboe, E.S. (2004) Faculty and the observation of trainees' clinical skills: Problems and opportunities. *Academic Medicine*, 79 (no. 1), 16–22.

Joint Royal Colleges of Physicians Training Board. (2014) *Recommendations for Specialty Trainee Assessment and Review* [WWW document]. URL http://www.jrcptb.org.uk/assessment/workplace-based-assessment.

Kluger, A. & Djik, A. (2010) Feedback, the various tasks of the doctor, and the feedforward alternative. *Medical Education*, 44, 1166.

Kogan, J.R., Holmboe, E.S. & Hauer, K.E. (2009) Tools for direct observation and assessment of clinical skills of medical trainees: A systematic review. *JAMA*, 302 (no. 12), 1316–1326.

Lawlor, E.E. (1973) *Motivation in Work Organisations*. Wadsworth Publishing, Belmont, CA.

Lefroy, J., Gay, S.P., Gibson, S., Williams, S. & McKinley, R.K. (2011) Development and face validation of an instrument to assess and improve clinical consultation skills. *International Journal of Clinical Skills*, 5 (no. 2), 115–125.

Lefroy, J., Hawarden, A., Gay, S.P., McKinley, R.K. & Cleland, J. (2015) Grades in formative workplace-based assessment: A study of what works for whom and why. *Medical Education*, 49 (no. 3), 307–320.

Matthews, D. & Feinstein, A. (1989) A new instrument for patients' ratings of physician performance n the hospital setting. *Journal of General Internal Medicine*, 4, 14–22.

McKinley, R.K., Fraser, R.C., der Van Vleuten, C.P.M. & Hastings, A.M. (2000) Formative assessment of the consultation performance of medical students in the setting of general practice using a modified version of the Leicester assessment package. *Medical Education*, 34 (no. 7), 573–579.

Miller, A. (2010) Impact of workplace-based assessment on doctors' education and performance: A systematic review. *BMJ*, 341, c5064.

Norcini, J. (2010) The power of feedback. *Medical Education*, 44, 16–17.

Norcini, J. & Burch, V. (2007) Workplace-based assessment as an educational tool: AMEE Guide No 31. *Medical Teacher*, 29 (no. 9–10), 855.

Norcini, J.J., Blank, L.L, Duffy, F.D. & Fortna, G.S. (2003) The mini-CEX: A method for assessing clinical skills. *Annals of Internal Medicine*, 138 (no. 6), 476–481.

Pascoe, G.C. (1983) Patient satisfaction in primary health care: A literature review and analysis. *Evaluation and Programme Planning*, 6, 185–210.

Rethans, J.J., Norcini, J.J., Baron-Maldonado, M., Blackmore, D., Jolly, B.C., LaDuca, T., Lew, S., Page, G.G. & Southgate, L.J. (2002) The relationship between competence and performance: Implications for assessing practice performance. *Medical Education*, 36, 901–909.

Royal College of General Practitioners. (2014a) *Direct Observation of Procedural Skills (DOPS) and Clinical Examination and Procedural Skills (CEPS)* [WWW document]. URLhttp://www.rcgp.org.uk/training-exams/mrcgp-workplace-based-assessment-wpba/dops-tool-for-mrcgp-workplace-based-assessment.aspx.

Royal College of General Practitioners. (2014b) *PSQ for Workplace-Based Assessment*. URL http://www.rcgp.org.uk/training-exams/mrcgp-workplace-based-assessment-wpba/psq-for-workplace-based-assessment.aspx.

Smither, J.W., London, M. & Reilly, R.R. (2005) Does performance improve following multisource feedback? A theoretical model, meta-analysis, and review of empirical findings. *Personnel Psychology*, 58, 33–66.

Swanick, T. & Chana, N. (2009) Workplace-based assessment. *British Journal of Hospital Medicine*, 70, 290–293.

VandeWalle, D., Cron, W.L. & Slocum, Jr., J.W. (2001) The role of goal orientation following performance feedback. *Journal of Applied Psychology*, 86 (no. 4), 629–640.

Veloski, J., Boex, J., Graserger, J., Evans, A. & Wolfson, D.B. (2006) Systematic review of the literature on assessment, feedback and physicians' clinical performance. BEME Guide No. 7. *Medical Teacher*, 28 (no. 2), 117.

Violato, C., Lockyer, J. & Fidler, H. (2008) Changes in performance: A 5-year longitudinal study of participants in a multi-source feedback programme. *Medical Education*, 42, 1007–1013.

Wensing, M., Vingerhoets, E. & Grol, R. (2003) Feedback based on patient evaluations: A tool for quality improvement? *Patient Education and Counseling*, 51, 149–154.

Whitehouse, A., Hassell, A., Wood, L., Wall, D., Walzman, M. & Campbell, I. (2005) Development and reliability testing of TAB a form for 360 degree assessment of Senior House Officers' professional behaviour, as specified by the General Medical Council. *Medical Teacher*, 27 (3) 252–258.

Wilkinson, J.R., Crossley, J.G.M., Wragg, A., Mills, P., Cowan, G. & Wade, W. (2008) Implementing workplace-based assessment across the medical specialities in the United Kingdom. *Medical Education*, 42, 364–373.

Wood, L., Hassell, A., Whitehouse, A., Bullock, A. & Wall, D. (2006) A literature review of multi-source feedback systems within and without health services, leading to 10 tips for their successful design. *Medical Teacher*, 28 (no. 7), 185–191.

Wragg, A., Wade, W., Fuller, G., Cowan, G. & Mills, P. (2003) Assessing the performance of specialist registrars. *Clinical Medicine*, 3 (no. 2), 131–134.

PART 4

Afterword

CHAPTER 37

Afterword

Jo Brown, Lorraine M. Noble, Alexia Papageorgiou and Jane Kidd

We started the journey to create this book six years ago. As the leads for teaching clinical communication in our respective institutions, we needed to draw upon the ever-increasing evidence base about effective doctor–patient communication and how to teach clinical communication effectively to our students and trainees. There were, and are, many books providing guidance for learners of clinical communication and also many books summarising the research evidence from diverse disciplinary fields. However, there was no single volume that synthesised the theoretical, evidential and pedagogical basis of this discipline. Drawing inspiration from the landmark publication *The Medical Interview* (Lipkin *et al.* 1995), the community of practice of clinical communication in undergraduate medical education in the UK – the *UK Council* – came together to fulfil this objective.

We believe that clinical communication is a constantly evolving subject and that this book is just a stop on a continuing journey. Clinical communication must serve the society in which it is situated. It is informed by, reflects and in turn changes the expectations and practice of healthcare. Not only is there international variation in the definition and acceptance of what constitutes effective clinical communication, but even within a small country like the UK there is variation both within and between institutions. This poses a challenge for our students in preparing for their careers as effective and sensitive practitioners.

One of the key messages arising from this project is that the future of clinical communication lies in greater integration in all aspects and at all stages of the curriculum. This requires integration across teaching, research and practice – but not just within medicine; rather, encompassing all of the health-related disciplines that work together to deliver patient-centred care.

Reference

Lipkin, M., Putnam, S.M. & Lazare, A. (eds) (1995) *The Medical Interview: Clinical Care, Education and Research*. Springer Verlag, New York.

Index

Clinical Communication in Medicine, First Edition. Edited by Jo Brown, Lorraine M. Noble, Alexia Papageorgiou and Jane Kidd.
© 2016 John Wiley & Sons, Ltd. Published 2016 by John Wiley & Sons, Ltd.